THE MUSCLE LADDER

GET JACKED USING SCIENCE

JEFF NIPPARD

VICTORY BELT PUBLISHING INC.
LAS VEGAS

First published in 2024 by Victory Belt Publishing Inc.

ISBN-13: 978-1-628604-86-3

The author is not a licensed practitioner, physician, or medical professional and offers no medical diagnoses, treatments, suggestions, or counseling. The information presented herein has not been evaluated by the U.S. Food and Drug Administration, and it is not intended to diagnose, treat, cure, or prevent any disease. Full medical clearance from a licensed physician should be obtained before beginning or modifying any diet, exercise, or lifestyle program, and physicians should be informed of all nutritional changes.

The author/owner claims no responsibility to any person or entity for any liability, loss, or damage caused or alleged to be caused directly or indirectly as a result of the use, application, or interpretation of the information presented herein.

Cover design by Crizalie Olimpo

Interior design by Kat Lannom and Justin-Aaron Velasco

Illustrations by Crizalie Olimpo and Elita San Juan

TABLE OF CONTENTS

01 SETTING UP THE LADDER | 4

02 SUSTAINABILITY
Will This Work Long Term? | 12

03 MINDSET
Thinking Your Way to Gains | 30

04 TECHNIQUE
How to Lift the Weights | 58

05 EXERCISE SELECTION
What Are the Best Exercises? | 144

06 EFFORT
Am I Training Hard Enough? | 178

07 PROGRESSIVE OVERLOAD
Am I Actually Progressing? | 192

08 VOLUME
How Much Work Should I Do? | 206

09 TRAINING SPLITS & TRAINING FREQUENCY
How Often Should I Lift? | 220

10 LOAD & REP RANGES
How Heavy Should I Lift? | 234

11 REST PERIODS
How Long Should I Rest Between Sets? | 248

12 ADVANCED TECHNIQUES
How Do I Keep Driving Progress? | 256

13 PERIODIZATION
How Do I Organize Training Over Time? | 268

14 NUTRITION, CARDIO & SUPPLEMENTS
How Do I Manage the Other Stuff? | 290

15 TRAINING PROGRAMS
How Should I Structure My Programs? | 316

354 ACKNOWLEDGMENTS

355 GLOSSARY

358 REFERENCES

371 INDEX

CHAPTER 1
SETTING UP THE LADDER

Welcome to *The Muscle Ladder*! As the name implies, it's a series of steps making progress in your quest to achieve your best physique possible—the strongest, leanest, and most muscular body your time, energy, and genetics will allow. The ladder is based on scientific principles and organized according to their importance. Once you fully grasp these fundamentals, you'll know what matters most for muscle growth and what isn't worth worrying about.

One thing I notice in my lifting community: Many people ask the wrong questions. They aren't necessarily "bad" questions, but they aren't the ones they should be asking at their stage of development. The questions aren't relevant to someone with their experience level, which means the answers won't get them any closer to their goals. It's like they're trying to jump to the roof of a building without using a ladder—the one tool designed to get them there safely and efficiently.

My goal is to help you understand and use that ladder. Each rung gives you deeper insight into the fundamentals of training. By the time you reach the top, you'll be answering questions instead of asking them.

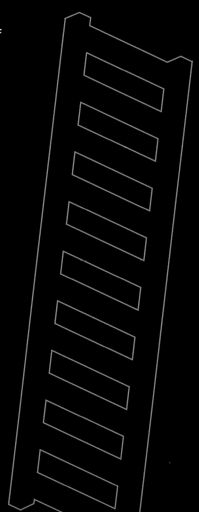

HOW I BUILT THE LADDER

Before I get to the specifics of the ladder, I want to share some of my experiences as I progressed from new lifter to national champion and professional natural bodybuilder. I currently use what I've learned to create videos, interviews, and articles that reach hundreds of millions of people across the globe.

I spent the first four to five years of my training career searching for something—anything—that would work a little better than the last thing I'd tried. After I ran through every cookie-cutter training program from any magazine I could get my hands on, I picked up what I could from the more experienced (but not necessarily more knowledgeable) lifters I met at the gym.

It was, in retrospect, a sloppy, disorganized, and mostly unscientific approach. But that doesn't mean it didn't work. I made enough progress from random programs and well-meaning advice to win the junior championships at a local bodybuilding show. Despite not really understanding what I was doing on a fundamental level, I had three important advantages:

- I was a newbie.

- I worked my butt off.

- I had good genetics for what I was trying to do.

Let's take the last one first. With some people, you can just look at them and predict what they'd be able to do better than the rest of us. If you see someone who has to stoop to avoid hitting their head on the door frame when they walk into a room, you automatically think, "Basketball." You'd never confuse me with a basketball player, but what I lack in height, I more than make up for in width. I was born with a solid frame for bodybuilding: short, with naturally wide shoulders and thick legs. My genetic baseline was like a cheat code, allowing me to get maximal results with minimal knowledge.

A ROUGH GUIDE TO TRAINING STATUS

Beginner (newbie): Anyone in their first year of serious, dedicated training. At this stage, most trainees can make strength progress from workout to workout.

Intermediate: Anyone with two to five years of serious, dedicated training experience. Most trainees can make weekly or monthly progress at this stage but can expect occasional plateaus—periods where they make little to no improvement.

Advanced: Anyone with five to ten years of serious, dedicated training experience. Progress occurs over months or even years rather than weekly or monthly. Training plateaus are often the norm rather than the exception.

Elite: An advanced lifter who's reached the limit of what they can achieve without highly individualized programming from a professional coach.

Maybe you've heard the adage that hard work beats talent when talent doesn't work hard. Long before I understood the potential I was born with, I committed myself to working hard. I showed up every day, ready and willing to train as long and hard as necessary to achieve my goals.

Then there's the famous "newbie period." As every musclehead eventually figures out, your biggest gains will come in your first few years of lifting. It's analogous to a honeymoon. You just need to get a few basic things right and enjoy it while it lasts.

These three factors allowed me to succeed *despite* what I was doing rather than *because of* what I was doing. Over the next decade, I came to understand the problems with my scattershot approach in those early years:

- **My results could have been even better!** Yes, I made excellent gains by almost any standard. But I now see how much more I could have achieved with a better understanding of what actually drives muscle growth.

- **My short-term gains didn't set me up for long-term success.** When you randomly try different things, you eventually find something that works. But without a fundamental understanding of *why* certain things work and other things don't, you can't predict what will and won't work in the future. Building a physique without a firm grasp of foundational principles is like making an ice cream sundae without ice cream. You end up with a big pile of toppings and nothing underneath.

- **It's more than the training variables.** It's also diet, supplements, and lifestyle choices. The longer you train, the more important it is to understand not only what to adjust but what to leave alone.

I eventually found a way to blend my passion for lifting with my passion for science. I completed a science degree, conducted countless interviews with leading researchers in the fitness industry, and wrote training programs for thousands of people, from complete beginners to competitive bodybuilders. I've presented at international conferences and coached professional natural bodybuilders and powerlifters on the biggest stages those sports have to offer. This combination of education and experience has enabled me to distill nearly unlimited information into a handful of core principles determining muscle growth. Focusing your training on these principles will help you ignore the many distractions.

THE STRUCTURE OF THE LADDER

My goal in creating this ladder is to equip you for times of uncertainty in your training. When you question something, you can immediately ask, "What rung of the ladder does this question apply to?" That tells you where to look for an answer.

If you still can't find what you need, you at least know how much it matters. In the big picture, is this something you truly need to figure out? Does your progress depend on knowing it *now*? Or is it less urgent, something interesting to consider but not worth obsessing over?

As you might expect, the ladder has rails (side supports) and rungs.

THE SIDE RAILS

I've referred some to the ladder's rungs but haven't said much about the vital pieces holding the rungs in place. Without those two side rails—sustainability and mindset—you're not even getting off the ground, much less climbing to your destination. For the ladder to function properly, each rung must be securely attached to both rails:

- **Sustainability:** Regardless of how well your program is put together, it won't take you very far if it's not sustainable over the long term.

- **Mindset:** Without the proper mindset, you'll be less likely to follow through, especially when challenges arise.

Sustainability and mindset matter equally to beginners at the bottom rungs and the advanced and elite trainees at the top. Trust me on this: The higher you climb, the more tempting it will be to overlook one or the other, but sustainability and mindset become even more important as your body gets closer to its genetic potential. You won't make gains without the proper mindset, and there's no point in making those gains if they aren't sustainable.

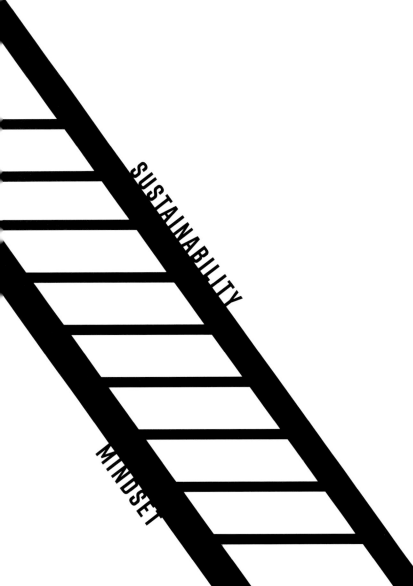

THE 10 RUNGS

Now that our ladder has the side rails it needs to hold it together, let's look at the rungs:

① TECHNIQUE

Before anything else, you must learn to lift weights properly.

② EXERCISE SELECTION

Once you know how to do the exercises, your next step is to choose which ones are best for your goals.

③ EFFORT

Now that you've chosen your exercises and your form is strong enough to do them safely, you're ready to push yourself. The next eight steps won't matter without the appropriate effort.

④ PROGRESSIVE OVERLOAD

Effort isn't something you apply once. Results depend on progressively increasing your strength, skill, and capacity in the gym.

⑤ VOLUME

Training volume is a moving target. Too few sets and reps, and you won't make your best gains. Too many sets and reps, and you risk injury and burnout. But what constitutes "just right" varies from person to person.

⑥ SPLITS AND FREQUENCY

You don't have to worry about a training split at the bottom of the ladder. You can train your entire body two or three times a week, using the same basic exercises, and still get stronger from workout to workout. But eventually, you'll need to think about how you should split up your training, emphasizing different muscles on different days. Which split you choose will depend on how frequently you want to train each muscle and how deep you are into your training career.

⑦ LOAD AND REP RANGES

Again, these are easy choices for a beginner. Three sets of ten, four sets of eight. You can do pretty much the same thing for every exercise and workout. But on the ladder's seventh rung, it takes a lot more calculation. Sometimes, you'll want to use heavier weights. That means fewer reps per set and more time to warm up. Other times you'll want to use lighter weights, which means higher reps. You'll need to make different choices for different exercises at different times.

⑧ REST PERIODS

These decisions are closely related to your exercise choices and rep ranges. Certain exercises and certain rep ranges require more rest time. For example, you'll want more time to recover between sets when you're doing heavy barbell squats for low reps. Most people think short rest periods are better for muscle growth, but new science challenges this.

⑨ ADVANCED TECHNIQUES

When plateaus become frequent, you may need to spice up your training with selective use of long-length partial reps, myo-reps, drop sets, and other hypertrophy techniques to spark new growth.

⑩ PERIODIZATION

This refers to how you organize and balance your program over time. As you step off this final rung, you'll have all the knowledge you need to create a long-term training plan.

You may notice that the two side rails and some lower rungs aren't particularly "sexy." They certainly don't receive the same attention as the rungs toward the top of the ladder. But just because you hear about something more often doesn't mean it's more important—or that it's something you need to concern yourself with at all. I'm not saying that the things on the higher rungs don't matter; I wouldn't have included them if they didn't. But without the components from the side rails and the lower rungs, they won't be especially effective.

It's also important to remember that the training ladder isn't the *only* way to think about your training. Like any science-based model, it doesn't fully capture every possible detail. In this book, I organize the most important training information available, chunk it down into discrete concepts, and show you how to apply them to your goals. As such, your climb on the ladder will focus more on the practical elements of training than the theory.

Each of the next twelve chapters focuses on a side rail or rung of the ladder. When you reach Chapter 13, you'll understand the entire ladder. In Chapter 14, you'll see a brief overview of nutrition, cardio, and supplementation. Finally, in Chapter 15, you'll find some sample training programs.

I recommend reading the book in order because each rung builds on the previous one, and the rungs are organized in order of importance. If you skip a rung, you risk falling off the ladder. That said, if you're like me, you're probably more curious about some topics than others, and I won't hold it against you if you skip ahead to get that information into your brain ASAP. All I ask is that you circle back to the chapters you jumped past to get the proper context for the most compelling information. Additionally, if you're a more experienced and educated trainee who's already familiar with the fundamentals, I give you permission to skim past those chapters so you can focus on the higher rungs. Just don't blame me if you slip on your way to the top.

CHAPTER 2

SUSTAINABILITY

WILL THIS WORK LONG TERM?

If we were building an actual ladder, we wouldn't start with the rungs. We'd start with the two vertical side rails, which must be sturdy enough to hold the individual rungs in place securely. In our Muscle Ladder, those two rails are sustainability and mindset.

Let's kick things off with sustainability. For someone new to the gym, the importance of sustainability becomes apparent once they reach the tail end of the newbie phase, after about six to twelve months of lifting. The closer they get to the end of that period, the slower their gains will be. Now they have to find a way to continue training over the following months and years without feeling the rush of near-constant improvements. Many people simply lose interest at that point. Beginning with a sustainable approach rather than searching for one a year or two down the road is crucial to avoiding this situation.

Sustainable training needs to be enjoyable, safe, and properly paced. If your training isn't enjoyable, you'll quickly lose your motivation. If it isn't safe, you're more likely to get injured. If it isn't properly paced, you'll either lose interest because the gains don't come fast enough or burn out because you've tried to do too much, too soon. Let's take a closer look at each aspect of sustainable training.

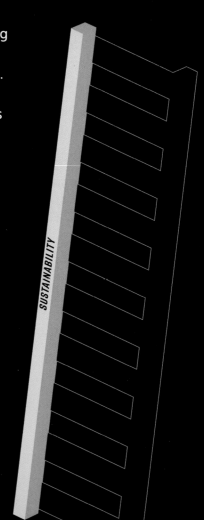

SUSTAINABILITY

ENJOYMENT

One maxim that I think applies to just about anything in life is the more you enjoy it, the more likely you are to stick with it. The less you enjoy it, the more likely you are to head for the exit. That's especially true for a voluntary activity like a training program. I'm not saying every workout will be a barrel of laughs. Some will actually suck. What's important is that you make training as engaging as possible and you look forward to your workouts more often than not.

We all recognize this principle when we're talking about diet. Very few people can stick to a bland, monotonous meal plan. But when you have a more flexible diet, with enjoyable and varied food options, your adherence improves.

For some reason, people are less likely to embrace this principle of enjoyment in the context of training. I think it goes back to the outdated idea that training won't work if it's not painful. "No pain, no gain," right? Not exactly. Sure, training should be challenging. Sometimes you need to push yourself beyond your comfort zone. But if you dread going to the gym, that's a sure sign your program isn't right for you. This principle is especially important for beginners. You don't need to grind yourself down with grueling training methods. In fact, in the early stages of lifting, you'll almost certainly make better progress without them—and enjoy the process a whole lot more.

Some people argue that focusing on enjoyment is incompatible with successful training. "Pushing yourself hard, *truly* hard, isn't supposed to be fun," they say. "If you want it to work, it has to *feel* like work." I disagree. In my experience as both a trainer and a trainee, increased enjoyment goes hand in hand with increased effort. People almost always push themselves harder when they're enjoying what they're doing.

Of course, some people simply don't like strength training at all. There isn't a program on earth they'll enjoy enough to stick with. I get it, truly. I don't like cleaning my house, and I don't think I'll ever find a house-cleaning program I'll look forward to doing.

Other people are somewhere in the middle. They don't love lifting, but they don't want to quit either. If that applies to you, rather than thinking of ways to make your training more enjoyable, it might be better to come up with ways to make it suck less.

The simplest and most practical way to un-suck your training is to streamline your program and minimize the parts you find the most annoying. If the gym isn't your happy place, spend as little time there as you can without compromising your results. Instead of asking, "What's the most *effective* way to train?" you should be asking, "What's the most *efficient* way to train effectively?" I call this the minimalist approach.

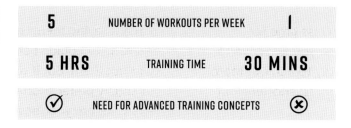

OPTIMIZE TRAINING	5	NUMBER OF WORKOUTS PER WEEK	1	OPTIMIZE EFFICIENCY
	5 HRS	TRAINING TIME	30 MINS	
	✓	NEED FOR ADVANCED TRAINING CONCEPTS	✕	

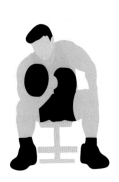
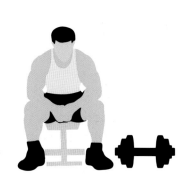

TRAINING MINIMALISM

My younger brother, Bradley, absolutely hates weight training. He likens the experience of lifting to plucking needles from a cactus for an hour...without gloves. However, when he started experiencing hip pain as a result of long workdays, he decided to consult his big bro for a training program.

The last thing he needed was a classic bodybuilding program. He would've given up within a week. So instead of prioritizing *effectiveness,* I focused on *efficiency.* I gave him the most minimalistic program I've ever written. It consisted of just three exercises, done once a week, on Sundays.

Here it is:

Goblet squat: 3 sets × 10 reps

Push-up: 3 sets × 6 reps (try to add 1 rep each week)

Dumbbell row: 3 sets × 12 reps

That's it.

No, this program wasn't going to make him the next Mr. Olympia, but it was very effective at reducing his hip pain and increasing his total-body strength for work. Since those were his goals, I'd call that a success. Even though my instinct was to give him a program that would've built far more muscle, it would have been so unsustainable that I might as well have not given him any program at all. Another plus: My brother now had an entry point for strength training.

In fact, he recently decided to commit to a full year of training with me, bodybuilding-style. We began a scientific study to investigate the difference between someone with nearly two decades of training experience (me) and someone completely new to lifting for muscle gain (Bradley). The full results aren't available yet (we're part way through the experiment as I write this), but I can say that he gained 12 pounds of lean mass and lost 3 percent body fat in the first month. Absolutely incredible results!

Maybe you're in a situation similar to where Bradley was at first. Maybe you have a demanding job or a young family or other priorities that leave you with less time for training. You still want results; you just have to find a more time-efficient way to achieve them. These are your two best options: shorten your workouts or train less often.

MAKING WORKOUTS SHORTER

The simplest way to tighten your workouts without sacrificing gains is to prioritize compound exercises over isolation exercises.

Compound exercises involve multiple joints and activate larger muscles along with smaller ones. The classic examples are squats, deadlifts, and lunges for the lower body and presses, rows, and pull-ups or pulldowns for the upper body. Isolation exercises involve a single joint and typically focus on training just one muscle or muscle group. These include curls for your biceps, extensions for your triceps, lateral raises for your shoulders, and calf raises for your calves.

Because compound exercises work so many different muscles at the same time, you don't need to spend as much time on isolation exercises for each muscle. Consider the dumbbell bench press, for example. You hit your chest, shoulders, and triceps on every repetition. For variety, you can raise the bench into an incline position, which emphasizes different parts of those muscles. If you tried to work those muscles with isolation movements, you'd do something like a fly for the chest, a lateral raise for the shoulders, and an extension for the triceps. It takes a lot longer to do three exercises compared to one. Even then, you might not get the same results because people tend to gain strength faster with compound exercises.

I'm not saying there isn't a place for isolation exercises. I couldn't be a successful bodybuilder without them. But if you're pressed for time, or simply prefer shorter workouts, compound exercises are your best bet.

Another way to streamline your workouts is to use machines instead of free weights. You won't need as much time to warm up, and it's a lot easier to increase or reduce the weight. I'll return to the choice of machines versus free weights later in the book. For now, I'll only note that using machines typically shaves precious minutes from your workout.

Keep in mind there's no "minimum" time required to make progress. Strength-training adaptations involve complex processes. But none of them are set to a timer. Any training is far better than no training. In fact, a 2022 meta-analysis (a study combining the results of many other studies) found that as little as 30 to 60 minutes of resistance exercise per week was enough to reduce the risk of cancer, cardiovascular disease, diabetes, and death from any cause by an estimated 10 to 20 percent.[1] Only 30 to 60 minutes per *week!* Granted, as much as I wish it were true, you won't max out your muscle growth with such little training. But you also don't need to spend hours a day in the gym to achieve measurable and visible results. Most of the time, for entry-level lifters, 30- to 60-minute workouts done two to three times a week will be enough for you to make consistent progress.

More experienced lifters generally require longer workouts. That isn't because longer workouts are inherently better but because intermediate and advanced trainees typically need more exercises and more total sets than they did when they were starting out.

If you're a newer lifter, you don't need to worry about that just yet. For you, it's unequivocally smarter to prioritize sustainability by making your workouts fit your preferences and schedule.

TRAINING LESS OFTEN

Because most bodybuilders spend five to seven days per week in the gym (me included), beginners sometimes get the impression that's what it takes to make progress. Not only is that not true, it's hard to think of a worse way to start out. A new lifter needs to focus on the first three rungs of the ladder: Are you lifting with good form? Are you doing the best exercises for your goals? Are you putting in enough effort to make progress? In addition, you need to make sure you recover properly between workouts. As long as you have those bases covered, you're free to structure your training schedule to make it work for you.

If you prefer to train twice a week, I recommend a schedule like this:

Monday	Full body
Tuesday	Rest
Wednesday	Rest
Thursday	Full body
Friday	Rest
Saturday	Rest
Sunday	Rest

If you prefer to work out three times a week, you could try something like this:

Monday	Full body
Tuesday	Rest
Wednesday	Upper body
Thursday	Rest
Friday	Lower body
Saturday	Rest
Sunday	Rest

You can make significant progress with either routine. And remember what I said a moment ago: Any training is better than no training.

PICKING AN APPROACH

I assume most readers of this book are genuinely interested in weight training. (I can't imagine why you'd be reading it if you aren't.) You may already have a passion for it. If you're anything like me, the idea of spending less time in the gym doesn't resonate much. I love training, and I don't worry about making my workouts shorter. I focus on what's most effective for me. In fact, if anything, I'd choose to spend more time in the gym. That's how much I enjoy being there.

But I understand that many people don't have the option to take an effectiveness-first approach. No matter how much or how little they enjoy training, they can't schedule their life around their workouts the way I can. Their only choice is an efficiency-first approach. And that's perfectly fine! The Muscle Ladder works well with either approach.

The efficiency-first approach may be especially appropriate if you're just starting out or if you're returning to the gym after a long layoff. As long as you climb the Muscle Ladder, the quality of your training in the first year matters much more than how much time you spend doing it.

MAKING WORKOUTS MORE FUN

To someone who hates training, the idea that any part of a workout can be "fun" might be hard to process, but it really can be. Whether the gym is the best part of your day, the worst part, or something in between, you can always find ways to improve the experience.

I say that knowing you and I may have completely different ideas of what we consider fun. So I'll say up front that I'm not talking about the kind of fun you expect to have on a night out with your friends or a night in with someone special. I'm simply talking about increasing the enjoyment factor of your workouts. Try doing these things:

- **Prioritize exercises you enjoy.** For virtually any fitness goal, there's always more than one way to get the job done. Once you've determined which exercises are roughly comparable— they work the same muscles through a similar range of motion—you can narrow them down according to how much you like doing them. Workouts work better when you're doing exercises you enjoy!

- **Prioritize rep ranges you enjoy.** While higher-rep workouts with relatively light weights are more appropriate for some goals, and lower-rep workouts with relatively heavy weights are more appropriate for others, research shows that all rep ranges can be used to build muscle.[2] Therefore, if you really enjoy the challenge of lifting heavier weights with lower reps but despise the burn of lifting lighter weights for higher reps, design your program accordingly. And if you're one of those freaks who actually enjoys grinding out tons of reps with lighter weights, make sure to include them in your routine.

- **Find a fun training environment.** The more comfortable you feel in your gym, the more likely you are to show up and do the work. If you don't like the atmosphere or people or energy in your current gym, try to find one with vibes that come closer to your own. And if you can't find a gym like that, consider investing in some basic equipment and training at home. You can set up the space however you like, wear anything you want, and listen to anything you like at whatever volume you prefer (and your family, roomies, or neighbors will tolerate). You don't even need to go all out on the home gym. As a new lifter, you can get in some great workouts with just a few dumbbells and some bodyweight exercises.

- **Consider finding a good training partner.** Not only is a gym buddy great for accountability, but establishing rapport with someone who shares your goals can make training more enjoyable for both of you. However, if you prefer to train alone, that's fine too!

- **Listen to music, podcasts, or audiobooks while training.** I constantly update my gym playlist, which helps keep my workouts feeling fresh and fun.

- **Keep your mental state light.** Some people train hardest when they adopt a hardcore, stone-cold state of mind. And that's okay if it works for you. Personally, I've found that people who take a more lighthearted approach seem to do better over the long haul. That's especially true for people whose default setting is to put pressure on themselves. A little humor can sometimes take you further than a more extreme mindset.

- **Get results.** Training is more fun when you're getting those sweet, sweet gains. And the more fun you have training, the more likely you are to train consistently and get those results.

- **Stay healthy.** Injuries are by far the least enjoyable aspect of training. Even the mildest tweaks can slow you down. The more serious strains and tears can set you back for months. A sustainable program is a safe program, and safety is the subject of the next section.

SAFETY

Have you seen that episode of *The Office* where Michael tries to make safety training more exciting by threatening to jump off the building? Well, rather than threatening to jump off a squat rack to keep your attention, I'll instead make this section as brief as I can.

As you get deeper into your training career, you may be tempted to sacrifice safety for results. For some elite athletes at the highest levels of competition, this is an acceptable risk. Becoming the *best* at your sport—any sport—involves pushing yourself to the very edge of your abilities, and sometimes beyond. I can't speak for other athletes. But in my own experience as an elite-level bodybuilder, the extra 1 to 2 percent I might gain from a more risky training strategy won't be worth *anything* if an injury forces me to lose a month or more of training. That's even more true for noncompetitive lifters.

Even though safety isn't something you might think about a lot while lifting (and rightfully so), you can't put it out of your mind entirely. Your long-term success depends on staying healthy.

Too many lifters, unfortunately, get so caught up in chasing that extra 1 to 2 percent that they end up making poor decisions. Instead of getting 1 to 2 percent better, they get 10 to 20 percent worse because of an injury.

My intention here isn't to *scare you* out of getting hurt. In fact, the best research in this area shows that athletes recovering from an injury are more likely to re-injure themselves when they're in a state of fear.[3] Their fear, paradoxically, makes them too timid in their training, which can set them up for the next injury.

The best way to avoid getting hurt in the gym is to train with confidence rather than fear. If you think of your body as being fragile, you'll act as if your body is fragile. And that's exactly what your body will become.

Clearly, there's a middle ground you should aim for. You don't want to be so utterly obsessed with avoiding pain or discomfort that every workout begins with putting on a hazmat suit. But you also don't want to be totally blasé about safety concerns.

RISK OF INJURY FROM LIFTING

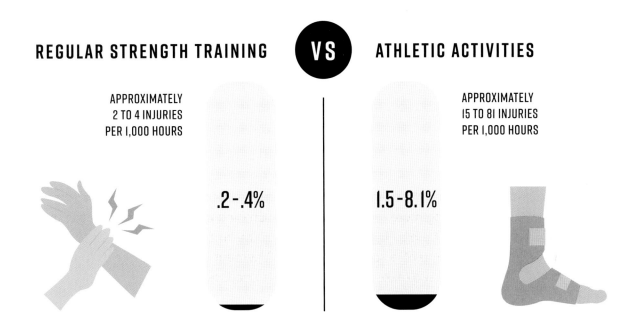

REGULAR STRENGTH TRAINING **VS** **ATHLETIC ACTIVITIES**

APPROXIMATELY
2 TO 4 INJURIES
PER 1,000 HOURS

.2-.4%

1.5-8.1%

APPROXIMATELY
15 TO 81 INJURIES
PER 1,000 HOURS

Luckily, weight training has a relatively low risk of injury compared to other sports. A 2017 systematic review examined twenty studies and found that most weight-training sports (including bodybuilding and powerlifting) have injury rates of approximately 2 to 4 injuries per 1,000 hours of training. For comparison, soccer, rugby, and cricket have rates of approximately 15 to 81 injuries per 1,000 hours—7 to 20 times the injury risk of weight-training![4]

These studies were conducted on athletes who compete at the highest levels and train extremely hard. You can assume they'd be more willing to risk injury than the average trainee, which means the studies may actually overestimate injury risk for noncompetitive gym-goers. In fact, regular strength training not only presents a very low injury risk compared to other athletic activities, it can also reduce your risk of injury while doing activities outside the gym. A 2023 systematic review on the safety and effectiveness of strength training in 604 children concluded that "strength training at an early age helps to reduce overuse injuries by 50 percent."[5]

That makes sense. Weight training makes you stronger and more capable of using your body for daily activities that involve strength. You're a lot less likely to pull a muscle bringing in the groceries if you can deadlift several hundred pounds with ease. Regular weight training has also been shown to improve bone mineral density, reduce the risk of fractures and breaks, and minimize muscle loss later in life.[6]

So while the data on training safety suggests there's no good reason to *fear* weight training, you should still look for ways to make your workouts as safe as possible.

I've distilled my injury prevention strategies down to three main principles: managing total workload, ensuring adequate recovery, and practicing proper technique, with the first two being most important (contrary to popular belief).

MANAGING TOTAL WORKLOAD

I believe that managing your total workload in the gym is the most effective way to prevent injuries. When you train hard, your muscles become damaged, and your body experiences fatigue. Normally, your body repairs the damage and recovers from the fatigue before your next workout—as long as you give it enough time to do those things. Pushing too hard for too long means you're accumulating damage and ultimately increasing your risk of injury.

Most injuries are preceded by clear warning signs. They're the body's way of telling you, "Hey, maybe you should chill out a bit."

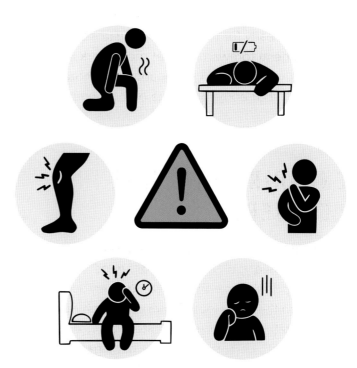

Common warning signs include

• Persistent joint aches

• Persistent loss of strength

• Feeling exhausted and run down

• Persistent extreme muscle soreness

• Loss of training motivation

• Difficulty sleeping

If you experience several of these warning signs concurrently, you should consider reducing your training load for a week or two to see if the signals decrease or go away. These lighter weeks, formally called *deloads,* can help reduce fatigue and give your body time to repair muscle damage. Later in the book, I'll show you how to set up a deload week, but for now, you can simply think of it as a light week where you train with a little less weight and a little less volume.

I can't tell you what your ideal workload is just yet. It's too early for that. For now, I'll leave you with a general forewarning that more work isn't necessarily better. You don't want to do more work than your body is capable of recovering from.

ENSURING ADEQUATE RECOVERY

Recovery is a complex and multifactorial process. While you'll find many different definitions in the scientific literature, they all kind of land on the same idea: Recovery is a physical and mental *return to baseline* after training. When you lift weights, you cause damage and fatigue. When you rest after lifting, you recover from that damage and fatigue.

The volume and intensity of your workouts generally determine how long it will take to recover. If you go longer than usual or push yourself harder than usual, you need more recovery time before the next workout.

Lifestyle factors also play a big role. Do you have a physically demanding job? How much stress do you have at work and home? How well do you sleep? Does your diet support your training and recovery? Because all of these factors play into recovery, it's important to consider not just the stress imposed on your body inside the gym walls but also the stress imposed on your body outside the gym walls.

How do you know when you've recovered? For beginner and intermediate trainees, a good gauge is when you no longer feel tired and sore from your last workout. If your vibe says you're ready to train again, you probably are.

Here's a quick example: Let's say you did a really hard arm workout yesterday, and it's hitting you today. Your arms feel heavy, tired, and sore, and when you pick up your three-year-old child, it's like they somehow turned into a six-year-old overnight. These are all signs that you're still recovering. The last thing you want to do is train your arms again.

Now let's jump ahead two or three days. You no longer notice any soreness, and when you pick up your child, they feel like your preschooler again. Collectively, everything points in the same direction: Your arms are fully recovered, and you can't wait to get in the gym and smash them again.

So far, I've described *local recovery* involving a single muscle. That's different from *systemic recovery,* which involves your entire body. An arm workout inflicts some microtears in the muscle fibers of your biceps and build up some metabolic waste, but it shouldn't impede your ability to train legs today, even though your biceps are still recovering.

Systemic recovery can be a bit trickier. For example, let's say you work legs today. You do deadlifts, leg curls, and (*wince*) Bulgarian split squats. By tomorrow, not only will your legs fail the vibe check, but the rest of your body will most likely be feeling some fatigue as well.

Some exercises and training methods take more out of you than others, and they require more total-body recovery. You have to keep that in mind when you put together your training program. Compound exercises like squats and deadlifts create a lot more systemic fatigue than isolation moves like curls and extensions. Same with full-body workouts compared to single body-part workouts. That's why you can train arms and legs on consecutive days without issue, but you may want to take a rest day after a high-volume lower body workout that includes heavy squats.

I have three more strategies for improving your overall recovery from training:

- Get enough sleep

- Eat a better diet

- Get enough rest between workouts

GET ENOUGH SLEEP

In my experience, people vastly underestimate the impact sleep can have on recovery. Part of it may be societal; people often boast about how little sleep they get as a signal of their ambition and work ethic. In reality, doing your best to get a good night's sleep doesn't mean you're lazy. It means you're smart.

The National Sleep Foundation recommends that adults get between seven and nine hours of sleep per night for overall health.[7] Weight training, however, imposes an additional recovery demand. This means you may actually need eight to nine hours per night to fully recover.[8]

Sleep deprivation is profoundly negative for training performance. In a classic 1994 study, researchers restricted subjects who normally slept eight hours per night to only three hours per night for three days in a row.[9] Then they did 20 reps of biceps curls, bench presses, leg presses, and deadlifts while sleep deprived.

As you'd expect, there was a significant and linear decline in the amount of weight they could lift for the three compound exercises—bench press, deadlift, leg press. It got progressively worse with additional sleep deprivation. The control group did not experience any decrease in performance.

Maximum strength on the biceps curl decreased as well, but not enough to reach statistical significance. The researchers speculated that missed sleep has a bigger effect on larger, more complicated exercises.

At the other extreme, several studies have shown that performance improves when athletes get more than the recommended amount of sleep. For example, a 2015 study by Schwartz and Simon found that with just one week of extended sleep duration—nine hours instead of seven—collegiate tennis players significantly improved the accuracy of their serve.[10]

A 2011 study from Mah and colleagues also showed impressive results by increasing sleep time in collegiate basketball players.[11] When the players were instructed to spend a minimum of 10 hours in bed per night, their sleep time increased from about 6.7 hours per night to about 8.5 hours. This resulted in significantly improved sprint speed, free throw shooting, three-point shooting, and reaction time. The sleep-loaded athletes also reported improved mood, less fatigue, and better well-being.

Although these sleep-extension studies didn't focus on resistance training, their results strongly suggest that getting more sleep can substantially improve performance and recovery.

I realize not everyone can get eight to nine hours of sleep per night. That's okay. I've coached bodybuilders whose demanding jobs make hitting these sleep targets nearly impossible. Still, their competitive success shows it's absolutely possible to make great progress despite suboptimal sleep.

I prefer to think of it this way: Any increase in sleep duration, even if you still fall short of eight to nine hours, is a move in the right direction and should give you tangible benefits.[12] On the next page are a few of my best tips for improving the quality and quantity of your sleep each night.

- Have a sleep schedule. Try to go to bed and wake up at the same time every day, including weekends and holidays.

- Avoid rigorous exercise within an hour of going to bed.

- Avoid alcohol and caffeine in the evening.

- Establish a relaxation routine before bed—taking a bath, reading, and so on.

- Design a sleep-friendly environment with a comfortable mattress and pillows, dimmable lights, and a room temperature that's a bit cooler at night than during the day.

- Avoid tackling big jobs or stressful tasks right before sleep.

- If you find yourself stressing out over a task you haven't finished (or haven't even started), write it down on the next day's to-do list. That will help get it off your mind so you can relax and fall asleep.

- Naps are your friend, as long as they don't affect how long or how well you sleep at night. Research shows that napping can be especially beneficial for those who work night shifts or have sleep disorders.[13]

If you continue to struggle with sleep after trying some of these suggestions, make an appointment with your family doctor to see if you have a sleep disorder. Most disorders are treatable, and your doctor can help you find the best options available.

EAT A BETTER DIET

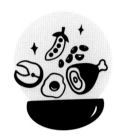

Truly poor nutrition can derail your recovery. (I hope that's not a surprise.) But you have to work pretty hard to get there. For example, a very low-calorie crash diet compromises your recovery for two fairly obvious reasons. It depletes energy reserves that are already depleted by your workouts, and it adds stress on top of the stress of training.

Fortunately, "good" nutrition, *in the context of recovery,* is incredibly simple. Your main concern is eating enough calories to replenish your energy stores and enough protein to build new muscle tissue. Then, as long as your meals provide a variety of vitamins and minerals, you're good to go.

I'll do a deeper dive in Chapter 14 on how many calories you should eat for fat loss and/or muscle gain. For now, just keep in mind that aggressive cuts aren't ideal for recovery and can make you more susceptible to burnout.

You should aim to consume a minimum of 1.2 to 1.8 grams of protein per kilogram of body weight per day (0.6 to 0.8 gram per pound).[14] There are circumstances when it makes sense to go above these protein standards. (I'll cover them in Chapter 14.) But these amounts are sufficient for recovery for the majority of beginner- and intermediate-level lifters.

Beyond getting in enough calories and protein, try to eat a well-balanced, healthy diet most of the time. Broadly speaking, this means eating plenty of fruits and vegetables and prioritizing minimally processed, nutrient-rich whole foods.

GET ENOUGH REST BETWEEN WORKOUTS

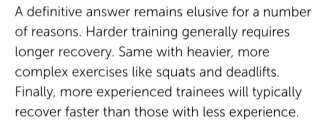

Even with optimized sleep and nutrition, your muscles still need time to repair the damage caused by weight training. Exactly how much time you need between sessions is hotly debated among exercise scientists. (I'll revisit the topic when we discuss training frequency in Chapter 9.)

A definitive answer remains elusive for a number of reasons. Harder training generally requires longer recovery. Same with heavier, more complex exercises like squats and deadlifts. Finally, more experienced trainees will typically recover faster than those with less experience.

For example, let's say I go to the gym today and do just one relatively light set of biceps curls. That's it. Very little muscle damage would occur, and my arms would easily recover in time for tomorrow's workout. Now let's imagine I do barbell back squats, and I really get after it: 5 sets of 5 reps, using near-maximum weights. It would probably take three to five days for my quads to fully recover. And if it had been a while since I used that exercise, and even longer since I trained with such heavy loads, I would probably need a full week or more before I was ready for another trip to the squat rack.

So while recovery times are highly context dependent, as a very general guideline, you should give a muscle two to four days of rest before training it again. Training a muscle before it's completely recovered slows down your rate

of progress and increases your risk of burnout or injury.

That said, there are circumstances where training the same muscle on consecutive days is a perfectly viable approach. But for most lifters, most of the time, your goal is to give your muscles as much time as they need for proper recovery.

WHAT ABOUT SAUNAS, MASSAGE, ICE BATHS, AND FOAM ROLLING?

You may have noticed that I haven't mentioned saunas, ice baths, massage, or foam rolling, all of which are reputed to speed up recovery. That's because their popularity is well ahead of the evidence—which, so far, isn't strong enough to support practical recommendations.[15] Saunas, massage, and foam rolling may help a little with recovery but probably won't help a lot, especially compared to sleep, nutrition, and rest. The only one I caution against is ice baths. They may help with recovery, but high-quality research suggests they impair muscle growth, especially if done post-workout or for longer than five to ten minutes.[16] Not ideal for an aspiring bodybuilder!

PRACTICE PROPER TECHNIQUE

You would expect that proper exercise technique, with joints in their ideal alignment, is absolutely crucial for preventing pain and injury. That's what fitness experts have been telling us pretty much forever. But it's a surprisingly contentious topic. Some evidence-based strength coaches argue that "proper technique" is poorly defined, largely subjective, and not definitively linked to injury prevention. They say our bodies are more resilient than we tend to give them credit for, and we can tolerate a broad range of exercise techniques without an increased risk of harm.

I won't try to settle this debate here, but I will offer my opinion. While I believe the link between technique and injury has been overstated by many personal trainers, that doesn't diminish the importance of technique for training safely and productively.

Your body is incredibly adaptive. The more challenges you expose it to, the more durable and resilient it becomes. Instead of thinking about technique in a binary way—good or bad, safe or unsafe—it makes more sense to see proper form as a range of acceptable variations. Your goal is to be reasonably *consistent* with your technique with the understanding that minor deviations are normal, expected, and usually not a cause for concern.

I'll go into more detail about technique in Chapter 4. But as a taste, here are some general guidelines that apply to most exercises you would use to build muscle, starting with these two fundamental principles:

- **Control the negative.** Don't let the weight free-fall back to the starting position. Control it all the way down.

- **Move through a reasonably full range of motion.** On most exercises, you should work the target muscles through a deep stretch at the bottom and a full "squeeze" at the top. Emerging evidence suggests that the stretched aspect may be particularly important.[17]

DON'T LIFT HEAVIER WEIGHTS THAN YOU CAN HANDLE

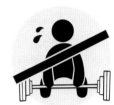

One easy way to identify beginners in the weight room: They try to use weights that are clearly too heavy for them. Each repetition looks different from the previous one. If you can't do all your reps with reasonably consistent form—whether you're doing five or fifty or anything in between—that means the weight you selected is inappropriate for you.

Keep in mind that technique is the first rung on the Muscle Ladder. New lifters need to master exercise form before worrying about how much weight they use. It's better to start too light than too heavy. Once you're confident in your ability to perform the exercises, it's time to increase the weight more assertively by applying progressive overload, the fourth rung on the Muscle Ladder, which I'll cover in Chapter 7.

DEALING WITH PAIN AND INJURIES

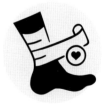

No matter how much you prioritize safety, you'll most likely experience pain or sustain some kind of setback in your training career. Accidents happen, and bumps and bruises are a normal part of lifting. Learn from them, laugh about them, and do what you can to avoid repeating your mistakes or missteps.

From time to time, you'll have to deal with an injury. Here are a few suggestions for how to proceed.

- **Avoid catastrophizing.** Just because you're in pain doesn't mean you're broken. Beware of negative spiraling thoughts. I guarantee they won't help.

- **Be patient.** Most aches and pains naturally subside. Give your body time to heal itself.

- **Find a new entry point.** If the problem persists, and you can no longer train normally without pain, the next step is to find a new way to work the same muscles without aggravating the injury. You can try an alternative exercise, the same exercise performed with less weight, or the same exercise with a limited range of motion that you can access without pain.

  For example, I injured my left shoulder while bench pressing. The flat bench press was consistently leading to shoulder pain, so I switched to an incline press instead. There was still some slight discomfort with the incline press initially, but my shoulder felt fine once I reduced the weight. That was my new entry point: I could use lighter weights with higher reps on the incline bench and still get a solid chest workout.

- **Work your way back to the baseline.** This usually means gradually increasing the weight and/or cautiously returning to the original exercise as things start to feel better. At this point, it's crucial to keep your ego from taking over. Avoid the temptation to jump right back to your pre-injury weights. Plan a reasonable progression and stick to it.

For example, with my shoulder injury, after a few weeks of light incline pressing, I started loading incline presses with more weight. After a few weeks of this, I began doing flat bench again with very light loads and high reps. Over time, I simply added weight in small increments until I was back to where I started.

- **Stay positive.** Recovery won't always be straightforward and linear. Sometimes it feels like a constant cycle of taking two steps forward and one step back. It's frustrating, but it still represents progress. Be patient and work with your body, not against it.

- **Seek professional help.** If the problem persists, it's time to visit a medical or rehab professional. You need someone who's trained to address your specific issue.

DON'T SKIP YOUR WARM-UP

As a final note on safety, I'm giving you a quick crash course on how to warm up before your workouts. The limited research we have doesn't actually show a strong causative link between warming up and injury risk, so it isn't something to obsess over (as many trainees do).[18] Long, drawn out warm-ups are just wasting your time at worst or burning a few calories at best.

That said, there are a few things you really should get into the habit of doing before you start lifting. I start every workout with the same warm-up, no exceptions. I'm calling this type of warm-up a "general warm-up" because you can use it regardless of what muscle groups or exercises are being trained that day. Here is the exact general warm-up I do prior to each workout:

General Warm-Up	
Perform the following general warm-up before every workout (should take about 7 to 12 minutes max). You can save time by doing some of the dynamic stretches as you do warm-up sets for the first exercise.	
5 to 10 minutes	Light cardio on your choice of machine (treadmill, stair climber, elliptical, bike, and so on)
10 reps per side	Arm swings
10 reps per side	Arm circles
10 reps per side	Front-to-back leg swings
10 reps per side	Side-to-side leg swings

Like I said, this should only take you 7 to 12 minutes. After completing the general warm-up, you do an exercise-specific warm-up. Here, start with the first exercise of your workout and gradually build your way up in weight until you get to your working weight (the weight you'll use for your actual hard sets). Do 1 to 4 warm-up sets, depending on the exercise and how much weight you're using. Heavy compound exercises like squats and presses usually need more warm-up sets. Lighter isolation exercises like curls and calf raises usually don't need much, if any.

Here's a guide for how to perform an exercise-specific warm-up of up to 4 sets.

Exercise-Specific Warm-Up	
1 warm-up set	Use about 60% of your planned working weight for 6 to 10 reps (or until you feel warm and loose)
2 warm-up sets	Perform a mini warm-up pyramid: Warm-up set 1: About 50% of planned working weight for 6 to 10 reps Warm-up set 2: About 70% of planned working weight for 4 to 6 reps
3 warm-up sets	Perform a full warm-up pyramid: Warm-up set 1: About 45% of planned working weight for 6 to 10 reps Warm-up set 2: About 65% of planned working weight for 4 to 6 reps Warm-up set 3: About 85% of planned working weight for 3 to 4 reps
4 warm-up sets	Perform a full warm-up pyramid: Warm-up set 1: About 45% of planned working weight for 6 to 10 reps Warm-up set 2: About 60% of planned working weight for 4 to 6 reps Warm-up set 3: About 75% of planned working weight for 3 to 5 reps Warm-up set 4: About 85% of planned working weight for 2 to 4 reps

As a rule of thumb, the heavier the weight you're working up to and the more muscle groups involved in the exercise, the more warm-up sets you'll want to do. For example, dumbbell lateral raises may need only 1 warm-up set, whereas heavy barbell back squats may require 3 or 4 warm-up sets.

PROPER PACING

A bold promise is the oldest trick in fitness marketing:

- "Gain ten pounds of muscle with the secret pill doctors don't want you to know about!"

- "Lose twenty pounds of fat with this workout hack!"

- "Add an inch to your arms overnight!"

It works because enough people really believe in shortcuts to success. That belief leads to unsustainable approaches to nutrition and fitness. Trainees get into the game expecting overnight results, only to get frustrated and give up when their hard work doesn't deliver the promised results.

That's why proper pacing—allowing an appropriate rate of progress—is such an important aspect of sustainability.

Bodybuilding is a lifelong journey. While some results will come quickly, the most meaningful ones are those that take months and years rather than days and weeks. If you recognize this on the front end, you won't feel compelled to rush the process.

In the next chapter, I'll explain how fast you can expect to make progress based on how many years you've been training. For now, I'll conclude this section with a selection of quotes—some by a person trying to rush their fitness journey and others by someone with proper pacing.

Table 2.1: Rushing Versus Properly Pacing

Someone Rushing Their Journey	Someone Properly Pacing Their Journey
"I've been at this for a month already! How long does it usually take?"	"I've only been lifting for a month and I'm already feeling stronger! Let's keep it going!"
"I'm eating less than a thousand calories a day and still barely losing weight. My metabolism must be broken! I'm giving up."	"I'm eating 2,000 calories a day, and even though I'm not losing weight as fast as I'd like, my clothes are fitting better and I'm feeling healthier. This feels sustainable for me."
"If I don't set a new personal record on the bench press every workout, what's the point? Go hard or go home, baby!"	"If I don't set a new personal record every workout, that's fine. Some days I'm stronger than others. The overall trend line is what really matters."
"Even though my elbow is bothering me, I'm not modifying my workout. I want this more than anyone else. No excuses!"	"Since my elbow is bothering me on dips, I'll switch them out for a decline press instead. That way, I'll allow my elbow to heal while still getting a similar workout. I'll return to dips when I'm ready."
"My training partner is making gains faster than me. Now I have to cheat to use the same weights. I can't let them lift more than me!"	"Because everyone has different genetic abilities, I can't compare my progress to anyone else's. I'm just happy to see how much I've gained."

Now that you understand the importance of enjoyment, safety, and proper pacing in building a sustainable training plan, Chapter 3 shifts your attention to mindset, the second vertical rail of the Muscle Ladder.

CHAPTER 3

MINDSET

THINKING YOUR WAY TO GAINS

Now we turn to mindset, the second rail of the ladder:

Every rep you ever go for in the gym either happens or doesn't happen because of your brain. When you decide it's time to lift a weight, the motor cortex in your brain sends a signal through your spinal cord to your muscles, telling them it's time to go to work. At this point, your muscles contract, trying to lift the weight. If your muscles sense that the weight might not be movable, they send such advice back up to your brain. Your brain can then decide if it wants to override the muscle's counsel and go for the rep anyway or listen to the muscle's guidance and put the weight down. Sometimes, the weight is just physically not movable, whether the brain likes it or not. In these cases, despite the override from the brain to go for it, the rep is failed.

Your brain also decides how you feel about the workout. When you have a good one, it releases natural painkillers and euphoriants. You remember that feeling, and it makes you more likely to show up for the next training session, the one after that, and the one after that. The more you show up, the better your results. And the better your results, the greater your feeling of accomplishment. You feel good about what you're doing and trust that feeling.

That's why one of the most important questions you can ask yourself is, "How should I *think* about my training?"

What are you trying to accomplish? Is what you want realistic? If it is, how do you get there? What habits do you need to establish? And when you hit a rough patch, how will you navigate it?

I'll begin with the biggest question for someone reading a bodybuilding book.

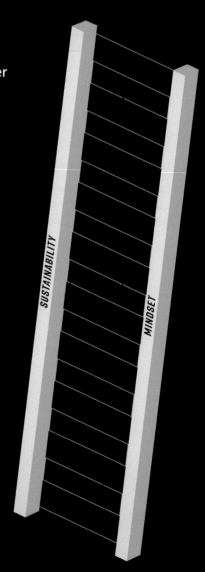

HOW MUCH MUSCLE CAN I BUILD, AND HOW LONG WILL IT TAKE?

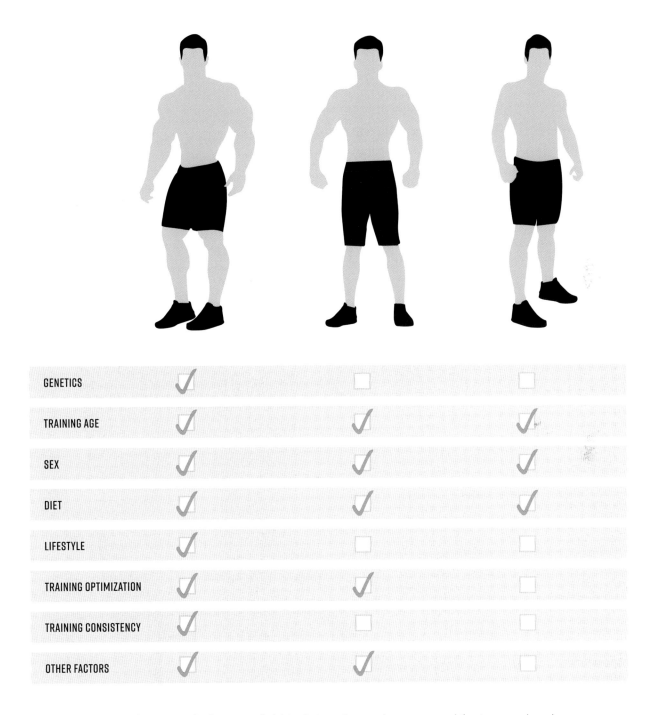

GENETICS	✓	☐	☐
TRAINING AGE	✓	✓	✓
SEX	✓	✓	✓
DIET	✓	✓	✓
LIFESTYLE	✓	☐	☐
TRAINING OPTIMIZATION	✓	✓	☐
TRAINING CONSISTENCY	✓	☐	☐
OTHER FACTORS	✓	✓	☐

How much muscle you gain from weight training depends on several factors and varies widely from person to person. Table 3.1 includes a list of the main factors impacting your rate of muscle growth:

Table 3.1: Factors Influencing Rate of Muscle Gain

Factor	Effect
Genetics	Some people are simply wired to build more muscle and to build it faster than others.
Training age	New lifters build muscle faster than people who have been training for some time.
Sex	Men and women build muscle at a similar *relative* rate. However, men usually start with more muscle at baseline, so they tend to build muscle faster on an *absolute* scale and end up with higher total lean mass, on average.
Diet	Eating in a caloric surplus generally allows for faster muscle growth (up to a point) than eating in a caloric deficit or at caloric maintenance. Eating a higher-protein diet (up to a point) results in more muscle gain, too.
Lifestyle	People who stress less and sleep better tend to build more muscle.
Training optimization	People who train intelligently build muscle faster than those who train suboptimally.
Training consistency	People who train consistently tend to build more muscle than those who skip workouts and are inconsistent with their program adherence.
Other factors	Age, use of supplements, drug use, injuries, athletic background, equipment access, and psychological factors can also impact your rate of muscle gain.

Given the incredible range of possible outcomes, you can appreciate the challenge of offering predictions for how much muscle any individual can expect to build and how fast they can expect to build it. However, I can share ranges for realistic rates of muscle development that apply to *most* people. I do this with the understanding that outliers are always at both ends. Some people will pack on muscle even faster than the high end of my estimates, and a rare few may struggle to reach the low end, especially if they skip workouts often. Chances are, you'll land somewhere in the middle.

Tables 3.2 and 3.3 offer muscle growth guidelines for what most people can expect to gain in each year of their training journey, assuming their diet is conducive to muscle-building (that is, enough calories and protein); they've optimized their training (the main topic of this book); they aren't using steroids (which accelerate muscle growth but not without side effects); and they have no obvious extenuating circumstances such as a serious illness or injury, a sleep disorder, or extreme stress at work or home.

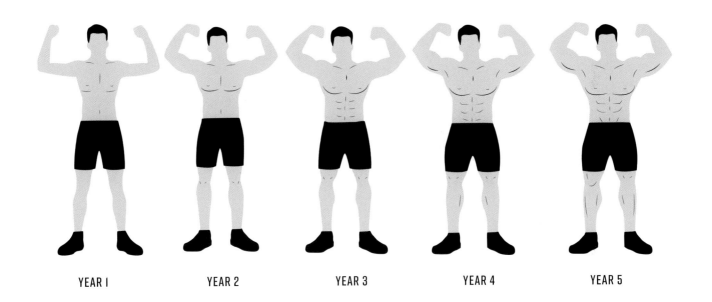

YEAR I YEAR 2 YEAR 3 YEAR 4 YEAR 5

Table 3.2: Realistic Rates of Muscle Gain (Men)[1]

	Realistic Muscle Gain (Per Year)	Realistic Muscle Gain (Per Month)
Year 1	10 to 25 lb (4.5 to 11 kg)	0.8 to 2.1 lb (0.4 to 1 kg)
Year 2	5 to 10 lb (2 to 4.5 kg)	0.4 to 0.8 lb (0.2 to 0.4 kg)
Year 3	2.5 to 7.5 lb (1 to 3.5 kg)	0.2 to 0.6 lb (0.1 to 0.25 kg)
Year 4	1 to 5 lb (.5 to 2 kg)	0.1 to 0.4 lb (0.05 to 0.2 kg)
Year 5 and on	0.5 to 1 lb (0.25 to 0.5 kg)	0 to 0.1 lb (0 to 0.05 kg)
Total Muscle Gained (Lifetime)	20 to 50 lb (13.5 to 23 kg)	

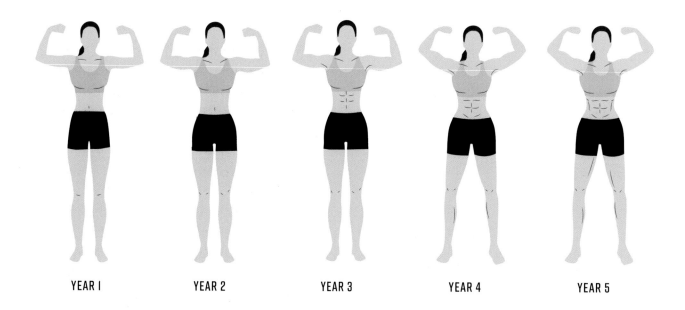

YEAR 1   YEAR 2   YEAR 3   YEAR 4   YEAR 5

Table 3.3: Realistic Rates of Muscle Gain (Women)[2]

	Realistic Muscle Gain (Per Year)	Realistic Muscle Gain (Per Month)
Year 1	6 to 15 lb (2.5 to 7 kg)	0.5 to 1.25 lb (0.2 to 0.6 kg)
Year 2	3 to 6 lb (1.5 to 3 kg)	0.25 to 0.5 lb (0.1 to 0.25 kg)
Year 3	1.5 to 4.5 lb (0.5 to 2 kg)	0.1 to 0.4 lb (0.05 to 0.2 kg)
Year 4	0.5 to 3 lb (0.25 to 1.5 kg)	0 to 0.25 lb (0 to 0.125 kg)
Year 5 and on	0.25 to 0.5 lb (0.1 to 0.25 kg)	0 to 0.05 lb (0 to 0.02 kg)
Total Muscle Gained (Lifetime)	12 to 30 lb (5.5 to 14 kg)	

As you can see from the tables, most men can expect to gain 10 to 25 pounds of muscle in their first year of lifting, and most women can expect to gain 6 to 15 pounds. That's the newbie-period honeymoon. Once you're past it, growth tends to slow down, assuming you were training hard and smart from the jump. By the time you reach year five, gains may only be visually noticeable with a very dedicated training approach.

We don't fully understand why muscle growth slows down, but it makes perfect sense that it would. Even the Incredible Hulk didn't Hulk out to infinity. He stopped at "monstrously huge."

In case you're feeling discouraged by the idea of getting close to maxing out your gains after just five years of lifting, I'll add this: Very, very few lifters, no matter how dedicated, reach their genetic potential on that timeline. It would take serious, intelligent training, optimized nutrition, and a lifestyle built around training to get everything right. It would also mean nothing went wrong. No serious accidents, injuries, or illnesses. No major changes to your work or family life. No distractions that take the edge off your motivation.

Most of us, including me, spend our first few years searching for the ideal approach to training and nutrition. The younger you are, the more likely you are to blow off sleep, eat whatever looks good, and experience big changes in your career and relationships. All those factors affect your results in the gym. You could reach your fifth year of training with plenty of unrealized potential. And even if you think you've hit your genetic ceiling, you may surprise yourself with the gains you can make with the advanced training techniques I'll show you in Chapter 12.

Now, when we talk about changes in muscle mass, we're also usually talking about changes in body weight. It's very uncommon to change one without also changing the other. To maintain your body weight while gaining muscle, you'd have to take off a pound of fat for every pound of muscle you put on. While this perfect match certainly can occur, especially in new lifters with significant fat to lose, it isn't the most common scenario.

Remember what I noted in Table 3.1: The fastest way to gain muscle is to create a caloric surplus—eating about 5 to 10 percent more food than you need to maintain your current weight. (I'll go into more detail about this in Chapter 14.)

Weight gain is rarely, if ever, 100 percent lean tissue. (Lean tissue includes muscle, bone, connective tissue, organ mass, and everything else that isn't fat.) Nor is weight loss ever 100 percent fat. You always put on or take off a combination of the two. A genetically average lifter who builds 15 pounds of muscle in their first year of training might also add 5 pounds of fat for a total weight gain of 20 pounds.

But it's hard to predict. A new lifter who's relatively lean and gains weight slowly will probably add a higher percentage of muscle, whereas a larger individual who gains weight quickly will probably add a higher percentage of fat alongside their muscle.

Some of you, I expect, will want to build muscle and lose fat at the same time, a pursuit known as *body recomposition.* The good news is that "recomp" is a very realistic goal for beginners, especially if you have a lot of fat to lose. (More experienced trainees can still experience recomp, but it comes at the cost of slower muscle gain.) For body recomposition, you want to keep your calories right around maintenance as you eat a high-protein diet and dial in your training. Just keep in mind that when going the recomp route, your muscle gains will be in the neighborhood of 40 to 75 percent of the rates shown in the tables. Again, that's because muscle gain is slower without a caloric surplus. But if you're simultaneously losing fat, that may be a fair trade-off.

And if fat loss is your primary goal? You'll need a caloric deficit of around 10 to 20 percent. That means you eat 10 to 20 percent fewer calories than you need to maintain your weight. As long as you don't go crazy with the calorie cuts, you can still gain muscle, especially if you're new to training. You may not quite reach the rates in the tables, which are based on a caloric surplus. But again, that's a good trade-off if you look and feel better after losing fat. (As I mentioned, I cover all this in more detail in Chapter 14.)

One final note about realistic expectations for muscle growth: You don't know how your body will respond to training until you actually train. And even then, you won't *really* know how much your physique can improve until you've put in years of training. Bodybuilding is a long game. Celebrate and appreciate any gains as they come!

STOP COMPARING YOURSELF TO OTHER PEOPLE

It's perfectly fine to draw inspiration from someone else's physique; that's why so many lifters put up posters of Arnold before they even touch their first barbell. Just make sure it comes from a place of appreciation rather than envy. You never want to stand on the ladder's first rung and compare yourself to someone who's already reached the top. The view from below is butt-ugly.

"Compare and despair" is a surefire way to deny yourself a happy, fulfilling life. It's especially destructive in fitness and bodybuilding. There are just too many factors outside our control to make truly fair 1:1 comparisons.

The biggest one is genetics. You don't know what your body can do until you start training and have trained consistently for years. And you have no idea how your genetics compare to someone else's. Trust me on this: You can always find someone with genetic potential superior to yours. And your potential is almost certainly superior to someone else's.

You don't know how long someone has been training or what advantages they enjoyed along the way. Maybe they got a head start because of their access to coaching or facilities. Maybe they had more social support from family, friends, or teammates. Maybe they figured out their nutrition years before you tasted your first protein shake. Maybe they have less stress at home or work. Maybe they sleep like a rock while you toss and turn much of the night. Finally, you have no idea what "special sports supplements" they take or may have taken in the past.

All these details are ultimately irrelevant to you. Your journey is *your* journey. The only comparison that matters is your current place versus your starting place. Think of your training as an ongoing scientific experiment. The control group is your untrained self, which has identical genetics to yours. Every workout and every meal are part of the experiment. You'll enjoy the process a lot more when you focus 100 percent on what you've gained and what you can do to build on those gains.

SETTING SCIENCE-BASED GOALS FOR BUILDING MUSCLE

Now that you have a sense of how much muscle you *can* build, it's time to decide how much you *will* build by setting some science-based muscle-building goals. To help you establish and pursue those goals, I'm borrowing from the vast research on the psychology of goal setting.

YOUR GOAL HIERARCHY

Researchers at the University of Bern in Switzerland introduced the concept of a goal hierarchy in a fantastic 2018 paper.[3] The authors argued that long-term success improves when you pursue a goal at three distinct levels.

At the top is your superordinate goal—the thing you want to achieve. At the bottom are your subordinate goals. These are the small, specific habits and behaviors you need to establish. In the authors' words, "They define precisely what to do and how to do it." In between are intermediate goals—what happens after you achieve your subordinate goals but before you reach your primary objective.

Figure 3.1 illustrates my current goal hierarchy.

Figure 3.1

My superordinate, intermediate, and subordinate fitness goals

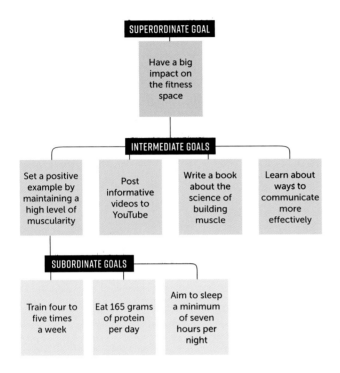

Superordinate Goals (Your "Why")

I sometimes think of superordinate goals as "fuzzy" because they're typically vague, if not abstract. They describe something you want to achieve or become in the future. Goals like these are often frowned upon in self-help guides, which encourage you to focus on extremely specific and detailed goals. The evidence, however, is that such precise goals probably aren't enough on their own. They're important, but they're also constrained. They don't offer any insight into *why* you would bother achieving them.

For me, the superordinate goal is to "have a big impact on the fitness space." It motivates me to stick with my subordinate and intermediate goals—one of which is writing this book.

You can think of superordinate goals as your "why." Why do you want to build muscle? Is it to

be healthier and live longer? Is it to look more **attractive**? To be more confident? To improve your overall well-being? To be stronger and more capable in day-to-day tasks? To set a good example for your kids? To raise your profile in the fitness industry?

Understanding *why* you want to build muscle means you're more likely to follow through, especially when you encounter challenges and setbacks.

Intermediate Goals

Intermediate goals are neither short-term nor long-term. They're the bridge between your extremely specific subordinate goals and the loftier ambition of your superordinate goals. Yours might include increasing your strength on the squat, bench press, and deadlift; lowering your body-fat percentage; or launching or expanding a fitness-related business.

Ideally, they help you build *from* your subordinate goals and *toward* your superordinate goals.

Subordinate Goals

Subordinate goals are unambiguous. They're the hierarchy's most actionable, detailed, and specific components. They tell you exactly what to do and how to do it, so they provide the foundation for everything you want to achieve.

Each subordinate goal supports an intermediate goal. So, a subordinate training goal (working out three days a week for forty-five to sixty minutes per session) would help you achieve the intermediate goal of increasing your strength on the three power lifts. A subordinate nutrition goal (tracking your protein consumption on an app to ensure you get 150 grams per day) supports the intermediate goal of getting leaner. And a subordinate business goal (post at least twice per **week** on your primary social media platform) gets the attention of future coaching clients.

Rolling with my own example again, I broke down the intermediate goal of "writing a book about the science of building muscle" into the subordinate goal of "doing a ten-day writing retreat in a remote location away from home." (I rented a cabin just outside Mont Tremblant, Québec, where I managed to write the better part of eight chapters.)

Here are some of the subordinate goals I am currently using to support my intermediate goal of "set a positive example by maintaining a high level of muscularity":

- Train five or six times a week on a push/pull/legs split

- Eat 165 grams of protein per day using the MacroFactor app to track

- Aim to sleep a minimum of seven hours per night

OUTCOME-ORIENTED GOALS VERSUS PROCESS-ORIENTED GOALS

How you frame goals also matters. Your language reveals how you think about your goals and how you'll interpret challenges along the way. Psychologists divide goals into two general categories: outcome-oriented and process-oriented.

Most of us in fitness and bodybuilding gravitate toward outcome-oriented goals, which, as the name suggests, focus on a specific result. Here are some examples:

- I will lose 22 pounds by March 1.

- I will bench press 315 pounds this year.

- I will win the Mr. Olympia contest!

The problem with outcome-oriented goals is that the result you want often depends on things you can't control. And if you fall short, you'll feel like you failed.

Take the 22-pound weight-loss goal, for example. Let's say you lose 10 pounds by March 1. Did you fail because 10 pounds is less than half your weight-loss goal? I would say you succeeded because it's hard to lose 10 pounds, and you've clearly moved in the right direction. On top of that, you probably encountered some unexpected challenges along the way: Maybe you rolled your ankle, making it harder to do cardio. Maybe something came up at work or home that added stress and interfered with your sleep. Maybe your metabolism adapted faster than you expected, making progress slow down. These things aren't excuses. They're illustrations of why outcome-oriented goals usually aren't ideal.

Process-oriented goals, on the other hand, specify actions and behaviors rather than exact results. More often than not, those things are much more within your control.

Let's return to our weight-loss example. Instead of focusing on an outcome, let's say you established process-oriented goals like these:

- Eat at least two servings of vegetables and two servings of fruit per day.

- Do thirty minutes of cardio three days a week.

- Track food intake in a nutrition app six days a week.

For bench press strength, instead of specifying an outcome, you could set process-oriented goals like these:

- I will bench press twice per week.

- I will increase my caloric intake to support my strength goals.

- I will check in with my coach weekly to assess my progress and adjust my program as needed.

You've not only set yourself up to make progress, but you're much more likely to view any progress as a win (which it is). Equally important, without fixating on an arbitrary outcome goal, there's no reason to think you've failed. Your process-oriented mindset helps you enjoy the journey as much as the outcome.

HOW DO I MEASURE PROGRESS?

In this section, I focus on two goals—building muscle and losing fat—and three tools to monitor your movement toward those goals: strength performance, progress photos, and body weight. Learning to use these tools appropriately is crucial in establishing a productive mindset toward your goals by avoiding misleading feedback and recognizing true progress.

STRENGTH PERFORMANCE

Muscle gains are notoriously hard to monitor in real time. What you see in the mirror doesn't always reflect what's going on below the skin. That's why, in my opinion, strength is the single best gauge of your progress. If you're getting stronger, you're almost certainly gaining muscle.

To be clear, "getting stronger" doesn't refer to your maximum strength on any specific lift. Nor does it imply that lifting heavy is the key to muscle growth. It refers to the amount of weight you train with. You want to increase your strength within the parameters of your program. If your program calls for 4 sets of 10 reps of biceps curls, you want to be able to use progressively heavier weights for that rep range. Let's say you start the program using 15-pound dumbbells. You can get all 10 reps on the first

2 sets but fall a couple reps short on the next 2 sets. When you hit 10 reps on all 4 sets, you increase the weight for subsequent workouts. Within a year, you're using 30-pounders for 10 reps, and after two years, you need 40-pounders to feel challenged. Assuming you kept your lifting form consistent, your biceps aren't just significantly stronger. They're also significantly bigger. You wouldn't be able to handle those weights if they weren't.

Similarly, if you go from doing two assisted pull-ups in your first week of training to 12 assisted pull-ups ten weeks later, I guarantee your back will look significantly more jacked than when you started. The same goes for any other exercise. You might make some early strength gains without adding muscle simply by improving your technique on more complex exercises like squats and deadlifts. But over months and years, your ability to handle heavier weights across a variety of rep ranges means you're gaining muscle mass.

To ensure strength progression, I recommend tracking your results for every workout— exercises, sets, reps, weights. If that's too cumbersome, you should at least be aware of your trends, especially for major compound lifts like presses, rows, and squats.

PROGRESS PHOTOS

Most people who get into lifting do it at least partly for the aesthetics—to look more fit, jacked, powerful, or athletic. Progress photos are the most direct and reliable way to see how you're doing.

It's a simple process. Your smartphone's camera should work well enough. You just need to get a few things right:

- Use the same background and similar lighting for each photo. That makes it easier to compare photos taken months apart.

- Position the camera between you and the light source, as shown here:

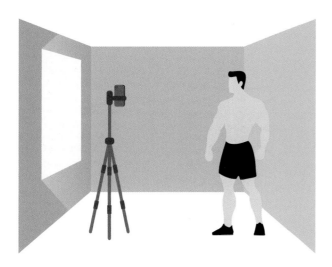

- Include your entire body, head to toe, in the photos.

- If you're male, wear underwear, bodybuilding trunks, or short shorts in your photos. If you're female, wear a bikini or shorts and a sports bra. You want a clear view of every major muscle group.

- Take at least three photos: front, side, rear.

- If you have bodybuilding goals, you can hit the mandatory poses: abdominals and thighs, front lat spread, front double biceps, front relaxed, most muscular, rear lat spread, rear double biceps, rear relaxed, side chest, and side triceps.

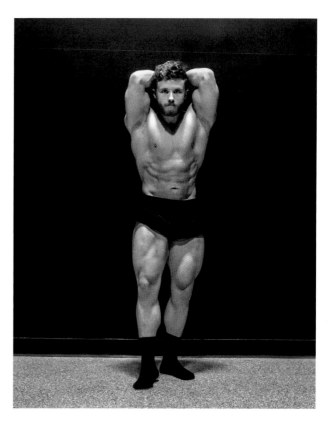

ABDOMINALS AND THIGHS

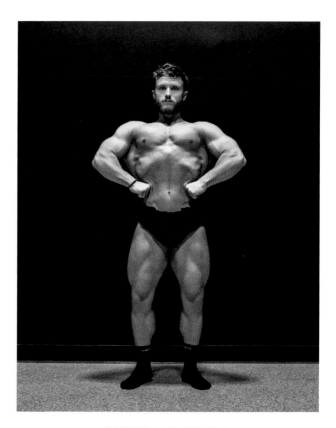

FRONT LAT SPREAD

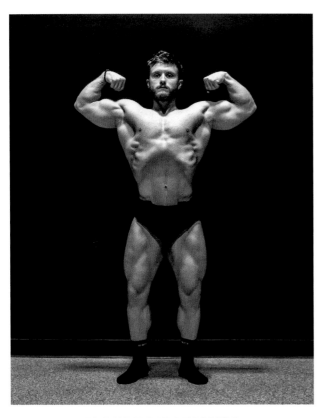

FRONT DOUBLE BICEPS

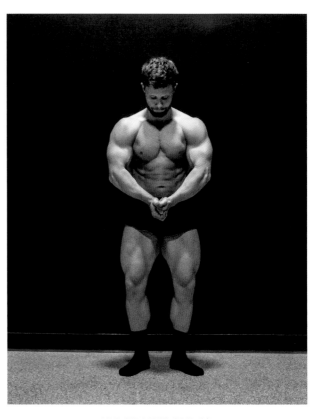

MOST MUSCULAR

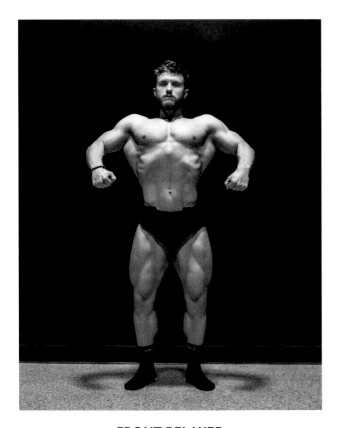

FRONT RELAXED

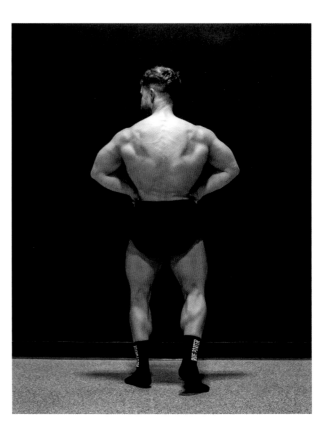

REAR LAT SPREAD

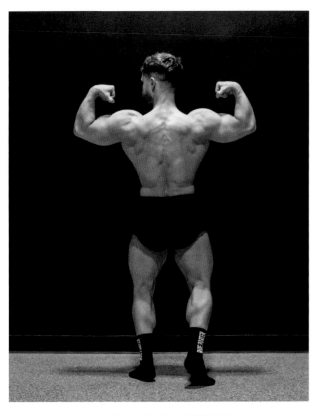

REAR DOUBLE BICEPS

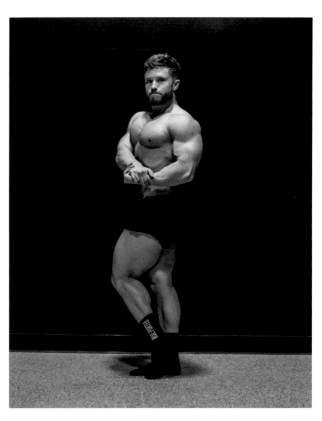

SIDE CHEST

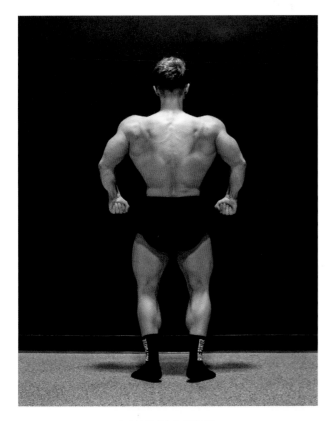

REAR RELAXED

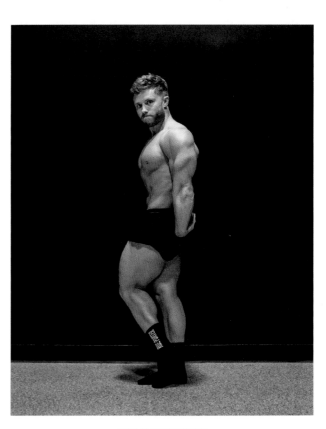

SIDE TRICEPS

I recommend taking progress photos at least once every two to three months and at most once a week. If you change up your program in a major way, be sure to take photos before you start and at regular intervals in the future. They'll help you decide if the changes are working.

One caution: Visual changes aren't like strength improvements. It's hard to detect them in real time. It's easy to get discouraged if you take photos too frequently. Once a month should give you all the information you need when you're starting out.

After that, the frequency depends on what you need to know and when you need to know it. For example, if you're training for a physique contest or a special event like a beach photo shoot, you may want to take photos more often as you get closer to the date.

What if you don't want to take photos at all? I strongly recommend taking them anyway, especially at the beginning of your journey. You wouldn't believe how many people have mind-blowing transformations but can't actually blow any minds because they didn't document what they looked like at the start. "Before" pictures give context to the "afters," even if you're the only person who ever sees them.

Trust me: Your future self will thank you for taking progress photos.

BODY WEIGHT

The final tool to measure progress is often the only tool used to monitor a physique transformation. Someone focused on muscle gain looks for the number on the scale to go up. Someone focused on fat loss wants to see that number go down.

Body weight obviously gives you important data for both of those goals, but it shouldn't be your only source of information. I'll return to this idea in a moment.

If your main goal is to add bulk to your physique, your specific rate of weight gain depends on all the factors I mentioned earlier in this chapter. Generally, I recommend increasing your weight by about 1 to 2 percent per month. In my experience, that allows you to maximize muscle growth while minimizing fat gain. So, if you currently weigh 160 pounds, your rough goal is to add 1.5 to 3 pounds per month. In six months, if you can maintain that rate, you'll pack on 9 to 18 pounds. Your gains will eventually slow down if they haven't already. But the difference will still be substantial by the end of the year.

The bigger you are and the more training experience you have, the more you should focus on the lower end of the range to prevent excess fat gain.

To maximize fat loss while minimizing muscle loss, I generally recommend losing about 0.5 to 1 percent of your body weight per week. So, if you currently weigh 220 pounds, you would try to lose 1 to 2 pounds per week. The leaner you are now, the slower you should go. Faster weight loss will cost you too much muscle.

And if you want to lose fat while building muscle—a goal that, as I've noted, is entirely possible for a new lifter but progressively more challenging with increasing experience—you generally want the number on the scale to stay about the same.

A digital scale is useful for any of these goals. It's a simple and accessible way to see if you're gaining, losing, or maintaining weight. Over time, you can calculate both the size and rate of any weight change.

That's fine, as far as it goes. What a scale can't tell you is *what* you're gaining, losing, or maintaining. Are you gaining fat? Losing muscle? The scale can't say.

You can buy a scale that purports to measure body fat. But the margin of error with those devices means their numbers aren't particularly helpful. Even if they were accurate, I'm not sure how enlightening the data would be.

If you're gaining at the recommended rate (that is, not too quickly), and you're being smart and consistent with your training, you're probably adding a lot more muscle than fat. And if you're losing at the recommended rate (not too quickly), and you're being smart and consistent with your training, you're probably shedding a lot more fat than muscle.

When you use your scale in combination with strength performance and progress photos, it tells you what you need to know. When your weight gain tracks with your strength increases, and your photos show visual progress, you're on the right track. When your weight goes down while your strength stays the same, and you like what you see in your photos, your program is clearly working. And if your weight stays the same while your strength increases and your photos show a leaner, more muscular physique, what more do you need to know?

I recommend taking body weight measurements two to seven days per week and calculating a weekly average. Then you can compare your body weight average from week to week to get a better idea of whether you are gaining, losing, or maintaining your weight over time.

PUTTING THE THREE MAIN TRACKING TOOLS TO USE

While each tracking tool gives you important information, none gives you *enough* information to assess your progress. It's only when you combine their feedback that you get an accurate picture. Let's look at what the tracking tools can tell you in five common scenarios, which are summarized in Table 3.4.

Scenario 1: Lean Muscle Gain

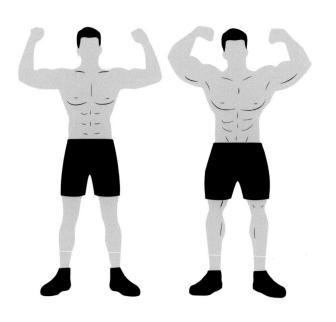

You're likely gaining lean muscle* if you're getting stronger in the gym, you're looking more jacked in your progress photos, and the number on the scale is increasing at the desired rate. This is an ideal scenario if your main goal is to lean bulk.

---

*Technically, there's no such thing as "lean muscle," just as there's no such thing as "muscular fat." Muscle is "lean" by definition, just as fat is "fat" by definition. I could be *really* pedantic by adding that adipocytes (aka fat cells) contain some lean tissue in the structural network that encases them. And small amounts of ectopic fat infiltrates muscle cells, especially as you get older or less fit. In this book, I use "lean muscle gain" to signify muscle gain that isn't accompanied by excess fat gain.

Scenario 2: Fat Loss (with Muscle Maintenance)

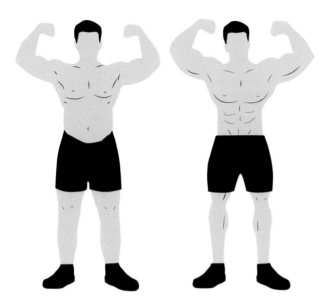

When your strength is holding steady, you look leaner in your progress photos, and the number on the scale is decreasing at the desired rate, you're very likely losing fat while maintaining muscle. This is obviously ideal if that's your main goal.

Scenario 3: Body Recomposition

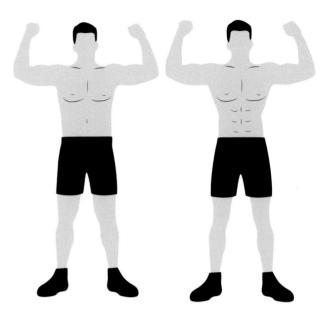

Losing fat while gaining muscle—"recomp" in fitness parlance—is one of the hardest things to pull off. The trifecta of building strength, gaining muscle, and getting leaner is a more likely outcome when any of the following apply:

- You're a new lifter.

- You're training with a well-designed program for the first time.

- You're returning to the gym after a long break from training, possibly due to an illness or injury.

- You're "skinny-fat"—a high body-fat percentage on a relatively small frame.

- You're using one or more anabolic, ergogenic drugs (steroids, peptides, growth hormone, etc.).

The more you've trained and the more progress you've made, the less likely you are to pull off impressive recomp. For faster results, highly experienced lifters should generally focus on one or the other goal at a time—building muscle *or* losing fat.

Scenario 4: Muscle Gain (with Excess Fat Gain)

Scenario 5: Fat Loss (with Excess Muscle Loss)

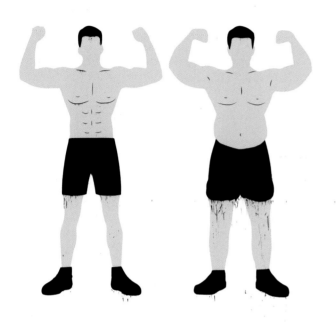

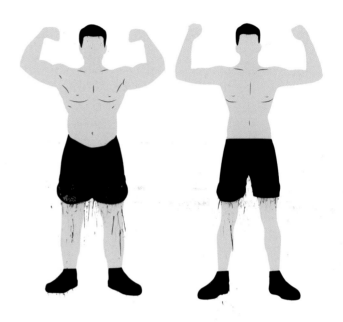

It's a good-news, bad-news situation: You're getting stronger. Possibly a *lot* stronger. And your body weight is going up alongside the loads you train with. You love the way your newly enlarged muscles strain your sleeves. But any definition you had in your "before" pictures is now smoothed out.

For some, that's an acceptable trade-off. A "dirty bulk" is better than no gains at all. But eventually, you'll have to decide what to do about the "dirty" part. Maybe you like being bigger and stronger and decide not to change anything. However, if you're primarily focused on aesthetics, you might want to switch to a fat-loss phase to trim off some excess bulk.

Or you can choose a middle path: Continue bulking at a slower pace and a smaller caloric surplus. More like Scenario 1, in other words.

Another good-news, bad-news situation: You're losing weight fast. However, your progress photos show a body that looks smaller but not necessarily more fit, lean, and healthy. And in the gym, your workouts are disappointing. You're losing strength and feel drained of energy.

For most lifters, the bad-news consequences of a crash diet outweigh the benefits of losing a lot of weight. Your progress photos and declining strength performance show that you're losing a lot of muscle and fat.

The solution is to slow your weight loss by modestly increasing calories. This creates a smaller caloric deficit and should bring you back to Scenario 2.

As you can see, these three basic tools give you a lot of information. It may be all the information you need or want to assess your progress and tweak your program if necessary. But for some lifters, in some situations, it helps to have more specific data. Let's look at a few additional tools.

Table 3.4: Interpreting Strength Data, Progress Photos, and Body Weight Changes

	Scenario 1	Scenario 2	Scenario 3	Scenario 4	Scenario 5
Strength	↑	↔	↑	↑	↓
Progress Photos	Looking more muscular	Looking leaner	Looking leaner and more muscular	Looking bigger but much less lean	Looking leaner but less muscular
Body Weight	Increasing at the desired rate	Decreasing at the desired rate	Maintaining	Increasing faster than desired	Decreasing faster than desired
Interpretation	You're building muscle without much fat gain. If your main goal is to add lean mass, you're doing it! Nice work!	You're losing fat while maintaining muscle. If your main goal is to get leaner without losing muscle, you're doing it! Good job!	You're losing fat while building muscle. If your goal is body recomposition—getting leaner and more jacked at the same time—you're doing it! Well done!	You're building muscle but also adding a lot of fat. Some might call this a "dirty bulk." Unless you're comfortable with the fat gain, you may want to slow down the weight gain by reducing your caloric surplus.	You're losing fat but also losing muscle mass. To limit muscle loss, you most likely need a smaller caloric deficit and may require smarter training and/or more protein.

Waist and Body-Part Measurements

Sometimes your progress is tricky to decipher, even when using the main three tools. For example, let's say you've started a new program to build muscle and lose fat simultaneously. But because you've been training long enough to get past your newbie period, you aren't an ideal candidate for speedy recomp.

So far, the scale shows your weight is within a few pounds of where you started. Your strength is improving but not dramatically. And while you think you see improvements in your progress photos, it's hard to be sure. What you need is a tiebreaker.

Waist measurements are a pretty good tool for assessing body fat. Like body weight, waist circumference can fluctuate for several reasons—temporary bloating, hydration status, menstrual cycle. But if your waist is getting smaller *over time*, you've most likely lost fat, even if your weight has increased. If it's bigger, you've probably gained some fat. In both scenarios, it's unlikely that you would gain or lose enough muscle in your abdominal area to change the circumference by more than a centimeter. Any larger difference is almost certainly because you've gained or lost fat.

The key to getting an accurate measurement is to measure in the same place—above, below, or at your belly button—at the same time of day. Like body weight, it's best to measure first thing in the morning, ideally after using the toilet but before eating or drinking anything.

Some lifters like to assess progress with direct measurements of their chest, arm, thigh, and calf circumference. Obviously, the goal is to see which muscles are growing and which aren't.

I find body-part measurements tedious and unnecessary for most lifters. Detecting differences in measurements can be cumbersome and even discouraging, especially if you notice the rate of gain decreasing beyond the first year or two of your lifting journey. Your progress will more reliably show up in your gym performance and progress photos. That's why you're more likely to get asked about your max bench press or squat rather than how big your chest and thighs are.

Body-part measurements are especially unreliable when you're cutting. Your thigh circumference might decrease, leading you to the incorrect conclusion that you're losing muscle, when in reality, you're losing fat. If your progress photos show the muscles looking full, with deepening separations, the circumference doesn't matter.

All that said, I don't want to dissuade you from taking body-part measurements if you like having more data and find the measurements motivating. Just avoid taking them too often. Once a month should capture your gains in your first year of training. After that, I suggest taking measurements no more than a few times a year.

Body Fat Assessment

If you have access to higher-grade devices like DEXA or BodPod to measure body composition, feel free to use them periodically. They're among the most accurate ways to assess your fat-to-lean mass ratio.

Your gym may have other options for measuring body fat, like bioelectrical impedance analysis (BIA) devices or skinfold calipers. However, because they have a relatively high margin of error and do not offer valuable insight beyond the more basic tools I've covered, I consider these tools optional. (If you do decide to use calipers, make sure the same person does the measurements each time, using the same equipment. Different users can come up with very different numbers.)

Again, I don't think these measurements are necessary to assess progress. When you're playing a long game, you rarely need a higher level of precision than you'll get from your three primary measurement tools (strength, progress photos, and body weight).

THE TREND IS *ALL* THAT MATTERS

It's easy to get derailed by a disappointing weigh-in, a bad workout, or a missed attempt at a PR. But those things simply don't matter—at all—in the grand scheme of things. Instead of micromanaging your progress, you should focus entirely on the trend line.

If your goal is to lose weight, is the number moving down over time? If the answer is yes, you're golden. Daily fluctuations will always occur due to an undigested meal, water retention, or any other factors I've mentioned. Those blips aren't important. The trend is all that matters.

If your goal is to increase your bench press strength, are your lifts trending up over time? If the answer is yes, you're golden. A single workout where you move less weight than usual simply doesn't matter. Maybe you're still fatigued from a previous workout, or you've lost sleep, or you're dealing with unexpected stress. The trend is all that matters.

If your goal is to gain muscle, do your progress photos show improvements? If the answer is yes, you're golden. A single day where you look a little off doesn't matter. Maybe the lighting was less than optimal, you were unusually tired, or you were a little bloated. Again, the trend is all that matters.

A NOTE ON SUBJECTIVE FACTORS

So far, I've focused on objective measurements. But subjective factors can be equally valuable for gauging progress. For example:

- Do you feel more confident and optimistic?

- Do you have more energy for your day-to-day tasks?

- Do you feel stronger and more capable?

- Do you have less pain or discomfort?

- Do your clothes fit better?

Your answers to these questions won't give you data you can track over time. Instead, they give you insight into how your program is working for you as a person. Every "yes" is a win.

HOW DO I BUILD HABITS AND ROUTINES?

"How do you stay motivated?"

It's one of the most common questions I hear, especially from discouraged lifters. It's a fair question, but I don't think the answer will help anyone who feels compelled to ask.

The truth is, I'm *not* always motivated. Even though I genuinely enjoy training, there will always be days when I don't feel like going to the gym. Motivation comes in waves, and I've learned not to count on it to pull me along. You shouldn't either. It's much smarter to focus on building the habits and routines that allow you to stick to your program—especially when, if you stop to think about it, you'd rather do almost anything else. It's like operating on autopilot.

For the rest of this chapter, I'm highlighting some of my favorite habit-building techniques. They've made my fitness journey much easier, and I hope they do the same for you.

BUNDLE TEMPTATIONS

Temptation bundling means linking an activity you enjoy (the "temptation") with a less enjoyable activity that's aligned with a long-term goal.

For example, for some reason, I love watching videos on YouTube where someone shows their reaction to listening to a new album for the first time. I can easily kill thirty to forty minutes just watching someone else listen to music. I know it's not the most productive use of my time, but that's why I call it a "temptation," instead of "a vital part of my daily routine." Conversely, I find cardio monotonous and boring and not at all tempting.

So, I hold off on my temptation (watching album reactions) until I can bundle it with something I don't enjoy (cardio). Because I can look forward to the videos, I'm much less likely to skip the cardio altogether.

A 2014 study by Milkman and colleagues found that people were more likely to go to the gym and exercise when they were given an audiobook to listen to.[4] The researchers described it as bundling an instantly gratifying "want" behavior (enjoying audiobooks) with a valuable "should" behavior (exercising).

Here are a few more temptation bundles you can try:

- Save new music you're excited about for gym-time listening.

- Play your favorite video game while doing cardio on your machine of choice.

- Have your favorite podcast ready to listen to while cooking healthy meals for the week.

- Allow yourself to watch a mindless livestream during your at-home leg day.

STACK HABITS

Habit stacking is when you pair an existing habit with a new behavior that you want to make a habit. Let's say you have someone in your life you want to check in with more often, but you can never quite find the time. And let's say you have a fifteen-minute commute to your gym. If you use that drive (an existing habit) to make those calls (a new behavior), they become a stacked pair of habits. Habits are stronger when they're stacked together.

Another example: Stack a consistent pre-workout meal with training. For the last year or two, I've been eating the same meal of ground turkey and rice, plus some blueberries and a kiwifruit, before my afternoon workout. It's gotten to the point where eating that meal *without* training afterward would feel weird.

Here are a couple more examples of habit stacking:

- If you're a competitive bodybuilder, stack your existing habit of brushing your teeth at night with the new habit of practicing poses in the mirror.

- Stack your existing habit of packing your gym bag in the morning with watching an informative fitness video on YouTube.

- Stack the existing habit of watching sports highlights every morning with the new habit of scanning an informative fitness article.

MODIFY YOUR ENVIRONMENT

Your surroundings play an enormous role in how likely you are to change your eating behaviors or follow through on your training plan. Modifying your environment is a powerful but underutilized way to make actions more automatic and less dependent on motivation.

Here are three simple home modifications that may help you break counterproductive nutrition habits and develop new ones:

- Is there a food you're likely to overeat? The easiest solution is to keep it out of your home. You can't eat what isn't there. If that's not an option because someone in your home can't live without it, ask if they'll store it somewhere where you can't see it and aren't likely to stumble across it.

- Do you struggle to find time to cook healthy meals or find the process overwhelming? Try this: Make Sundays your meal prep day. Collect your recipes, write a shopping list, stock your fridge with everything you need, and make all the meals simultaneously or sequentially. (Notice these are also examples of habit stacking.) Divide them into portions, label them for your weekday meals, and store them in the fridge or freezer. If you have the means to do so, you can make things even easier by using a prepared meal delivery service.

- If you stress-eat at night, try giving yourself easy access to alternative stress relievers, such as enjoyable video games, books, or puzzles.

Here are some ways to modify your training environment to improve your workout habits:

- The people, music, lighting, and overall vibes at your gym can make a massive difference in how motivated you feel. If you find your gym environment dull and unmotivating, consider switching to a better facility. Even if it's a little more expensive or a little farther from home, the investment will pay off if the new environment makes you more likely to show up for your workouts.

- The best training environment in the world won't matter until you get there. Lots of trainees cut into their workout time by mindlessly scrolling on their phones when they should be on their way to the gym. Or they're too tired to train because they mindlessly scrolled when they should've been asleep. If that's you, consider leaving your phone in another room. If you need an alarm to wake up, try a traditional alarm clock.

- Your phone can also be a distraction in the gym. If you find yourself paying more attention to incoming texts and social media notifications than to your sets and reps, try leaving your phone in your locker. Or switch to airplane mode for the duration of your workout. If you still find it distracting, try listening to music with an old-school MP3 player.

- If you train at lunch or after work, have your gym gear packed and waiting for you in your car. Same with a pre-workout drink or snack: have it ready so you don't need to go home before leaving work. This should decrease your likelihood of skipping the workout.

FIND A SUPPORTIVE COMMUNITY

Fitness, more often than not, is a solitary pursuit.

Yes, if you're lucky, you might find a training partner who's more or less at your level and has more or less similar goals and whose schedule is compatible with yours. A good training partner can help keep you accountable, push you through hard sets, provide constructive feedback on technique, and elevate the overall vibes of the workout. And, of course, you do the same for them.

Not everyone likes having company in the gym, though. I don't. I view workouts as my private time to disconnect from work and home, but I still have a supportive community that helps me stay committed to my goals. It includes friends and family who share my passion for bodybuilding and people from my online platforms who remind me why I do what I do.

It isn't always easy to connect with fitness enthusiasts in the real world, but there's a nearly endless supply of online fitness communities in the digital world. The most active and supportive communities are typically centered around an inspiring fitness personality or trusted brand. The members are pursuing similar goals, and the moderators keep conversations positive and civil for the most part.

Ideally, your online community is a place where you can upload progress photos, ask questions, swap training tips, and share weekly successes and challenges with other people on a similar journey.

BE MORE FLEXIBLE THAN RIGID

Many people who get into fitness and bodybuilding develop a rigid way of thinking about their daily routines and habits, which can be effective in the short term if it keeps you on track. Eating the exact same meals at the exact same time gives you fewer opportunities to deviate from the plan.

But what starts as a disciplined approach, which is admirable in the short term, can eventually turn robotic. Humans don't make good robots. We each have unique thoughts, feelings, and emotions. Rejecting those aspects of our personality not only robs us of the full range of human experience but is also unsustainable.

That's why a flexible mindset works best for most aspects of fitness.

Here are a few ways you can be flexible with nutrition:

- The specific timing of your meals: It doesn't matter if you eat meal four at exactly 5 p.m. every day.

- The specific foods you eat: Give yourself the freedom to mix and match a variety of foods.

- The exact number of calories you eat: You don't need to be 100 percent accurate with your caloric intake for your diet to be effective.

- The exact amount of protein, carbs, and fat you eat: If you track your macros, you don't need to hit them precisely to the gram.

- The intersection of your diet and social life: It's perfectly okay to enjoy parties and family get-togethers, even if the meals can't be perfectly tracked.

A 1999 study from Westenhoefer and colleagues found that a more flexible approach to nutrition was associated with less disordered eating behavior when compared to a rigid approach.[5] Moreover, the flexible approach was associated with lower body mass index (a ratio of weight to height) and more successful long-term weight-loss maintenance.[6]

Here are a few ways you can be more flexible with training:

- **The specific days you lift:** Your body doesn't know what day of the week it is. If something comes up on Monday, you can "borrow" a rest day and shift Monday's workout to Tuesday. Just try to get all your planned workouts in by the end of the week.

- **The specific exercises you do:** If the thought of doing barbell squats makes you resent working out, or if the squat racks are occupied, swap them out for something you would rather do or can do with the available equipment. You can return to squats next week.

- **The exact loads you use:** If you're not feeling as strong as you expected one day, you can train with lighter weights and higher reps. Or if you're feeling stronger than usual, you can train with heavier weights and lower reps. As long as you push the sets hard, results will be similar.

- **Your rest periods between sets:** There is no need to monitor your rest time down to the second.

- **The order of your exercises:** If your workout begins with leg presses but the machine is occupied, do the next exercise in your program and return to leg presses when you can. As long as you're generally prioritizing heavier compound lifts by putting them closer to the beginning of your session, being flexible with exercise order is perfectly fine.

Flexibility, like uncompromising rigidity, can still go too far. Your goal is to hit the sweet spot: enough structure to keep you on track and enough flexibility to make your journey sustainable. You won't reach your goals with a diet so flexible that you eat what you want, when you want it, in any quantity that feels good. Nor will you get very far with completely haphazard and unstructured workouts.

You need to strike a balance between structure and flexibility. Too much structure and the process becomes robotic and unsustainable. Too much flexibility and you lose direction and focus. In nearly two decades of training and coaching, I've found the sweet spot is somewhere in the middle, leaning toward the flexible side when the goal is more lifestyle-oriented and toward the rigid side when the goal is more competition-oriented.

For more information on the science behind the goal-setting techniques in this chapter, I recommend reading "An Evidence-Based Approach to Goal Setting and Behavior Change" at www.strongerbyscience.com/goal-setting. For more detail on the habit-building techniques I discussed in this chapter, I recommend reading *Atomic Habits* by James Clear.

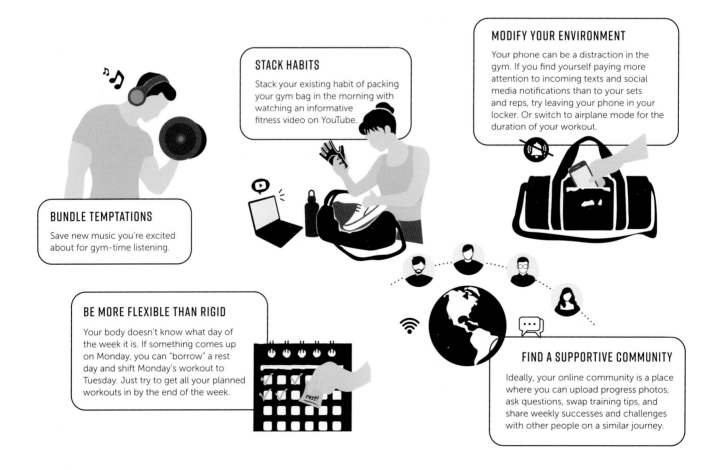

STACK HABITS
Stack your existing habit of packing your gym bag in the morning with watching an informative fitness video on YouTube.

MODIFY YOUR ENVIRONMENT
Your phone can be a distraction in the gym. If you find yourself paying more attention to incoming texts and social media notifications than to your sets and reps, try leaving your phone in your locker. Or switch to airplane mode for the duration of your workout.

BUNDLE TEMPTATIONS
Save new music you're excited about for gym-time listening.

BE MORE FLEXIBLE THAN RIGID
Your body doesn't know what day of the week it is. If something comes up on Monday, you can "borrow" a rest day and shift Monday's workout to Tuesday. Just try to get all your planned workouts in by the end of the week.

FIND A SUPPORTIVE COMMUNITY
Ideally, your online community is a place where you can upload progress photos, ask questions, swap training tips, and share weekly successes and challenges with other people on a similar journey.

WHAT ABOUT "NO PAIN, NO GAIN"?

I started this chapter with a neurological description of how your brain ultimately decides which reps you attempt. This raises the question of how to push through those difficult sets when you don't *feel* like doing that extra rep—when your muscles are begging your brain to give up.

For some lifters, a "no excuses, suck it up and get it done" mindset can be helpful. We say it in different ways: "Pain is just weakness leaving the body." "Never surrender." "No pain, no gain." Arnold Schwarzenegger talked about pushing through the "pain period"—that point in a set when your muscles are burning and you want to quit. Indeed, that's when most people do quit. But as Arnold said, that's where the best growth occurs.

I have two thoughts about this approach.

As with most platitudes, there's a kernel of truth. Some people are motivated by a militant "no excuses" mindset. It may get them to the gym regularly and help them crank out a few extra reps while they're there. They may even enjoy the pain on some level, similar to the pleasure someone might get from eating spicy food or getting a deep-tissue massage.

Early in my lifting career, this thinking helped me push through some brutal sets and probably got me to the gym a few times when I didn't feel like going. But as I grew as a bodybuilder, I saw the pitfalls of this attitude.

You can't reject physics; gravity doesn't care about your mindset. Gravity pulls an object toward the earth at 9.81 meters per second squared. If that object is in your hands and

you can't generate enough force to overcome gravity, you won't do that rep.

A refusal to accept the reality of physics can have negative consequences. Maybe you start using terrible technique to move a weight after your muscles have tapped out. You push through all types of pain, including the pain of an injury. You begin to resent your workouts because they're never satisfying.

Once you tell yourself you can always do a little more, how do you know when you've done enough? After you've puked? When your eyes turn red from burst blood vessels? If there's no logical stopping point, you can never do enough. And if no workout is good enough, you see yourself as a failure.

But you're not.

I've literally been carried out of a gym on a stretcher because I didn't accept excuses. Not just once but twice. (The second time was to prove my commitment to the character I was playing.) I've been so sore after leg day I had to use crutches to get around my house. I'd berate myself for missing reps I thought I should've hit, which led me to despise training at one point.

You can tell yourself that's just what it takes to be a champion. You can make a screen saver from that iconic image of Kobe Bryant practicing free throws with his left hand while his right hand is wrapped in a cast.

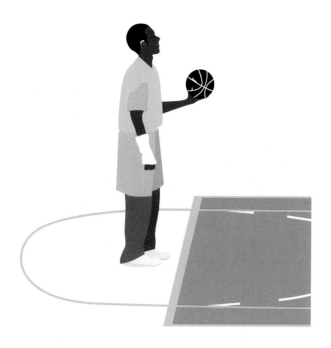

I don't deny the power of an image like this. It makes me want to run out and play basketball, and I'm five-foot-five. But when you apply a black-and-white, "no excuses" mindset to weight training, you're inviting an unsustainably high risk-reward ratio. I'm not saying it can't work. I'm saying it works in a potentially dangerous way.

That's why I now approach my training with two other mindset principles: self-trust and acceptance. They aren't inspiring enough to print on a T-shirt, but they can keep you training hard for years to come.

SELF-TRUST AND ACCEPTANCE

Self-trust means what it says: You trust yourself to follow through with your program. If the program calls for a tough workout, fine. You've done them before, and you're entirely capable of doing this one. If the plan calls for a light workout, that's also fine. Your ego won't push you to go harder. And if you need to modify a workout on the fly, that's cool too. You're mature enough to know you can't ignore that knee pain on your second set of squats, and your progress doesn't depend on you pushing through that injurious pain to complete your final two sets.

Live to fight another day, as the saying goes.

With self-trust comes self-compassion. Sometimes, you just need to do something else during your gym time. You trust yourself to

make the right choice, one that's aligned with your values, and you don't beat yourself up over it. An occasional missed workout doesn't mean you're no longer serious about lifting. It means you've balanced your passion for training and your responsibilities to your family, friends, colleagues, and community.

Acceptance is also important to a lifter. It means you accept your current reality without judging yourself harshly for inhabiting it. Not every workout will go the way you want. Some days, for no discernible reason, you just don't have it. You're weaker than you expected, or you feel like you're running on empty. Maybe the gym is busier than usual, or it's the normal crowd, but they're bogarting your favorite equipment. Whatever it is, your workout feels off, and you'd rather be anywhere but at the gym.

The "no excuses" lifter would refuse to see these things as legitimate reasons for a subpar workout. They'd blame themselves (while silently seething at people who don't read their mind and move away from the workout stations they planned to use). Not only does this unforgiving mindset make a bad workout worse, but it also sets them up for more bad workouts down the road.

The self-accepting lifter, by contrast, recognizes when things aren't within their control and realizes that everyone has bad days.

Now, if all that sounds a little too hippie-dippie, lovey-dovey for you, that's fine. I don't think one lifting mentality works best for everyone. But this is the training mentality that resonates the most with my brain, and it's gotten me through some rough patches throughout my lifting career.

These days, when I feel sluggish, I don't crank up my music or double-dose the caffeine. I don't tell myself to "go hard or go home." Instead, I ease my way into the workout, starting with my usual warm-up. I remind myself to take it one rep at a time. Who knows? Maybe I'll surprise myself and have a great workout. I often do.

Some people will tell you that too much acceptance leads to mediocrity and stagnation. "If I accept myself and my situation," you might ask, "how am I supposed to get better?" I understand your skepticism, but acceptance and improvement don't need to be at odds. You can accept your present circumstances and not judge yourself for them while still taking steps to improve things.

This is especially true if you understand your "why"—that is, you've defined your superordinate goal. If your highest-level goal is something that really matters to you, acceptance and self-trust don't threaten your chance of reaching it. When you trust yourself to follow your plan, you can accept the reality of your circumstances without weakening your desire to reach your goal.

PUTTING THE RAILS IN PLACE

As you begin climbing up the Muscle Ladder, remember how the two side rails, sustainability and mindset, interact with and support one another. Prioritizing sustainability over quick results sharpens your mindset, and having a sharp mindset leads to more sustainable results.

So, with this foundation in place, it's time to step onto the first rung.

CHAPTER 4

TECHNIQUE

HOW TO LIFT THE WEIGHTS

You don't buy a ladder for something just slightly out of reach. You need a step stool for that. A ladder is for climbing. For reaching the top. The first rung of the ladder gets you to the second rung, and so on.

That's also true of the Muscle Ladder. Technique is what allows you to train long enough and hard enough to reach your goals. But unlike the first rung of an actual ladder, technique isn't something you touch on and then move past.
Technique takes time to master and regular focus to maintain.

I start this chapter with some of the basic principles of technique, and then I follow up with detailed exercise instructions.

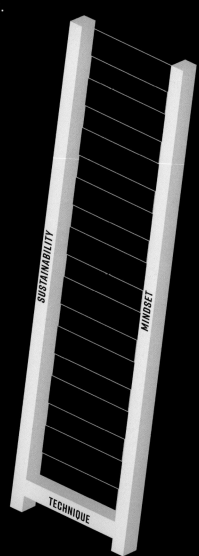

CONTROLLING THE NEGATIVE

Almost every exercise I discuss in this chapter has two parts: You lift the weight in the concentric (positive) phase, and you lower it in the eccentric (negative) phase. The order may change—sometimes you lower the weight before lifting and sometimes you lift first—but both phases are very important.

You probably wouldn't guess that the negative is at least as important as the positive—possibly even more important.[1] Far too many lifters just let the negative happen, succumbing to gravity rather than controlling the weight on the way down. That's a mistake.

Picture a dumbbell biceps curl. Which technique do you think is better for building muscle: Keeping tension on your biceps by actively resisting gravity on the negative, or letting your biceps go slack while the weight falls back to the starting position?

Some lifters go a step further by recommending a deliberately slow negative. It's an interesting idea, but in a 2024 research review, my coauthors and I didn't find any advantage with really slow repetitions.[2] As long as you control the negative, it doesn't matter whether the reps last two seconds, eight seconds, or anything in between. They all lead to similar muscle growth.

Even at eight seconds per rep, you're using such light weights that you're probably inhibiting your growth potential. The same is true with extremely fast, bouncy reps. If the positive and negative combined take less than two seconds, your muscles aren't generating tension for long enough to optimize growth.

Most of my reps last two to four seconds—one second to lift the weight and one to three seconds to lower it. That way I can be more explosive on the positive and feel my muscles stretch against resistance on the way down.

PROPER RANGE OF MOTION (ROM)

To keep things simple, you can think of your range of motion as how deep you go at the bottom and how far you go at the top.

There's a difference between a full ROM and the proper ROM. *Full* describes how far you *can* go in both phases. *Proper* means how far you *should* go. The optimal ROM will be a little different for each lifter and each exercise.

That's especially true for lower-body exercises like squats. The length of your limbs and configuration of your hips will help determine what is and isn't possible, but your fitness level, movement skill, health status, and injury history also play their parts.

It's OK if your ROM isn't as "full" as someone else's. You don't need to go glutes to calves to get the benefits of a squat. As long as you can work the targeted muscles through a reasonable ROM—feeling a stretch at the bottom and a squeeze at the top—you'll be fine.

Keep that in mind as I demonstrate exercises throughout this chapter. The photos showcase the proper ROM *for me.* That doesn't mean it's the optimal ROM for *you.* Figuring out your proper ROM will take patience and practice.

It may also evolve over time as your balance and mobility improve and as you become more confident in the weight room.

Once you find the proper ROM, your next challenge is to make it your *consistent* ROM. Your technique should look the same no matter how much weight you're lifting.

That's harder than it sounds.

Imagine it's Monday, and an eager young lifter starts their bench press routine with 135 pounds—one plate on each side of an Olympic barbell. They lower the bar all the way to their chest and press it back up until their elbows lock out at the top. You'd recognize what they've done as good technique.

However, instead of keeping their form constant, they let their technique change as they add more weight to the bar. With 225 pounds—two plates on each side—the bar stops an inch or two short of their chest. At 275 pounds, they lower it just halfway. At 315, their elbows barely bend before they push the bar back to the top. And even then, it looks like their spotter is doing most of the work.

OK, maybe I'm exaggerating a little, but the problem is real. At any moment in a crowded gym, you can find someone loading up the lat pulldown with so much weight they can't pull it anywhere close to their chest no matter how far they lean back or someone reducing their ROM on curls so they can use bigger dumbbells. If you start looking for this kind of thing, you'll see it everywhere.

The strongest lifters didn't get strong by compromising their technique. They did it by lifting progressively heavier weights with a consistent ROM.

SHOULD YOU EVER DO PARTIAL REPS?

For decades, experts have told lifters to use a full ROM for maximum muscle growth, with no exceptions.

I appreciate the simplicity, and I think it makes sense for most lifters in most situations. But

emerging evidence has added some nuance to the default recommendation.

A 2023 review from Wolf and colleagues pooled data from 24 studies on how ROM affects hypertrophy.[3] They found that full and partial ranges of motion were similarly effective for muscle growth as long as the partial reps were done with the muscle in a more lengthened position.

In fact, several studies showed lengthened partials outperformed the same exercises done with a full ROM, although the effects were small.

So, what is a "lengthened" partial? Think of the part of an exercise where the muscle is stretched—for example, the quads are stretched in the bottom of a squat. Same with the pecs in the bottom of a bench press, when the bar is on your chest. In a pulling exercise, it's usually the opposite. For example, in a lat pulldown, your lats are stretched in the top half of the movement, when your arms are extended overhead.

It's a relatively new area of research, and there's no consensus among experts about when and how much to use them, so I don't want to get too bogged down on lengthened partials. But I can say the following with some confidence:

- For most muscles, the stretched aspect of the ROM seems to be more important than the contracted portion.

- If you don't get the targeted muscles into a deep stretch, you're probably leaving some gains on the table.

- Partial reps can build muscle, as long as they're done in the stretched portion of the lift. But the evidence isn't yet strong enough for me to recommend them across all exercises.

- Partial reps in the shortened ("squeezed") part of the lift don't seem to build muscle as well as full-range lifts or lengthened partials.

- You really can't go wrong with a full range of motion. Since that includes the stretched portion of the lift, you're getting all the muscle-building stimulus the exercise offers.

I'll revisit lengthened partials, along with other advanced techniques, in Chapter 12. For now, assume that a reasonably full ROM, including a controlled negative, is the ideal way to do every exercise you'll see in this chapter.

The next few sections include a few more basic lifting technique principles to keep in mind.

MINIMIZE MOMENTUM

People talk a lot about the importance of using strict form, but there's surprisingly little evidence to support our admonitions. I'm not aware of a single study comparing strict to loose form. (I hope to conduct that study in the near future.)

So, although I can't prove that using tight, consistent technique will get you further than not using it, I'd be surprised if it's not true. Lifters who flagrantly use momentum usually aren't the biggest or strongest in the weight room (unless they have some serious pharmaceutical assistance).

One reason, I suspect, is that good form usually maximizes tension in the targeted muscles. Nonstandard form does the opposite: It gets other muscles involved, which means less work for the ones you're hoping to build.

Consider the barbell biceps curl. Sure, you can curl a lot more weight if you bend at your knees, swing at your hips and heave the weight up. It won't look pretty, but you'll get the weight moving a lot easier. That probably isn't a good thing, though, because it doesn't actually guarantee more tension is being applied to your biceps. Instead of swinging, if you maintain a more upright posture (chest up, hips straight), you'll not only direct more tension to your biceps, you'll have created a consistent technique standard to apply each time you repeat the exercise. If you're too lax with your technique, you'll have trouble knowing if you're moving more weight because your biceps are getting bigger and stronger or because your lower back muscles are taking over more and more.

BREATHE PROPERLY

Novice lifters are often surprised to find how hard it is to sync their breathing with new exercises. Some hold their breath through multiple reps, which they'll compensate for later in the set by taking two or three breaths per rep.

My recommendation is simple: Inhale during the eccentric (negative) and exhale during the concentric (positive). Do that for every rep, starting with your warm-up sets. It won't be long before it feels natural, and you do it automatically.

Stronger and more experienced lifters may want to experiment with the Valsalva maneuver, an advanced breathing technique used by powerlifters on heavy compound exercises like squats, deadlifts, and presses. Here's how it works: Take in a deep breath before starting a lift, hold it through the negative, and exhale about halfway through the positive.

At the top of a squat, for example, while your knees are still straight, you'd inhale while pressing your tongue against the roof of your mouth, which helps keep your airway closed. Hold your breath as you squat to the bottom position. Keep holding it until you're about halfway up. It takes longer to explain than to perform. You're only holding your breath for a couple of seconds.

The goal is to increase pressure in your abdomen, which stabilizes your core and maintains muscle tension during heavy lifts. That's why it's used by virtually every strength athlete.

Think of it as the equivalent of holding your breath while underwater, as shown in Figure 4.1.

Figure 4.1

The Valsalva maneuver on the squat (visualized with water)

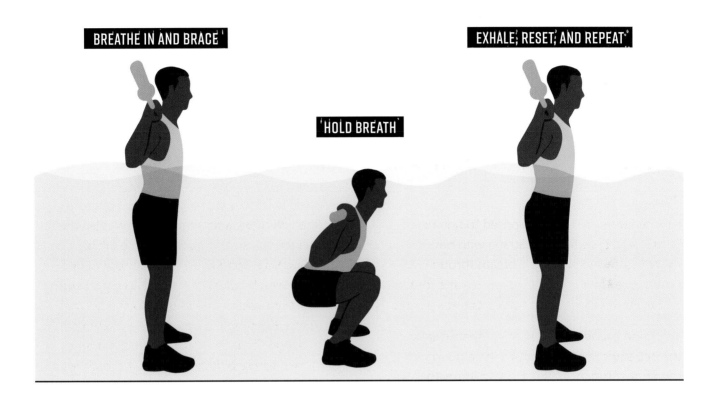

Research has shown the Valsalva produces a temporary increase in blood pressure.[4] I'm not aware of any evidence of long-term harm from the technique, but if you have high blood pressure or any other known cardiovascular risk factor, you should probably check with your doctor before using it.

Keep in mind that you should build a base of strength and lifting skill before it's smart for you to use the Valsalva. Most lifters need to spend at least a few months doing dedicated strength training. Remember, you generally only need to use the Valsalva on heavy compound lifts (squats, presses, deadlifts).

Until then, just keep it simple: Breathe in on the negative. Breathe out on the positive.

EXERCISE TECHNIQUE

I've described a handful of general principles that apply to good form on *most* exercises. Now it's time to dig into what constitutes good form on *specific* exercises.

How low should you go when you squat? Should you tuck your elbows in on the barbell bench press or flare them out? What about your grip on the lat pulldown? Should you go wide, narrow, or somewhere in between? Palms up or palms down?

I can't show you every variation of every exercise, but I will explain what you need to know about the most important and popular exercises. I'll focus mainly on free-weight exercises because machines, for the most part, are designed to be easy to use. Even if you need help figuring out the adjustments (some machines have a lot of them), the movements themselves are nearly foolproof.

For organizational purposes, I've sorted the exercises according to the primary muscles they target, even though most of them work multiple muscle groups.

HOW TO READ THIS SECTION

I won't be offended if you skim most of the content in this section. You don't need to read every technical detail about exercises you're already comfortable with. Focus on the ones that are new or unfamiliar. Return to this chapter for reference as needed. In some other chapters where I refer to specific exercises, I've cross-referenced the pages where you can find their descriptions.

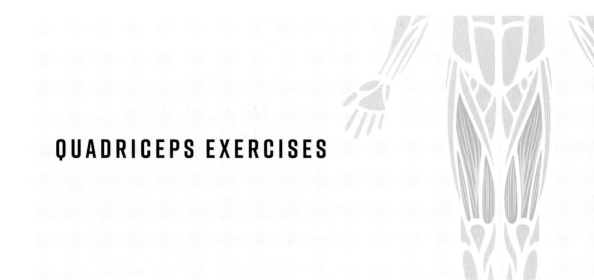

QUADRICEPS EXERCISES

BARBELL BACK SQUAT

PRIMARY MUSCLES TARGETED
Quads, glutes, adductors (inner thighs), spinal erectors (lower back)

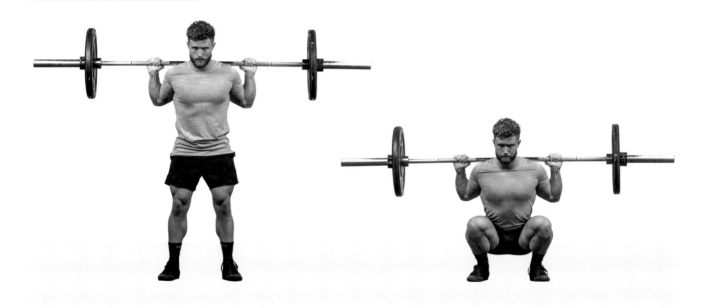

☑ Technique checklist

- Position the bar in a squat rack around armpit height.

- Grab the bar with your hands just outside shoulder width.

- Duck under the bar, placing it on your upper traps (high-bar position) or rear delts (low-bar position).

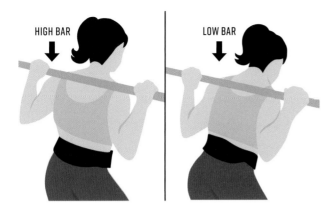

HIGH BAR   LOW BAR

- Stand up straight with the bar on your upper back; viewed from the side, the bar is directly over the middle of your feet.

- Take two or three steps back. Taking more than that is a waste of energy.

- Your feet should be at least shoulder width apart, and your toes should point out slightly.

- Take a deep breath.

- Push your hips back and squat down as far as you can without causing a lot of lower back rounding (a little lower back rounding is OK).

- Return to the standing position, exhaling when you're halfway up

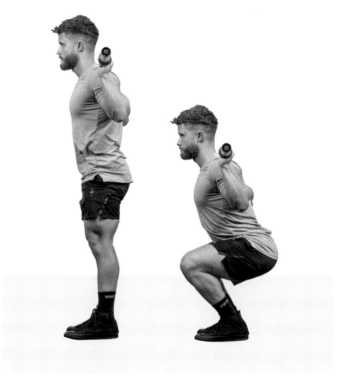

BARBELL FRONT SQUAT

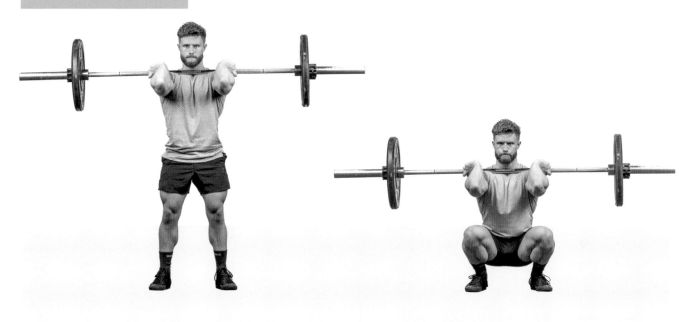

☑ Technique checklist

- Position the bar in a squat rack around armpit height.

- Secure the bar on top of your upper chest—the front rack position—using one of the three grip options shown in the photos: two-finger front-rack position, arms crossed front-rack position, or strap-assisted front-rack position.

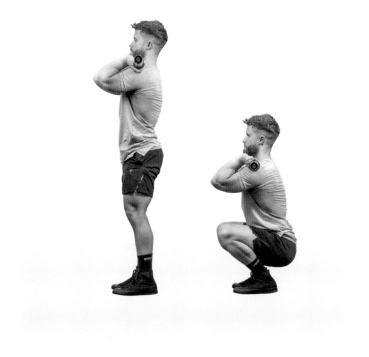

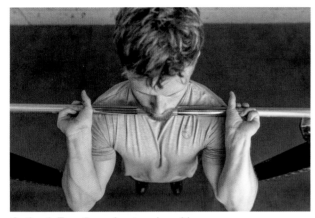

Option 1: Two-finger front-rack position

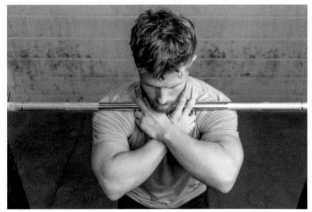

Option 2: Arms crossed front-rack position

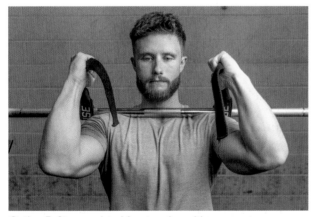

Option 3: Strap-assisted front-rack position

- Rotate your upper arms until they're parallel to the floor and perpendicular to your torso; that should secure the bar in the space between your deltoids and collarbones, just above your pecs.

- Stand up straight with your elbows pointing forward and your chin up.

- Follow the steps described for the back squat, with two differences:

  - Your torso should stay upright and your arms should stay up through the complete ROM (it's the only way to keep the bar in place).

  - You should be able to descend farther than you can in the back squat.

GOBLET SQUAT

PRIMARY MUSCLES TARGETED
Quads, glutes, adductors, spinal erectors

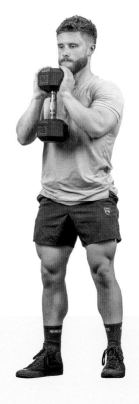 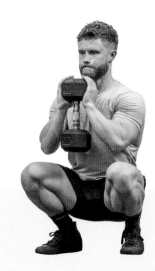

☑ Technique checklist

- Hold a dumbbell upright with your palms beneath the top head of the dumbbell and your fingers around the edges.

- Position the dumbbell in front of your chest just below your chin.

- Stand upright with your feet at least shoulder width apart.

- Point your toes out about the same as you did on the barbell squat variations.

- Take a deep breath, push your hips back, and squat; you should be able to achieve a similar or greater depth than you can in the barbell front squat.

- Exhale about halfway back to the starting position.

- Keep your chest high and chin up throughout the movement.

NOTE: *The goblet squat is a good beginner exercise. It's much easier to learn than the barbell squat variations.*

However, it has significant drawbacks for stronger and more skilled lifters. The first is strength itself. It's one thing to knock out sets with a 50- or 60-pound dumbbell. It's a much bigger challenge to squat with a 100-pounder. Even if your gym has one and you're strong enough to use it, it's incredibly awkward. That's why most lifters turn to barbell squats sooner or later.

Goblet squats can come back into play when rehabbing an injury and barbell lifts are giving you issues.

BARBELL LUNGE

PRIMARY MUSCLES TARGETED
Quads, glutes

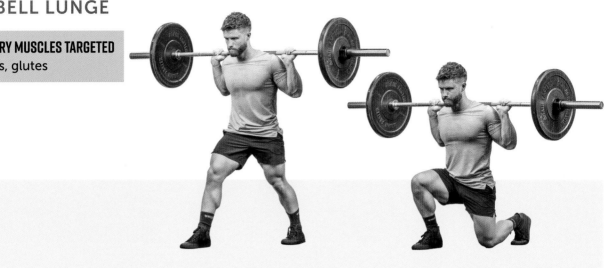

ⓥ Technique checklist

- Set up the bar inside or outside a squat rack at around armpit height.

- Grab the bar with your hands just outside shoulder width.

- Duck under the bar, placing it on your upper traps (high-bar position) or rear delts (low-bar position).

- Stand up straight so the bar lifts off the hooks.

- Take two to four steps back, creating enough space so you don't hit the rack when you lunge forward.

- Take one step forward to get into a split stance; this is your starting and finishing position.

- Keeping your torso upright, lower your body until your rear knee makes soft contact with the floor or gets as close to that position as you can without straining.

- Return to the starting position.

- Do all your reps and then switch legs and repeat the set.

NOTE: *If balance is an issue when maintaining the split stance, you can start and finish with your feet aligned and about hip width apart. Take a step back, lower your trailing leg toward the floor, and then return to the starting position. This variation is called the* reverse lunge *or* step-back lunge. *You can alternate legs on each repetition or do all your reps with the same leg stepping back and then repeat the set with the other leg stepping back.*

You can also do walking lunges *if you have enough free space. In this more advanced variation, you take a step forward on each rep and continue forward until you run out of room or complete the set. Make sure to propel the motion by pushing through the heel of your front leg.*

DUMBBELL LUNGE

PRIMARY MUSCLES TARGETED
Quads, glutes

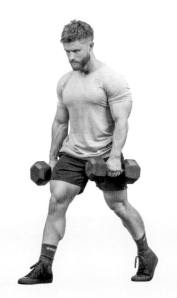
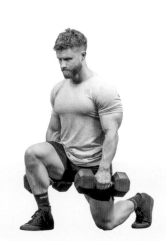

☑ Technique checklist

- The technique is the same as the barbell lunge, including the variations, except that you use a pair of dumbbells.

- If your legs are reasonably strong, you may need to use wrist straps so your grip isn't a limiting factor.

LEG PRESS

PRIMARY MUSCLES TARGETED
Quads, glutes

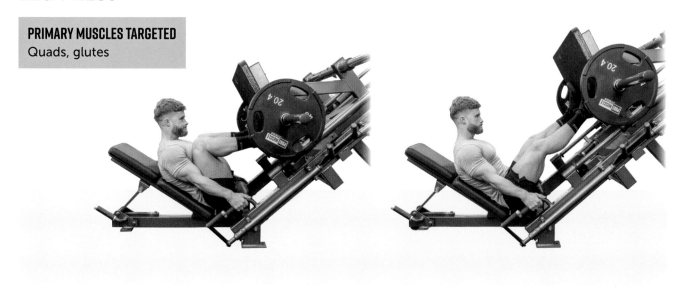

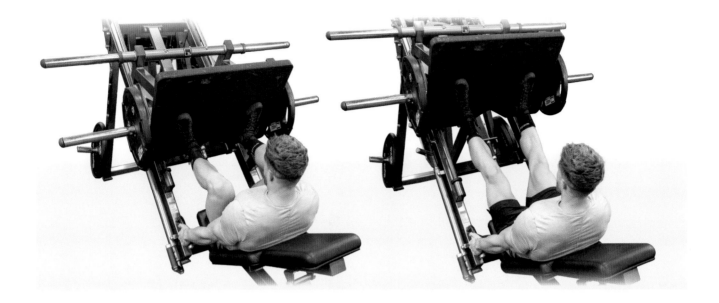

☑ Technique checklist

- Sit in the machine with your feet positioned on the footplate at least shoulder width apart and your toes pointed out slightly.

  - A higher foot placement shifts more work to your glutes.

  - A lower foot placement shifts more work to your quads.

  - A wider foot position shifts more work to the adductors.

- Push the platform to the top position and release the supports.

- Grab onto the fixed handles.

- Unlock your knees and lower the weight under control.

- Go as deep as you comfortably can while keeping your lower back and pelvis secured against the pad.

- Push through your heels to drive the platform back to the top position.

NOTE: *Locking your knees at the top doesn't pose an injury risk as long as you're in full control of the weight. If you prefer not to lock your knees, you can finish your reps with a slight bend.*

LEG EXTENSION

PRIMARY MUSCLES TARGETED
Quads

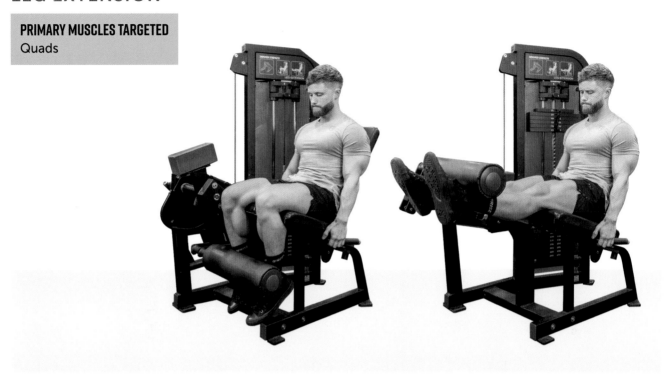

☑ Technique checklist

- Adjust the machine so the ankle pads rest on your shins just above your feet and allow the largest possible quad stretch in the bottom position.

- Point your toes in whatever direction feels most comfortable (usually straight ahead or slightly out).

- Contract your quads as you straighten your knees.

- Lower the weight under control, keeping tension on your quads.

NOTE: *It's generally safe to lock your knees out at the top. But if it causes discomfort, it's fine to finish with a slight bend in your knees.*

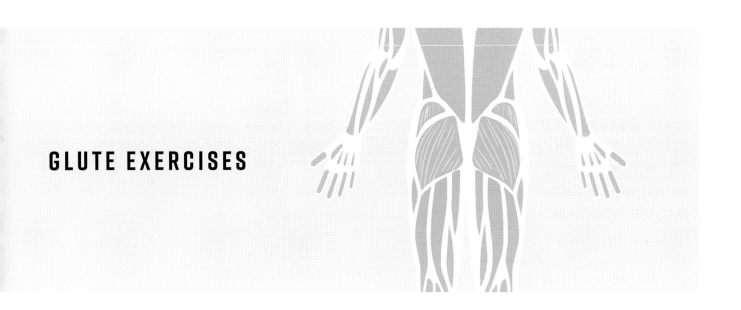

GLUTE EXERCISES

CONVENTIONAL DEADLIFT

PRIMARY MUSCLES TARGETED
Glutes, hamstrings,
spinal erectors, quads

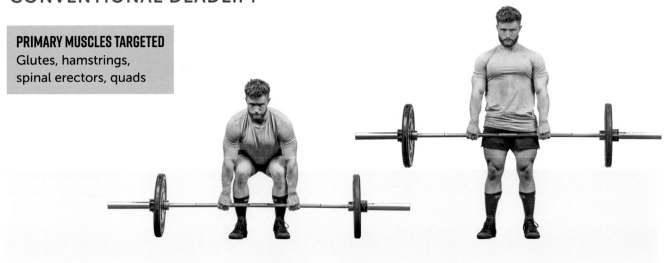

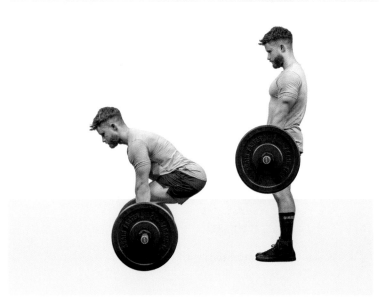

NOTE: *Because the deadlift is a more technical lift, I'm going into more detail with separate instructions for the setup and the pull.*

✅ Technique checklist

Setup:

- Load a barbell and stand with your shins about one inch from the bar, which should be over the middle of your feet.

- Set your feet about hip width apart and your toes pointed out slightly.

- Push your hips back and bend your knees just enough to grab the bar with your hands outside your legs and your feet flat on the floor; *don't* squat to pick up the bar.

- You can use one of three grip options:

  - Double overhand grip

  - Alternate grip (one palm up, one palm down)

  - Double overhand grip using wrist straps (or using chalk to improve your grip)

- Once you have a secure grip, push your knees forward slightly until your shins make soft contact with the bar without actually moving it.

- Your shins should be perpendicular or close to perpendicular to the floor.

You're in the starting position, and you're ready for the pull.

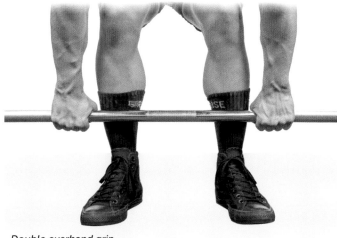
Double overhand grip

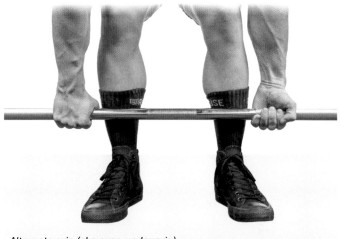
Alternate grip (aka over-under grip)

NOTE: *In the photos, I'm wearing Converse Chuck Taylor sneakers. Their flat soles make them ideal for deadlifting because you want your feet to be as close to the floor as possible. Some competitive powerlifters wear deadlift slippers, which is the closest you can get to lifting without shoes within the rules of the sport.*

At the other extreme, built-up running and walking shoes lift your feet farther from the floor, decreasing your stability while increasing the distance the bar has to travel.

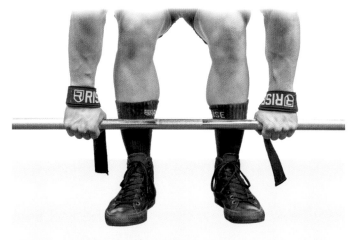
Double overhand grip using wrist straps

I have a few more grip tips:

- *Even with chalk, you'll eventually reach the point where your legs and back are stronger than your hands and forearms, and the double overhand grip will no longer work for your heaviest loads. That's when you'll need to switch to the alternate grip or use wrist straps.*

- *When using an alternate grip, you can periodically switch which hand goes over and which hand goes under to avoid creating an imbalance.*

- *Powerlifters will sometimes use a "hook grip" in which they mash their thumb between their fingers and the bar. It's an advanced technique, and it's as painful as it sounds the first few times you try it. If you aspire to competing as a powerlifter, you'll probably want to use it eventually. I rarely recommend it for anyone else.*

Execution:

- Tighten your body, from your grip to your shoulders, torso, hips, and lower body; you want total-body tension, with no slack anywhere in the movement chain.

- Pull the slack out of the bar by gradually pulling tension into it (rather than just gripping and ripping).

- Inhale as you thrust your hips forward and pull the bar off the floor. Keep the following things in mind:

  - Keep the bar in contact with your shins and thighs as you lift and lower the weight.

  - Wear high socks to protect your shins from scrapes.

- Exhale as the bar passes your knees.

- Finish the lift standing up straight, with your body forming a straight line from neck to ankles and the bar over the middle of your feet; don't pull your shoulder blades together or lean backward.

- Hold the lockout position for at least one second.

- To lower the bar, push your hips back, allowing your knees to bend after the bar passes them on its way to the floor.

- The descent should be a straight line, perpendicular to the floor, with the bar staying over the middle of your feet; it should end up exactly where it started.

- Don't bounce the weight off the floor; reset your grip, tighten your body, pull the slack out, and then begin the next lift.

SUMO DEADLIFT

PRIMARY MUSCLES TARGETED
Glutes, hamstrings, spinal erectors, quads, adductors

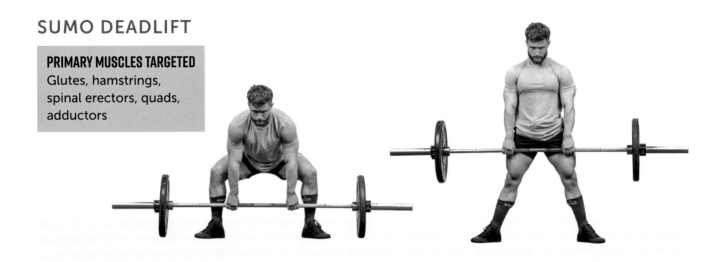

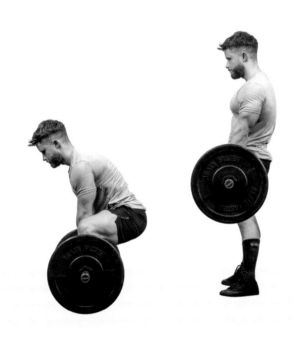

> **NOTE:** *There are two obvious differences between sumo and conventional deadlifts: You take a wider stance for the sumo, with your arms inside your legs instead of outside of them.*
>
> *The biomechanics and muscle activation of the two lifts are similar, with the conventional deadlift forcing the back muscles to work a little harder and the sumo shifting more work to the quads and adductors. Neither is "better"; use the one you're most comfortable with.*

☑ Technique checklist

Setup:

- Load a barbell and stand with your shins about one inch from the bar, which should be over the middle of your feet.

- Take a wide "sumo" stance. The exact width doesn't matter (it'll be a little different for each person based on their mobility and limb lengths), as long as it's comfortable and allows your shins to remain perpendicular to the floor (in the starting position from the front view).

- Point your toes toward the front edge of the plates; for most lifters that will be roughly 30 to 45 degrees.

- Push your hips back as you reach down to grab the bar; your knees will have to bend more in the sumo stance.

- Your grip options are the same as for a deadlift: double overhand, alternate, or double overhand with wrist straps.

- Your hips will be lower in the starting position than in a deadlift, but they should still be higher than your knees; remember, a deadlift isn't a squat.

Execution:

- Tighten your body and pull the slack out of the bar, as described for the deadlift (page 74).

- Initiate the pull by lifting your chest and thrusting your hips forward.

- Keep the bar in contact with your shins and thighs.

- Finish by standing up with straight hips and knees; don't pull your shoulder blades together or lean backward.

- Hold this lockout position for at least one second.

- To lower the bar, push your hips back, allowing your knees to bend as much as necessary.

- Again, the barbell should return to the floor in a straight line, centered over your feet, and end up exactly where it started.

- Reset your grip, tighten your body, and begin the next lift.

HIP THRUST

PRIMARY MUSCLES TARGETED
Glutes

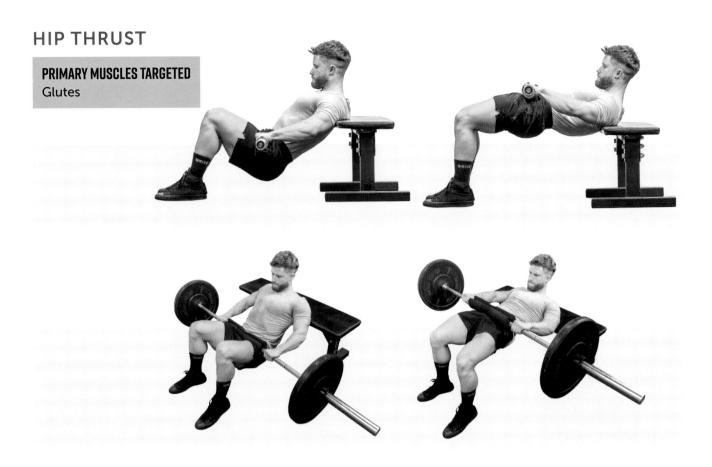

☑ Technique checklist

- Load a barbell on the floor in front of a flat bench or low box. If there's any chance the bench or box will shift around, anchor it against a wall.

- Wrap a soft pad around the barbell to cushion your hip bones.

- Slide underneath the bar, and roll it toward you until the pad is on your hips or the top of your thighs, whichever feels more comfortable.

- Set your feet hip width apart, with your toes turned out slightly.

- Grab the bar with your hands just outside your legs and your chin tucked toward your chest.

- Thrust your hips upward and squeeze your glutes hard at the top of the movement.

- Finish with your body straight from chest to knees and your shins perpendicular to the floor, while your chin remains tucked.

- Lower the bar under control until the plates and your glutes touch the floor.

- Don't "rebound" into the next rep; come to a full stop, reset, and repeat.

> **NOTE:** *If your shins aren't vertical at the top of the movement, shift your feet forward or back until you find the right placement. Remember the spot and use it for subsequent workouts.*

45-DEGREE BACK EXTENSION

PRIMARY MUSCLES TARGETED
Glutes, spinal erectors, hamstrings

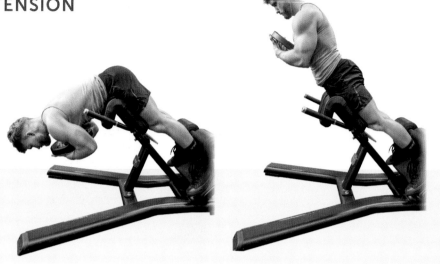

☑ Technique checklist

- Set up a back extension apparatus to fit your proportions; the top of the thigh pad should be at the top of your thighs with the ankle pad resting firmly on your lower calves. Your heels should be secured against the footplate.

- Bend forward until your legs and upper torso form a 90-degree angle, with your lower back in a neutral position.

- Contract your glutes and hamstrings to raise your torso until your body is straight from neck to ankles; squeeze your glutes hard at the top.

NOTE: *If you need an external load to increase the challenge, hold a weight plate or dumbbell to your chest, as shown in the photos.*

If you have a lot of experience with back extensions, you can try them with a rounded back. The goal is to shift some of the load from your back to your glutes. Start with just your body weight, and make sure you keep your back in the same position throughout the movement. Rounding and then straightening your back will put more load on your lower back rather than less.

HIP ABDUCTION

PRIMARY MUSCLES TARGETED
Gluteus medius

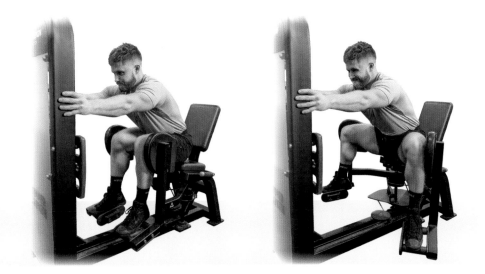

☑ Technique checklist

- Set up a hip abduction machine with the pads as close together as possible, leaving just enough room for your legs; the pads should press firmly against your outer thighs.

- Lean forward to maximize the stretch on your glutes.

- If there aren't any handles (there usually aren't), grab onto the machine.

- Press your thighs against the pads, using your glutes to move them as far as you can.

- Return to the starting position under control and repeat.

NOTE: *If you don't have access to a hip abduction machine, you can do cable hip abductions with an ankle strap, as shown in the next set of photos.*

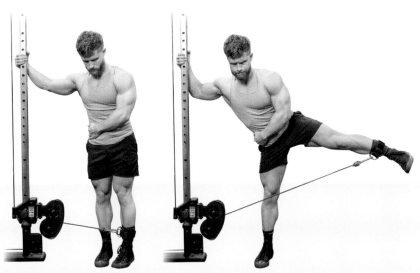

HIP ADDUCTION

PRIMARY MUSCLES TARGETED
Adductors (inner thighs)

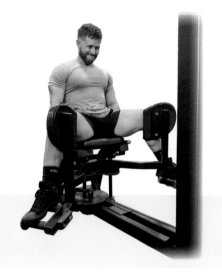 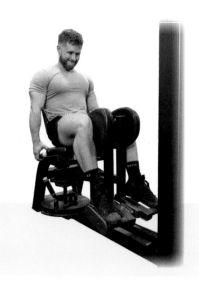

⊘ Technique checklist

- Set up a hip adduction machine with the pads as wide as you can comfortably get them. Over time, your flexibility will improve, and you may eventually max out the machine's width setting.

- The soft part of the pads should press firmly against the inside of your thighs.

- After selecting your weight, sit upright and hold onto the seat handles for stability.

- Press in against the pads, using your inner thighs to squeeze them in as far as you can.

- Return to the starting position under control and repeat.

NOTE: *If you don't have access to a hip adduction machine, you can do cable hip adductions using an ankle strap, as pictured below.*

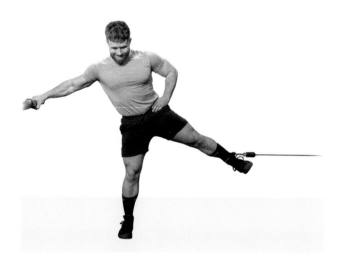

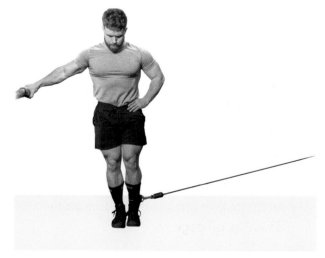

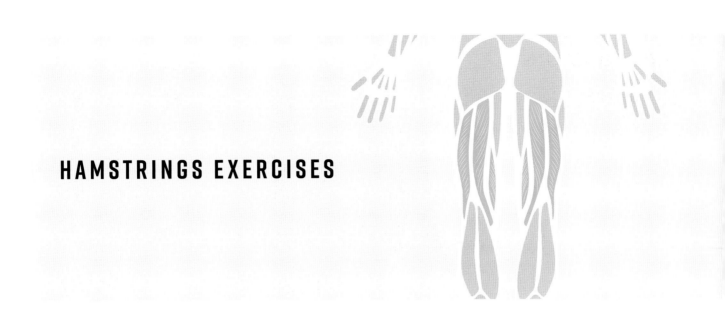

HAMSTRINGS EXERCISES

ROMANIAN DEADLIFT (RDL)

PRIMARY MUSCLES TARGETED
Hamstrings, glutes, spinal erectors

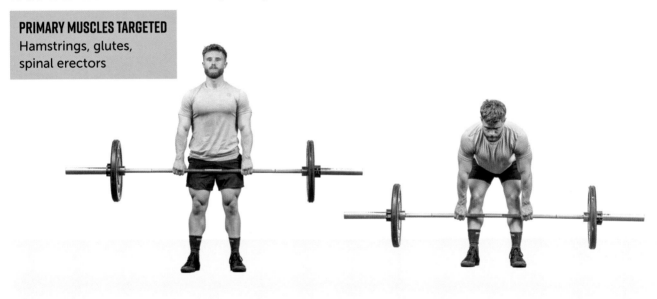

✓ Technique checklist

- Set up a barbell at about mid-thigh level. (You might want to use the squat rack for this.)

- Grip the bar just outside your thighs, using one of three grip options:

  - Double overhand grip (shown in the photos)

  - Alternate grip (one palm up, one palm down) as on page 75

- Double overhand grip using wrist straps (or using chalk to improve your grip) as on page 75

- Stand up straight, holding the bar against the front of your thighs. If you're using the squat rack, take two or three steps back to clear the rack.

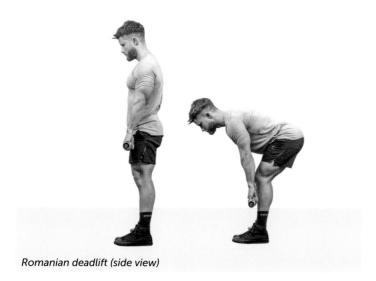

Romanian deadlift (side view)

- Set your feet about shoulder width apart, with your toes pointing forward or turned out slightly.

- Push your hips back, keeping your back straight, and allow a slight knee bend as you lower the bar past your knees.

- Keep the bar over the middle of your feet as you feel a stretch in your hamstrings.

- How deep you go depends on your limb and torso length and proportions, as well as your mobility; your goal is to maintain tension in your hamstrings and glutes while your lower back remains in the neutral position.

- Return to the starting position by lifting your chest up and thrusting your hips forward.

GOOD MORNING

PRIMARY MUSCLES TARGETED
Hamstrings, glutes, spinal erectors

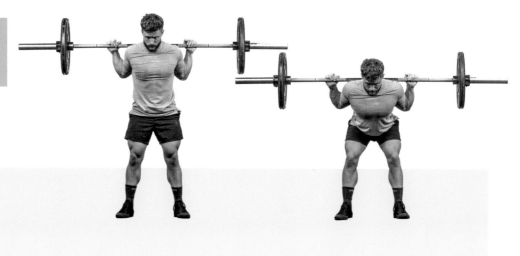

✅ Technique checklist

- Set up a barbell in a squat rack as you would for a squat.

- Grab the bar just outside shoulder width; some people are more comfortable with an even wider grip (up to double shoulder width).

- Duck under the bar, resting it on your rear delts; if you're used to a high bar position for squats (page 66), this one is about an inch or two lower.

- Stand up straight and lift the bar off the hooks.

- Take two or three steps back.

- Set your feet so they're parallel to each other and at least shoulder width apart with your toes pointed out slightly.

- Take a deep breath. From here, the movement is the same as the RDL except the barbell is on your upper back instead of in your hands:

  - Push your hips back while keeping your back straight and allowing a slight bend in your knees.

  - As you bend forward at the hips, try to keep the bar over the middle of your feet to avoid losing your balance.

  - Return to the starting position by lifting your chest up and thrusting your hips forward.

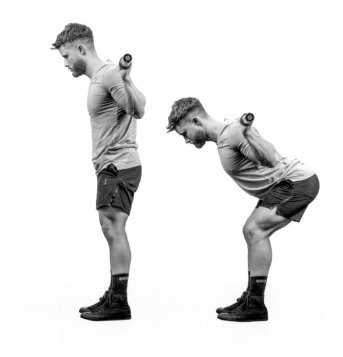

NOTE: *Don't worry if the ROM feels short. As long as you feel the stretch in your hamstrings and your lower back remains in the neutral position, you're doing it correctly.*

LYING LEG CURL

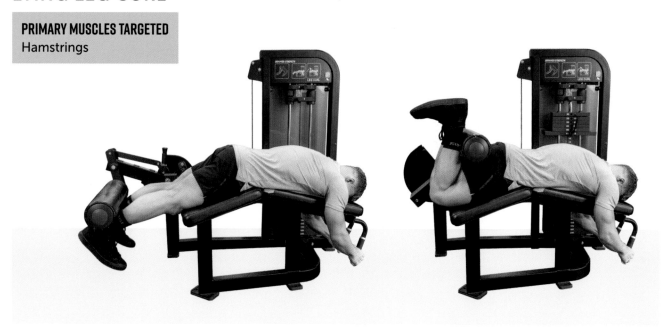

✓ Technique checklist

• Adjust the machine so the ankle pad rests just above your heels and allows the largest possible hamstring stretch in the bottom position.

• Point your toes in whatever direction feels most comfortable (usually straight ahead).

• Squeeze your hamstrings to curl the weight up as high as possible; ideally, the ankle pad will touch your glutes at the top.

• Lower the weight to the starting position while keeping tension on your hamstrings.

SEATED LEG CURL

PRIMARY MUSCLES TARGETED
Hamstrings

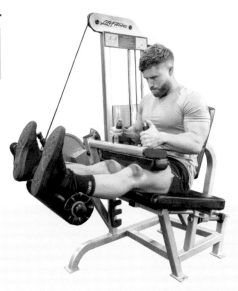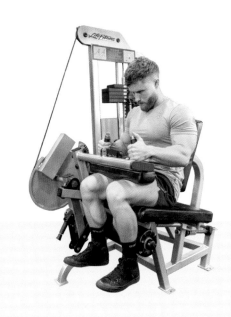

✓ Technique checklist

- Adjust the machine so the ankle pad rests just above your heels and allows the largest possible hamstring stretch in the top position.

- The top pad should rest firmly against your quads, just above your knees; there shouldn't be a gap between the pad and your quads.

- Point your toes in whatever direction feels most comfortable, usually straight ahead or slightly out.

- Squeeze your hamstrings to curl the weight down as far as you can.

- Allow the weight to move back up under control, keeping tension on your hamstrings.

GLUTE-HAM RAISE

PRIMARY MUSCLES TARGETED
Hamstrings, glutes

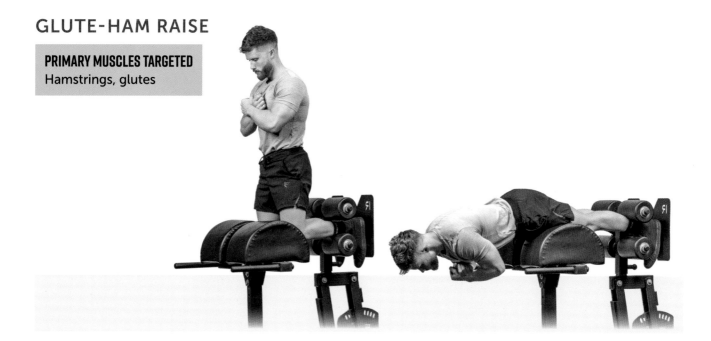

☑ Technique checklist

- After a thorough warm-up, adjust the machine so your ankles are firmly secured, your heels are tight against the footplate, and your knees are comfortably positioned at the bottom of the knee pad.

- Begin with your torso upright, your arms crossed on your chest, your knees bent about 90 degrees, and your hips and rib cage locked in place.

- Moving *only at the knees*, lower yourself until your body forms a straight line and your front thighs rest on top of the knee pad.

- Contract your hamstrings and squeeze your glutes as you lift yourself back to the starting position, again moving only at the knees.

NOTE: *If you can't return to the starting position, use the handles for assistance. On subsequent reps, find a ROM that allows you to lower and raise yourself using only your hams and glutes (you'll also feel your calf muscles pitching in).*

Try to increase your ROM by descending a bit deeper each week. Even if you never reach the full ROM, you'll still get the benefits of the glute-ham raise by keeping your body in a straight line from chest to knees and making the targeted muscles do all the work.

NORDIC HAM CURL

PRIMARY MUSCLES TARGETED
Hamstrings, glutes

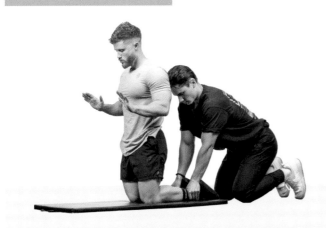 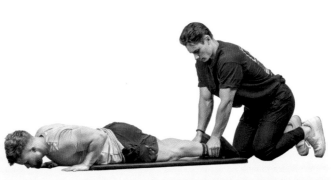

✓ Technique checklist

- After a thorough warm-up, kneel on a soft mat with a partner holding your ankles firmly against the floor.

- With your hips and rib cage locked in place, lower yourself slowly toward the floor, moving only at the knees.

- When you've gone as far as you can under control, allow yourself to fall the rest of the way, breaking the fall with your hands and stopping in the bottom position of a push-up.

- Push off the floor with your hands while squeezing your hamstrings and glutes and return to the starting position.

- Work to increase your ROM under full control in subsequent workouts. At the same time, try to minimize the push-off from the floor so your hamstrings and glutes do more work and your upper body does less.

CALF EXERCISES

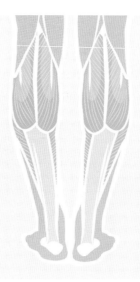

STANDING CALF RAISE

PRIMARY MUSCLES TARGETED
Calves

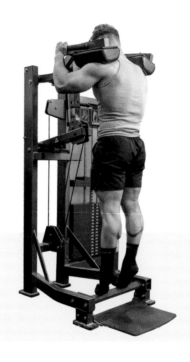 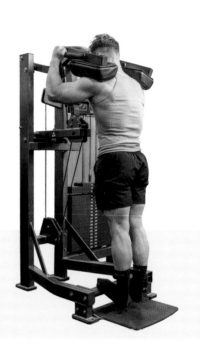

☑ Technique checklist

- Set the height of the calf raise machine so you have to bend your knees slightly to get your shoulders under the pads.

- Stand up straight and lock your knees out; if you've set the height properly, the weight should rise about 6 inches.

- Lower your heels, creating a big stretch in your calves.

- Pause for a second in this bottom position.

- Press down on the footplate with the balls of your feet without shrugging your shoulders or using your hips or knees to help your calves move the weight. How high you rise on your toes is up to you; the stretch is the most important part, so you don't need the ROM of a ballet dancer to get the benefits.

- After reaching the top of your ROM, lower your heels under control until you return to the fully stretched position.

SEATED CALF RAISE

PRIMARY MUSCLES TARGETED
Calves

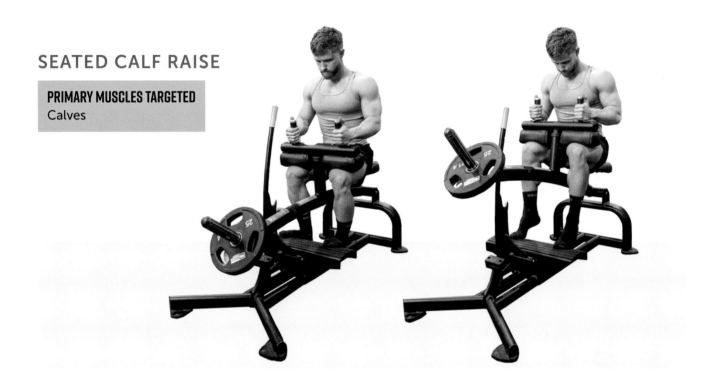

⊘ Technique checklist

- Set the knee pads to a height that puts firm pressure on your lower legs through the full ROM.

- Sit in the machine with the pads on your lower quads, just above your knees, and the balls of your feet on the footpad.

- Press up onto your toes and release the weight.

- Lower your heels, creating a big stretch in your calves.

- Pause for a second in the bottom position.

- Press down on the footplate with the balls of your feet while maintaining firm pressure against the knee pads.

- Lift your heels as high as you can.

- After reaching the top of your ROM, lower your heels under control until you return to the fully stretched position.

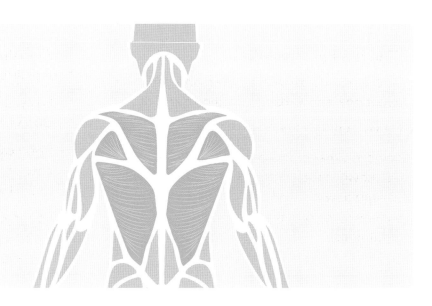

BACK EXERCISES

PULL-UP

PRIMARY MUSCLES TARGETED
Lats, middle and lower traps, rhomboids, biceps, forearms, rear delts

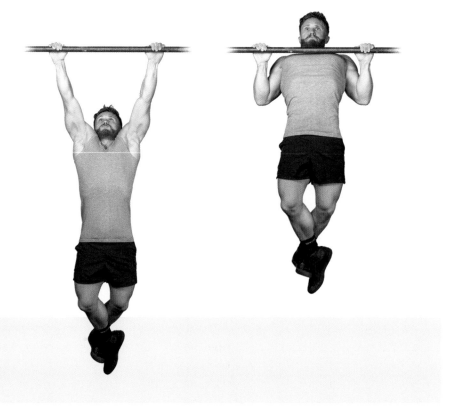

NOTE: *Your grip will be stronger with your thumbs wrapped around the bar (full grip), but most people experience a better mind-muscle connection with their thumbs behind the bar (false grip).*

✅ Technique checklist

- Grab a pull-up bar with an overhand grip that's about one-and-a-half times shoulder width.

- Let yourself sink into a deep stretch.

- You can either cross your legs behind you (as shown in the photos) or let them hang straight down; it won't affect the movement either way, so pick the one that feels more comfortable.

- From the full hang, arch your upper back slightly so your chest points toward the bar.

- Pull yourself up by thinking about driving your elbows down.

- If you can, touch the bar with your upper chest; if you can't, at least try to get your chin to the level of your hands.

- Lower yourself under control, hang in the fully stretched position just long enough to stop your momentum, and repeat.

NOTE: *If you can't do pull-ups with your body weight, start with machine- or band-assisted pull-ups.*

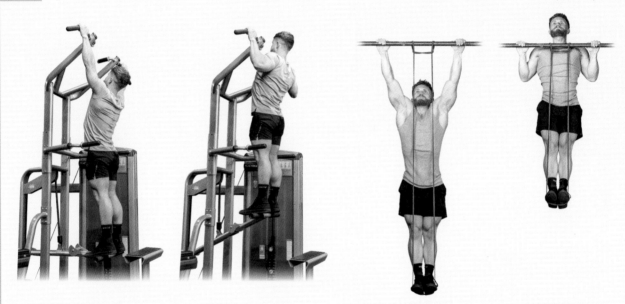

MACHINE-ASSISTED PULL-UP (REAR VIEW)

An assisted pull-up machine allows you to remove some of your own body weight by either standing on a footplate or resting your knees on a pad attached to a weight stack. The weight you select on the stack is how much you subtract from your body weight. The lower the selected weight, the more challenging the set will be. The higher the number, the more assistance you get from the machine.

BAND-ASSISTED PULL-UP (FRONT VIEW)

If you don't have access to an assisted pull-up machine, you can try looping a resistance band around the bar and stepping into it. The tension in the band will help pull you up, especially at the bottom of the range. (You may need a partner to help you get your feet into the band the first few times you try it.) The thicker the band, the more assistance it will provide.

CHIN-UP

PRIMARY MUSCLES TARGETED
Lats, biceps, middle and
lower traps, rhomboids

✅ Technique checklist

- Grab a pull-up bar with an underhand,
  shoulder-width grip.

- The technique is exactly the same as the
  pull-up; the only difference is that you
  work the biceps more directly.

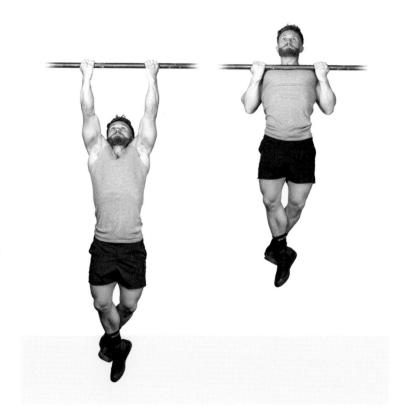

LAT PULLDOWN

PRIMARY MUSCLES TARGETED
lats, middle and lower
traps, rhomboids, rear
delts

✅ Technique checklist

- Attach a straight bar to the lat pulldown
  machine.

- Grab the bar with an overhand grip that's one
  to one-and-a-half times shoulder width.

- The straight bar and overhand grip are just
  one of the many options and combinations
  you have, but it's the most common and
  offers a solid mix of upper- and middle-back
  development.

- An underhand grip with a straight bar gets the
  biceps more involved.

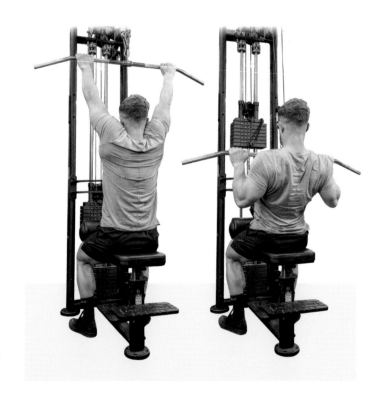

- A narrow, neutral grip using a V-handle allows you to target the lats more directly, especially if you focus on driving your elbows down rather than squeezing your shoulder blades back.

- Whichever option you choose, stick with it for several weeks at a time before mixing things up.

- As with pull-ups and chin-ups, you can use a full or false grip.

- With the bar in your hands, sit down with your thighs secured firmly under the knee pads; there shouldn't be a gap between your thighs and the pad when your feet are on the floor.

- Feel a stretch in your lats before beginning the first rep.

- Arch your upper back slightly to lift your chest.

- Pull the bar down to your upper chest as you push your chest out to meet the bar.

- It's okay to lean back slightly to get a deeper contraction in your middle back; just don't use it to generate momentum.

- Reverse the movement under full control; you should feel your shoulder blades pull apart and a deep stretch in your lats before you begin the next rep.

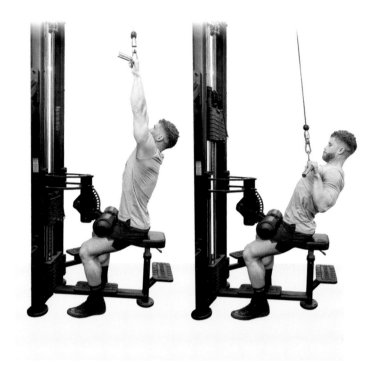

BARBELL ROW

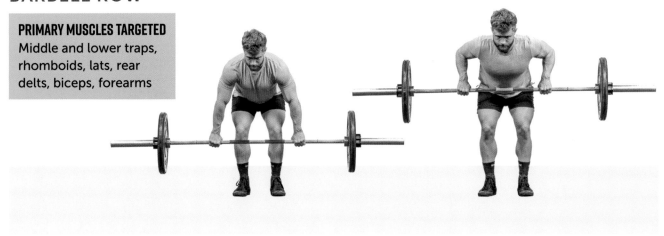

✓ Technique checklist

- Set up a barbell at around mid-thigh level as you would for an RDL. (You might want to use a squat rack for this.)

- Grab the bar with an overhand grip that's about one-and-a-quarter to one-and-a-half times shoulder width.

  - Use chalk for all your non-warm-up sets; you'll typically get at least one more rep per set with a more secure grip.

  - For your heaviest sets, you'll probably want to use wrist straps.

- Stand up straight with the bar in your hands and take two to three steps back.

- Bend forward about 45 degrees with your back flat and a slight bend in your knees; your hamstrings should be relaxed.

- Row the barbell to your upper abs, squeezing your shoulder blades together at the top of the ROM.

- Your elbows should be neither tucked in nor flared out; the sweet spot for lat and mid-back activation is about 45 degrees, relative to your torso.

- Lower the barbell under control to the starting position and repeat.

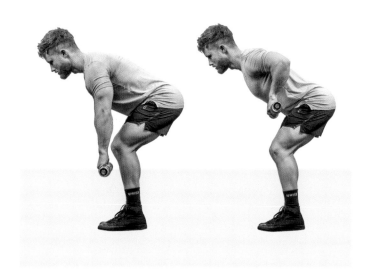

NOTE: *You'll have some hip movement as you raise the weight, but you should try to minimize it. If you need a lot of movement to complete your reps, reduce the load. Momentum means you aren't fully activating the targeted muscles.*

PENDLAY ROW

PRIMARY MUSCLES TARGETED
Middle and lower traps, rhomboids, lats, rear delts, biceps, forearms

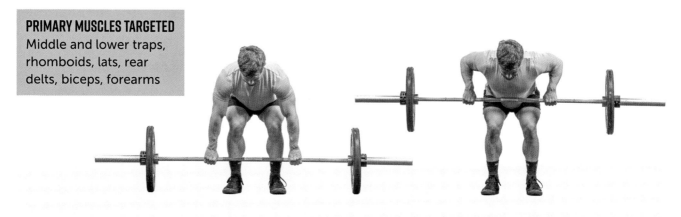

☑ Technique checklist

- Set up a barbell on the floor, as you would for a deadlift.

- Grab the bar as described for the barbell row; the big difference is that your torso is nearly parallel to the floor instead of diagonal to it.

- Row the barbell from the floor to the bottom of your chest, keeping your torso at the same angle throughout the ROM.

- Lower the barbell under control to the floor, pause long enough to eliminate momentum, and repeat.

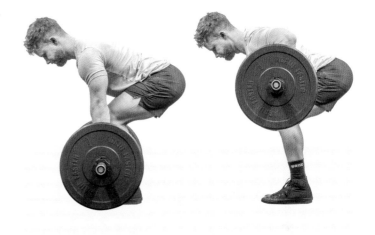

DUMBBELL ROW

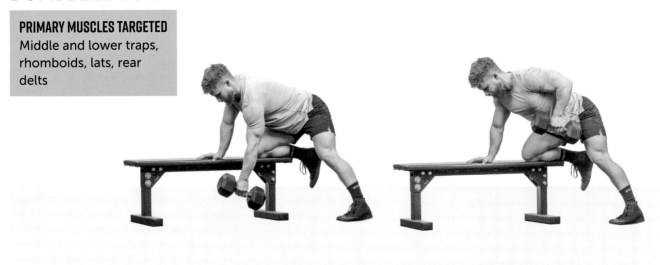

☑ Technique checklist

- Firmly plant your nonworking hand and same-side knee on a flat bench.

- Reach down and grab a dumbbell off the floor.

- Before initiating the first rep, allow the dumbbell to travel slightly forward, which will stretch your lat; this is your starting position (see the left photo).

- Row the dumbbell up and back as if you're starting a lawnmower.

- At the top of the row, the elbow of your working arm should be bent about 90 degrees; if your elbow bends a lot more than 90 degrees, you're probably not using enough weight.

- Follow the same path to lower the dumbbell under control to the starting position and repeat.

CHEST-SUPPORTED T-BAR ROW

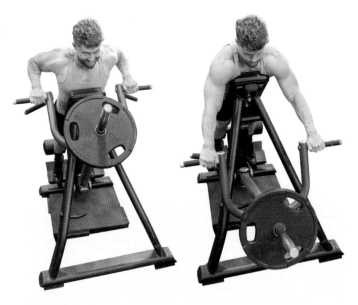

PRIMARY MUSCLES TARGETED
Middle and lower traps, rhomboids, lats, rear delts

☑ Technique checklist

- Position your chest against the pad with your heels anchored firmly on the footplate.

- Grab the handles with an overhand grip that's roughly one-and-a-quarter to one-and-a-half times shoulder width. Different machines and apparatuses offer different handle options; they all work the same muscles from slightly different angles.

  - Straight, horizontal handles are generally best for targeting your middle back.

  - Handles angled toward your torso give you a narrower grip and generally direct more work to your lats.

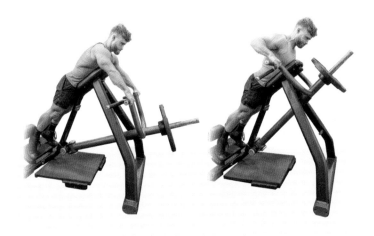

  - For muscle development, the differences are minor; use the handle and grip that give you the best combination of comfort and muscle activation.

  - It's good to keep your workouts fresh by mixing things up from time to time.

- Release the weight, let it hang for a moment with your arms fully extended, and then pull it up as far as you can by driving your elbows back and squeezing your shoulder blades together.

- Lower the weight under control to the starting position and repeat.

STRAIGHT-ARM LAT PULLOVER

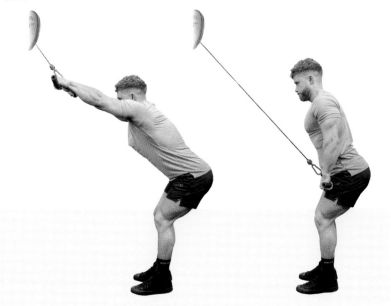

PRIMARY MUSCLES TARGETED
Lats, long head of triceps

⊘ Technique checklist

- Select a straight bar, EZ-curl bar, or rope attachment and set the cable pulley just above eye level.

  - The straight or EZ bar will probably give you a better feel for the movement, especially if you've never done it before.

  - The rope allows for a slightly longer ROM but might reduce the mind-muscle connection with the lats in some lifters (the triceps can take over more easily).

- Bend forward about 30 to 45 degrees and grab the attachment with an overhand grip.

- Step back from the cable stack far enough to allow a stretch in your lats when your arms are straight; your knees should be slightly bent and your feet shoulder width apart.

- From this starting position, pull the weight down with straight arms until the attachment reaches your thighs (if you're using a bar) or your arms are in line with your torso (if you're using a rope).

- As you pull, lift your chest up.

- Reverse the motion under control, feeling your lats stretch as you return to the starting position.

- Pause briefly and repeat.

CABLE LAT PULL-IN

PRIMARY MUSCLES TARGETED
Lats

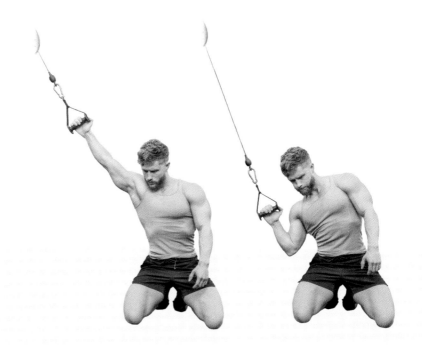

NOTE: *The pull-in works best as an activation exercise. It helps you feel your lats working in relative isolation, which in turn helps you feel them working in combination with other muscles on exercises like pull-ups and pulldowns. Use relatively light weights and high reps (15 to 20 per side) and focus on developing a mind-muscle connection.*

⊘ Technique checklist

- Attach a handle to a cable pulley and select a relatively light weight.

- Grab the handle, kneel on the floor perpendicular to the weight stack, and position yourself so your arm is positioned up and out to the side at a roughly 45-degree angle.

- Start with a nice stretch in your lat and then drive your elbow toward your torso; you can crunch slightly to the side as you pull if it helps you get a better feel for your lat in action.

- Return to the starting position under control while feeling a stretch in your lat.

- If it's difficult to keep your balance, take a half-kneeling stance with the knee closest to the weight stack on the floor and your non-working hand braced against your other knee.

CHEST EXERCISES

BENCH PRESS

PRIMARY MUSCLES TARGETED
Pecs, front delts, triceps

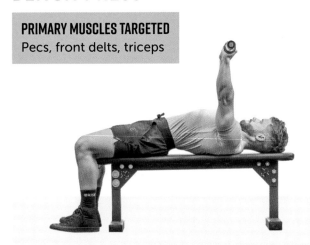

Bodybuilding-style bench press

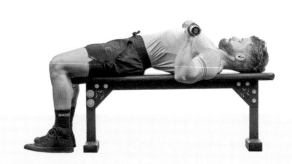

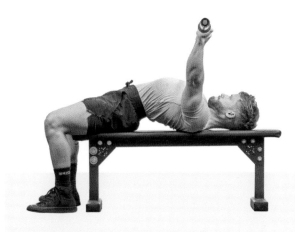

Powelifting-style bench press

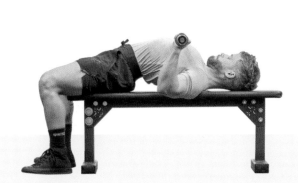

I teach bench press technique two different ways:

- The bodybuilding-style bench press when building muscle is the primary goal

- The powerlifting-style bench press when developing maximum strength is the goal

The main difference is that you'll have a flatter back and somewhat closer grip when using the bodybuilding style, as shown in the photos at the top of the facing page, but an arched back and wider grip for the powerlifting style, as shown in the bottom photos.

Because the bench press is a more technical lift, I'm providing checklists for both the setup and execution.

☑️ Technique checklist

Setup (bodybuilding style):

- With the bar on the rack hooks, lie flat on the bench with your head slightly behind the bar.

- Set your feet a comfortable distance apart with your shins roughly perpendicular to the floor and heels down.

- Grab the bar with your hands between one-and-a-quarter and one-and-a-half times shoulder width apart.

  - A closer grip gives a bit more work to your triceps.

  - A wider grip works your chest a bit more.

- Lift your chest, which creates a small arch in your upper back, and shift your head forward slightly; at this point, your eyes should be directly under the bar.

- Squeeze your shoulder blades together and tuck them down (imagine trying to stack as much of your back onto the bench as possible) to increase your stability on the bench.

- Your head, upper back, glutes, and feet should all be firmly planted and will remain that way.

Execution (bodybuilding style):

- Unrack the bar by pressing it straight up.

- With locked elbows, shift the bar forward slightly to clear the rack and line it up with your shoulders.

- Take a deep breath and hold it.

- Lower the bar by dropping your elbows at a 45-degree angle relative to your midline (see the next photo).

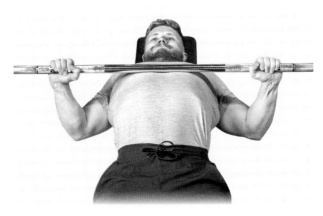

Elbow position on the bench press (top view)

- Maintain a straight wrist position as you lower the bar and bring it slightly forward.

- Touch the bar to the bottom of your chest but don't use your sternum as a trampoline.

- Press the bar along the same trajectory—up and slightly back; exhale as the bar gets close to the starting position.

NOTE: *It's okay if your elbows flare out as you lift, and it's also okay if you keep them tucked closer to your torso; if either style causes shoulder pain, do the opposite.*

Setup (powerlifting style):

- Lie on the bench as described for the bodybuilding style and grab the bar with your hands one-and-a-half to two times shoulder width apart; a wider grip, like the bigger arch, reduces ROM.

- If you plan to compete in powerlifting, the maximum grip width allowed in most federations is about 32 inches.

- The distance is marked on the barbell by smooth rings within the knurling.

- Your index fingers must be on or inside those rings when you lift.

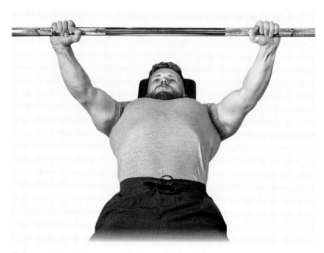

Grip position for powerlifting-style bench press

NOTE: *The bigger arch used in the powerlifting-style bench press decreases the ROM, which in turn increases how much weight you can lift. But with a shorter ROM, it may be marginally less effective for building muscle.*

NOTE: *On the next page, I describe the feet-up and feet-down arch setups. Most powerlifting federations require your heels to remain on the floor throughout the lift, and some powerlifting federations have banned the feet-up setup, which makes the feet-down setup your only choice.*

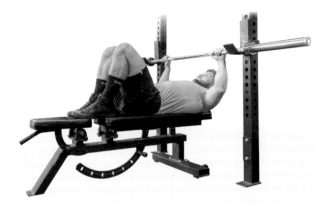

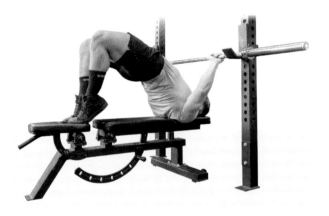

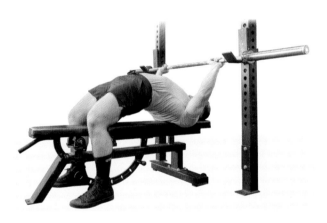

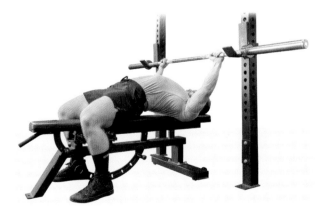

- Feet-up arch setup:
  - Place your feet on the bench (hence the name) and tuck them in close to your glutes.
  - Thrust your hips into the air and bring yourself forward on the bench until your eyes are directly under the bar. Think about pulling your shoulder blades to your glutes. You can go up on your toes if it allows for a better arch.
  - Drive your upper back into the bench while squeezing your shoulder blades together and tucking them down.
  - With your back firmly planted on the bench, set your feet on the floor one at a time.
  - Plant your feet comfortably with your heels on the floor.
  - Drop your hips down so your glutes are in contact with the bench.
- Feet-down arch setup:
  - With your feet on the floor, thrust your hips into the air and bring yourself forward on the bench until your eyes are directly under the bar. You can go up on your toes if it allows for a better arch.
  - Drive your upper back into the bench while squeezing your shoulder blades together and tucking them down.
  - Drop your hips down so your glutes are in contact with the bench.
  - Adjust your feet to set your heels on the floor. Some powerlifters prefer to move their feet farther back, whereas others keep them forward. Experiment with different positions to find where you can get the best leg drive while keeping your heels down. The further back you plant your feet, the more you'll need to point your toes out.

- The rest of the setup:
  - Your eyes should be directly under the bar.
  - Your head, upper back, glutes, and feet should all be firmly planted and remain that way through the lift.

Execution (powerlifting style):

- Unrack the bar by pressing it straight up.
- With locked elbows, shift the bar forward slightly to clear the rack and line it up with your shoulders.
- Take a deep breath, forcing the air into your midsection; you're going to hold this breath until you're about three-quarters of the way to lockout.
- Lower the bar by dropping your elbows at a 45-degree angle relative to your midline (see the next photo).
- Maintain a straight wrist position as you lower the bar down and slightly forward.
- Touch the bar to the bottom of your chest without bouncing it.
- Explosively press the bar up and slightly back to the starting position.
  - Drive your heels into the floor as you lift and think about pushing the floor away from you.
  - Exhale as the bar passes into the final 25 percent of the ROM.

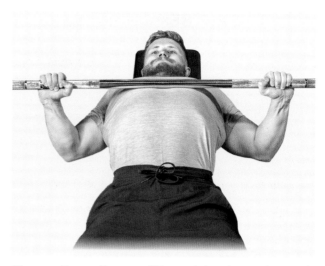

Elbow position on the powerlifting-style bench press (top view)

- The rep is complete once you lock your elbows out.
- Take another deep breath and begin your next rep.

CLOSE-GRIP BENCH PRESS

NOTE: *You can work your triceps and upper pecs a little harder with a grip that's between one and one-and-a-quarter times shoulder width. The close-grip bench press is mostly the same as the bench press (page 102), except for these differences:*

- *The closer the grip, the longer the ROM.*
- *With a longer ROM, you use about 15 to 25 percent less weight.*
- *You need to tuck your elbows closer to your torso.*

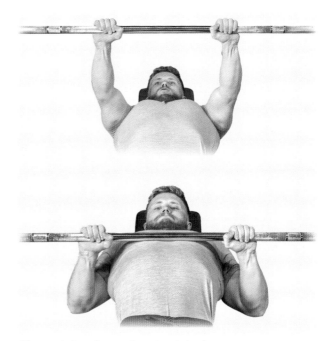

Close-grip bench press (overhead view)

INCLINE BENCH PRESS

PRIMARY MUSCLES TARGETED
Upper pecs, triceps, front delts

NOTE: *The technique is mostly the same on an incline bench press as for a bench press (page 102), but the differences are important:*

- *You can set the incline anywhere from 15 to 45 degrees; choose the angle that's most comfortable and feels as if it offers the best muscle activation.*
- *A higher incline shifts more work to the upper pecs and front delts.*
- *The contact point on your chest is a bit higher; if you touch too low, you may lose control of the bar.*
- *The bar path is more vertical compared to a flat press.*

DECLINE BENCH PRESS

PRIMARY MUSCLES TARGETED
Middle to lower pecs,
triceps, front delts

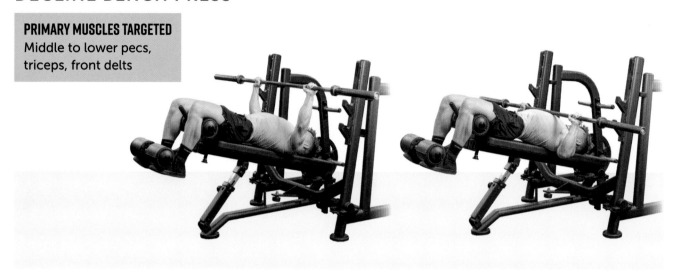

NOTE: *The technique is mostly the same as the other bench press variations, with these exceptions:*

- *Set the decline to 15 to 30 degrees. A steeper decline may reduce the ROM too much for the exercise to be effective.*
- *The contact point on your chest will be a bit lower.*

DUMBBELL BENCH PRESS

PRIMARY MUSCLES TARGETED
Pecs, triceps, front delts

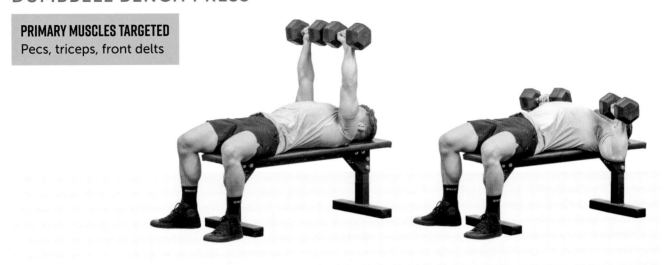

✓ Technique checklist

- Grab a pair of dumbbells and sit down on the edge of the bench with the dumbbells on your thighs, close to your knees.

- In one fluid motion, lean back onto the bench and use your legs to "kick" the dumbbells up so you're holding them over your shoulders with your arms straight.

- Your feet should be just beyond shoulder width, with your shins perpendicular to the floor and your toes pointed out slightly.

- Puff your chest up and squeeze your shoulder blades back and down; as with the barbell bench press variations, imagine you're trying to pack as much of your back onto the bench as possible.

- Your head, upper back, glutes, and thighs should all be firmly planted on the bench, where they'll remain.

- Take a deep breath and lower the dumbbells; your elbows and wrists should remain aligned throughout the movement, with your forearms perpendicular to the floor.

- Lower the weights until your hands are roughly level with your lower chest; if you feel any strain in your shoulders, shorten the ROM until it's pain-free.

- Press the dumbbells up and slightly back toward your face while driving your heels into the floor.

- You can flare your elbows out as you push or keep them tucked in, whichever feels most comfortable.

- Exhale as the dumbbells pass into the final 25 percent of the ROM.

DUMBBELL INCLINE PRESS

PRIMARY MUSCLES TARGETED
Upper pecs, triceps, front delts

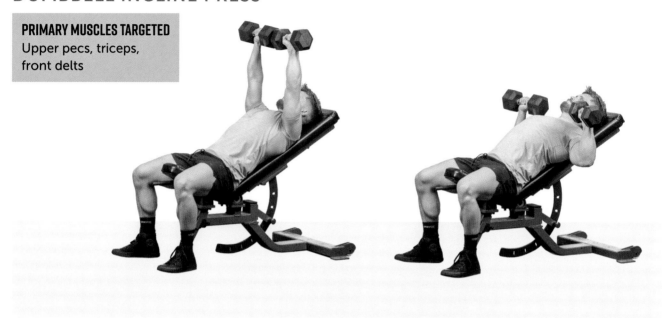

NOTE: *The incline press is mostly the same as what I described for the flat bench press (page 102), with these exceptions:*

- *You can set the incline anywhere from 15 to 45 degrees; a higher incline shifts more work to the upper pecs and front delts, but that's less important than your comfort and feel for the movement.*

- *The dumbbells move on a more vertical path compared to a flat bench press.*

DIP

PRIMARY MUSCLES TARGETED
Lower pecs, triceps,
front delts

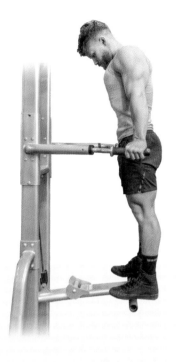
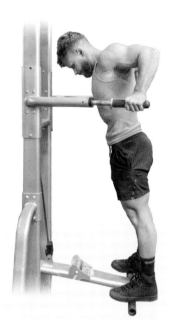

⊘ Technique checklist

- Take a comfortable grip just outside of shoulder width.
  - A closer grip hits the triceps more but also increases the ROM.
  - A wider grip works the pecs harder but may be less comfortable.
- Start with your arms straight and perpendicular to the ground.
- You can let your legs hang straight down or cross them at your ankles with a slight bend in your knees, whichever is more comfortable; your choice won't affect the lift either way. If you're using assistance from an assisted dip machine, as in the photos, your feet rest on the support bar. Some assisted dip machines may instead have a pad to kneel on.
- "Pack" your shoulders by pulling your shoulder blades together and down; keep them packed throughout the movement.
- Lean your torso forward slightly.

- Inhale as you slowly lower your torso until your elbows are bent roughly 90 degrees and you feel a pronounced stretch in your pecs and front delts.
  - If the stretch becomes painful, you've gone too far.
  - Shorten the ROM until you feel activation in your muscles without discomfort in your shoulders.
- Reverse the motion by driving your palms down into the handles as you keep your torso in the same position.
- Exhale as you near lockout.

DUMBBELL FLY

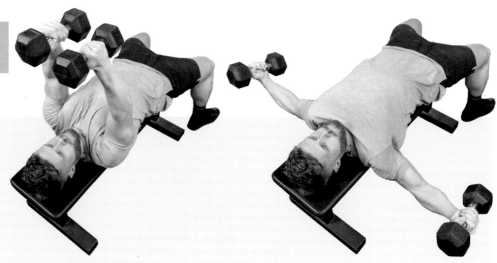

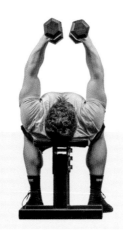
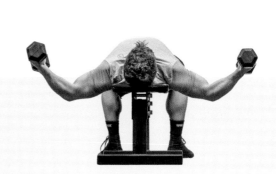

☑ Technique checklist

- Lie on the bench with the dumbbells over your shoulders and your palms facing each other; your elbows are bent slightly.

- Set your feet shoulder width apart and flat on the floor.

- As with the bench press variations, you want your shoulder blades back and down, with your head, upper back, glutes, and feet firmly planted, where they'll remain.

- Keeping a slight bend in your elbows, lower the dumbbells out to your sides while your arms remain perpendicular to your torso.

- When you feel a deep stretch in your pecs, reverse the movement and raise your arms back to the starting position, maintaining the same slight bend in your elbows throughout the ROM.

NOTE: *The closer you get to the top of the movement, the less resistance you'll get from gravity. So if you've mastered the full ROM and you're ready for something more advanced, try eliminating the top half. Go from the most stretched position to about halfway up. (I revisit this in Chapter 12.)*

CABLE FLY

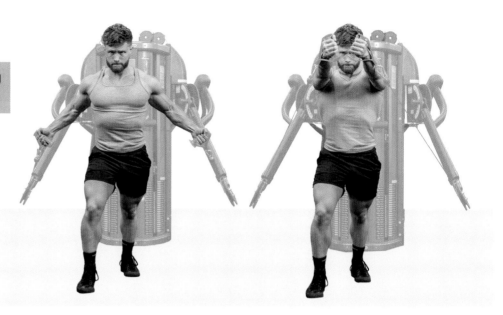

NOTE: *By changing the height of the cable pulleys, you can shift the focus to the upper, middle, or lower pecs. Use a lower setting (as shown in the photos) to target the upper pecs with a low-to-high lifting path. Set the pulleys around chest height to hit the middle pecs with a horizontal path. Or set the pulleys just above head height to work the lower pecs with a high-to-low path.*

☑ Technique checklist

- Grab the handles and stand between the two weight stacks.

- Take a step or two forward so you feel tension in your muscles; then set your legs in a staggered stance (one in front of the other) with both feet planted firmly on the floor.

- In the starting position, your arms are out to your sides with a slight bend in your elbows.

- Puff your chest up and squeeze your shoulder blades back and down, as you did on the bench press (page 102).

- Pull your palms toward each other, keeping the same slight bend in your elbows.

- Reverse the motion under control as you return to the starting position.

- You should feel continuous tension in your pecs, with a good stretch at the start of the motion.

PEC DECK

PRIMARY MUSCLES TARGETED
Pecs and front delts

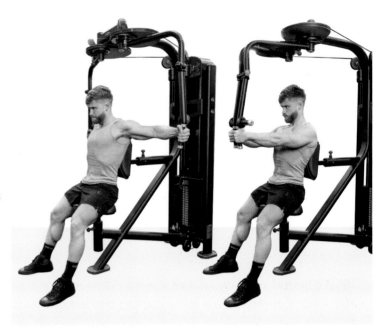

✓ Technique checklist

- Set the machine up so you start the movement with a deep stretch in your pecs and your arms roughly parallel to the floor.

- Grab the handles with a slight bend in your elbows.

- Puff your chest up and squeeze your shoulder blades back and down.

- Pull your palms toward each other, maintaining the same slight bend in your elbows throughout the ROM.

- Reverse the movement under control and begin the next rep with a deep stretch in the pecs.

PUSH-UP

PRIMARY MUSCLES TARGETED
Pecs, triceps, and front delts

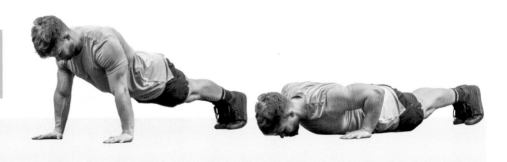

✓ Technique checklist

- Place your hands on the floor just outside your shoulders with your palms flat and fingers spread.

- With your arms straight and your weight supported on your hands and toes, externally rotate your upper arms, as if you're screwing your palms into the floor; that will help you set your shoulder blades back and down.

- Squeeze your glutes and tighten your core; your body should form a straight line from your neck through your ankles.

- Bend your elbows and slowly lower your torso until your chest is just above the floor.

- Reverse the motion by driving through your hands; keep your shoulder blades packed and core engaged throughout the movement.

BANDED PUSH-UP

PRIMARY MUSCLES TARGETED
Pecs, triceps, front delts

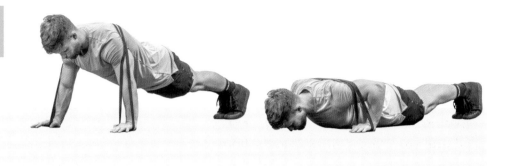

NOTE: *A banded push-up allows you to add resistance at the top, which is the easiest portion. That makes it a challenging exercise, even for intermediate to advanced lifters.*

To set it up, stretch a resistance band across your upper back, holding the loops between the floor and the middle of your palms. From there, the movement is the same as the push-up (page 114), although it'll take some practice to get the hang of it.

DEFICIT PUSH-UP

PRIMARY MUSCLES TARGETED
Pecs, triceps, front delts

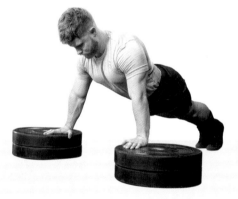
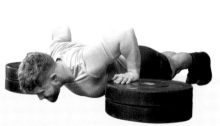

NOTE: *Deficit push-ups allow a deeper stretch in the pecs, making the exercise potentially more effective for hypertrophy but also putting more strain on your shoulder joints.*

To set it up, you need a matching pair of boxes, steps, or stacked bumper plates placed just beyond shoulder width apart. Set your palms on the boxes or steps at your normal width for push-ups. Perform the exercise as you normally would, only with a slightly deeper ROM.

When you feel a good stretch in your chest and front shoulders, pause for two to three seconds before you push back to the starting position. If you feel discomfort in either shoulder, you know you've gone too far. Shorten the ROM for subsequent reps.

SHOULDER EXERCISES

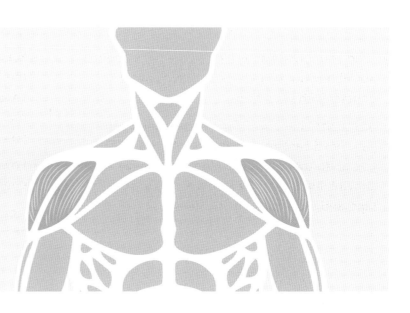

BARBELL OVERHEAD PRESS

PRIMARY MUSCLES TARGETED
Front and side delts,
upper pecs, triceps

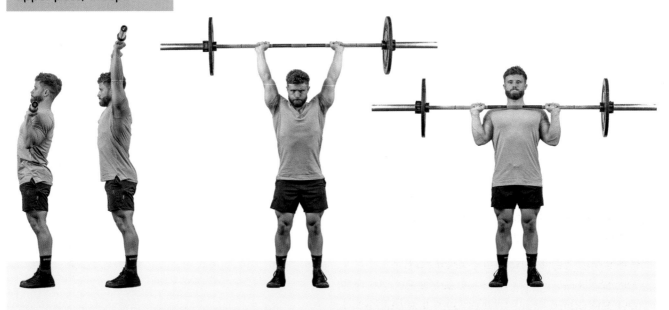

⊘ Technique checklist

- Set the bar up in a power rack around armpit height.

- Grab the bar with your hands slightly outside shoulder width and directly above your elbows.

- Unrack the weight, take two or three steps back, and set your feet about shoulder width apart with your toes turned out slightly.

- With the bar resting on your upper chest, flex your glutes, lift your chest, and take a deep breath.

- Hold your breath as you press the bar straight up, tilting your head back slightly to avoid contact with your chin.

- As the bar clears your face, exhale and push your head back to a neutral position; when you finish the movement, there should be a straight line from the bar to your shoulders, hips, and the middle of your feet.

- Your knees and hips should remain locked throughout the exercise; at no point should you use them to help you generate momentum. If you *need* their assistance, you're using too much weight.

- Lower the bar under control to your upper chest.

- Come to a complete stop, take a deep breath, and then begin your next rep.

DUMBBELL STANDING SHOULDER PRESS

PRIMARY MUSCLES TARGETED
Front and side delts

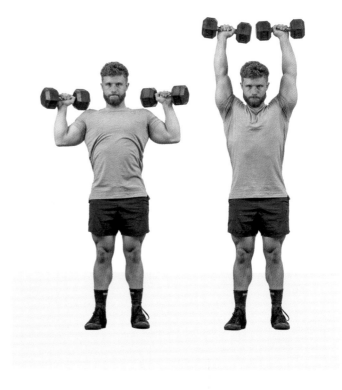

⊘ Technique checklist

- Grab the dumbbells and raise them to your shoulders. With heavier loads, start with the dumbbells resting on your thighs and then "kick" them up to your shoulders one at a time. This avoids wasting energy before you begin the exercise.

- Position your elbows wherever they feel most comfortable and allow the most friction-free ROM for your shoulders.

- The same goes for how you position the dumbbells relative to your shoulders—you can have the outer edges touching your shoulders or slightly above them; whatever you choose, that's your starting position

- Flex your glutes, take a deep breath, and press the dumbbells up and slightly in, with your hands, elbows, and shoulders aligned at the top.

- Exhale as the dumbbells clear the top of your head.

- Reverse the movement under control along the same path.

- Your knees and hips should remain locked throughout the movement.

DUMBBELL SEATED SHOULDER PRESS

PRIMARY MUSCLES TARGETED
Front and side delts

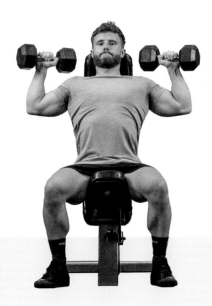
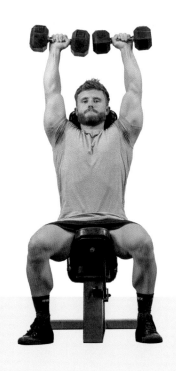

⊘ Technique checklist

- Grab the dumbbells and sit on a bench with the dumbbells resting on your thighs, close to your knees.

- Use your knees to help you lift one dumbbell at a time to your shoulders.

- Hold the dumbbells as described for the standing shoulder press (page 117); that's your starting position.

- Take a deep breath and press the dumbbells up and slightly in, with your hands, elbows, and shoulders aligned at the top.

- Exhale as the dumbbells clear the top of your head.

- Reverse the movement under control along the same path.

DUMBBELL LATERAL RAISE

PRIMARY MUSCLES TARGETED
Side delts and upper traps

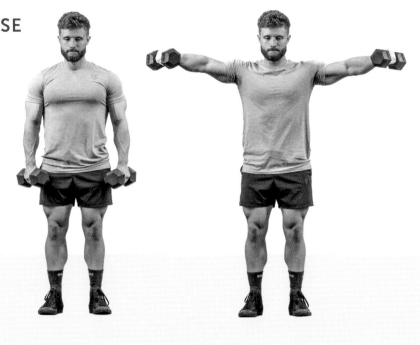

☑ Technique checklist

- Hold a pair of dumbbells at your sides.

- Squeeze your glutes and lift your chest up.

- Inhale and raise the weights up and slightly ahead of your torso; you're *not* lifting them straight out to your sides.

- Exhale as the weights rise past your upper abs and continue lifting until they reach shoulder height (or just above); your palms are facing the floor.

- If it feels comfortable, tilt your pinkie up slightly as you lift; this helps shift some work to your middle delts.

- Reverse the movement under control and come to a full stop before beginning the next rep.

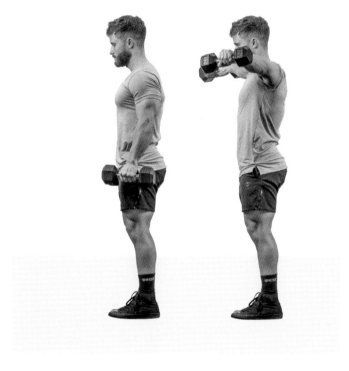

NOTE: *You can extend the ROM above shoulder level if you want to work your upper traps a little more. It's an advanced technique and not recommended if you have any history of shoulder pain.*

CABLE LATERAL RAISE

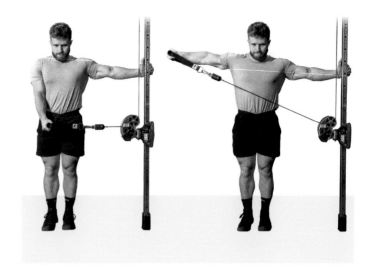

PRIMARY MUSCLES TARGETED
Side delts

✅ Technique checklist

- Set the cable pulley at wrist height and attach a D-shaped handle. This is a higher setting than you typically see for cable lateral raises; I find it allows you to isolate and apply more tension to the side delts, while the lower setting tends to bring in more supporting muscles.

- Stand perpendicular to the weight stack and hold the handle in front of your hips with your arm straight.

- Sweep the handle out and up, keeping your arm straight, until your hand reaches shoulder height, with your palm facing the floor.

- Once again, if it feels comfortable, you can tilt your pinky up slightly.

- Reverse the movement under control, keeping tension on the cable.

- Bring your arm past your midline and feel the stretch in your side delt before beginning the next rep.

BARBELL UPRIGHT ROW

PRIMARY MUSCLES TARGETED
Side delts, upper traps

✅ Technique checklist

- Grab the bar with your hands between one and one-and-a-half times shoulder width apart.

- Squeeze your glutes and lift your chest up.

- Initiate the movement by lifting your elbows out and up, keeping the bar close to your body.

- Stop when your elbows reach shoulder height or just above.

- Reverse the movement under control and come to a full stop before starting the next rep.

CABLE UPRIGHT ROW

PRIMARY MUSCLES TARGETED
Side delts, upper traps

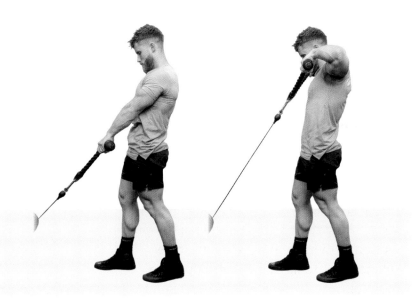

⊘ Technique checklist

- Set the cable pulley in its lowest position and attach a rope handle.

- Grab the rope overhand, with your pinkies touching the plastic ends; hold it at waist level with your feet in a staggered stance.

- Squeeze your glutes and lift your chest up.

- Lift your elbows out and up, pulling the rope toward your chin; stop when your upper arms are parallel to the floor and your hands are roughly level with your chin.

- Reverse the movement under control and pause before starting the next rep.

DUMBBELL BENT-OVER REVERSE FLY

PRIMARY MUSCLES TARGETED
Rear delts, rhomboids, traps

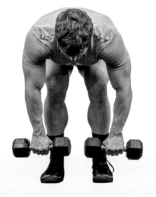

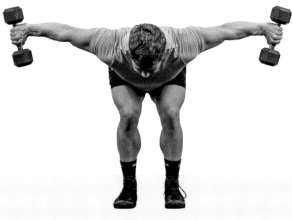

Technique checklist

- Grab the dumbbells with an overhand grip.

- Bend over until your torso is close to parallel to the floor. Keep a slight bend in your knees and hold the weights straight down from your shoulders with your palms turned toward your legs.

- With your shoulder blades back and down, pull the weights out and up, keeping your arms straight throughout the movement.

- Stop when your upper arms are at shoulder height and parallel to the floor.

- Reverse the movement under control and come to a complete stop before starting the next rep.

REVERSE PEC DECK

PRIMARY MUSCLES TARGETED
Rear delts, rhomboids, traps

Technique checklist

- Grab the handles with an overhand or thumbs up (neutral) grip, whichever gives you a better feel for your rear delts working.

- Sit up straight with your shoulders packed and chest up.

- Sweep your hands out, as if you're trying to create the largest half-circle possible.

- Squeeze your shoulder blades together at the end, with your arms even with or just past your torso.

- Reverse the movement under control, again creating the widest possible arc.

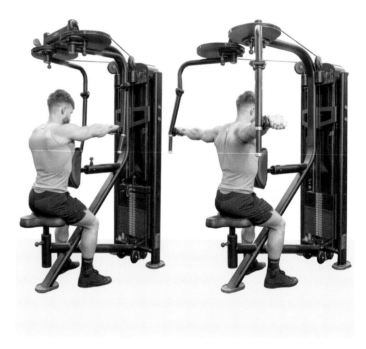

NOTE: *If you're trying to isolate the rear delts with minimal help from your traps, focus on sweeping your arms without squeezing your shoulder blades together at the end.*

BAND PULL-APART

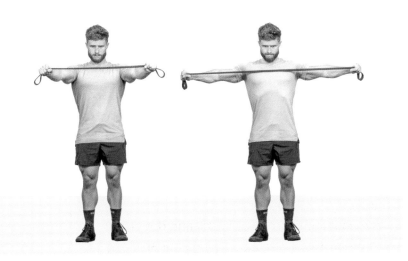

PRIMARY MUSCLES TARGETED
Rear delts, rhomboids, traps

☑ Technique checklist

- Grab the band with both hands and hold it straight out in front of your shoulders.

- Beginning with some tension in the band, sweep your hands out to your sides, keeping your arms straight.

- Squeeze your shoulder blades together at the end, when your hands are at or just past your torso.

- Reverse the movement under control, keeping some tension in the band, until your hands are back in front of your shoulders.

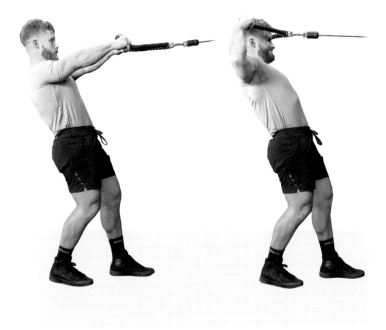

ROPE FACE PULL

PRIMARY MUSCLES TARGETED
Rear delts, rhomboids, traps, rotator cuff

☑ Technique checklist

- Set the cable pulley to shoulder height and attach a rope.

- Grab the rope with your thumbs in contact with the plastic ends.

- Step back from the machine, stand with a staggered stance, and hold the rope with straight arms and tension in the cable.

- Drive your elbows straight back as you pull the rope toward your forehead.

- Squeeze your shoulder blades back and down at the end of the movement, with your upper arms parallel to the floor.

- Reverse the motion under control, keeping tension in the cable as you return to the starting position.

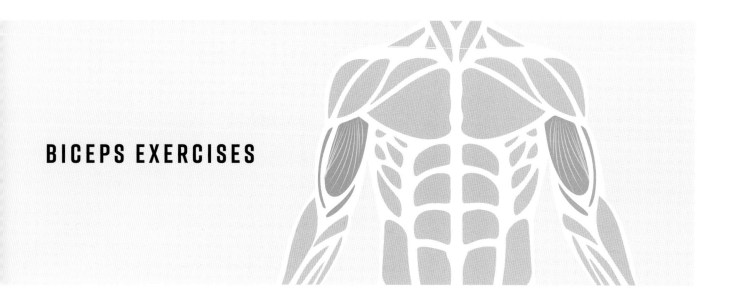

BICEPS EXERCISES

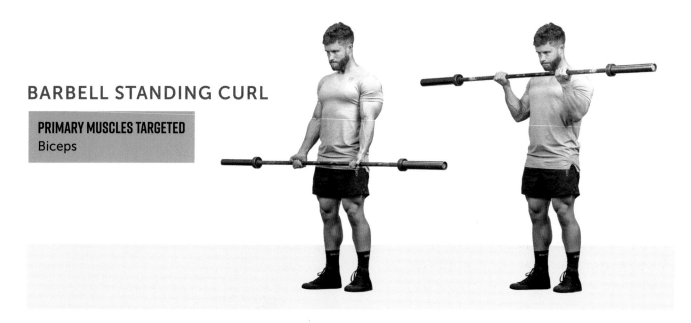

BARBELL STANDING CURL

PRIMARY MUSCLES TARGETED
Biceps

ⓥ Technique checklist

- Grab the bar with an underhand grip with your hands about shoulder width apart. Hold the bar with a loose grip and your elbows at your sides; the tighter your grasp, the more your forearm muscles will take over.

- Stand with your feet shoulder width apart, your core braced, and your knees bent slightly (not locked).

- Curl the bar up and out in a semicircle, rather than pulling it straight up your torso, while your elbows move forward slightly. Keep your wrists in a neutral position (neither curled forward nor bent backward) and apply pressure through your ring and pinky fingers, which will increase tension in your biceps.

- Minimize movement at your ankles, knees, hips, and back, and squeeze your biceps at the top, when the bar is around shoulder level.

- Reverse the movement under control and come to a full stop before starting the next rep.

NOTE: *Since lots of curl variations follow the same basic steps, I'm just covering the highlights for each.*

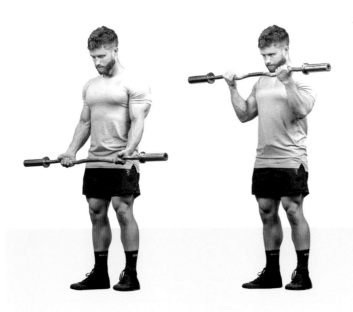

The cambered bar allows you to curl with your pinkies lower than your thumbs, which makes it easier on your wrists than a straight barbell.

Dumbbells are even easier on your wrists than the EZ-curl bar. I generally recommend curling with both arms at once because it's a more efficient use of time. However, if you prefer working one arm at a time, start with your weaker side and then match the reps with your stronger arm.

To get the most from either option, think about driving your pinky finger into the edge of the dumbbell on the way up, which will help you maximize tension on your biceps.

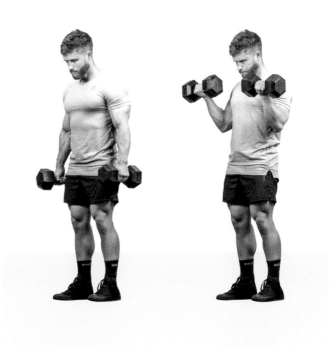

The incline curl puts your biceps into a stretched position at the start of each rep, which may be useful for hypertrophy. Keep your upper back pinned to the bench and don't let your shoulders travel forward as you lift.

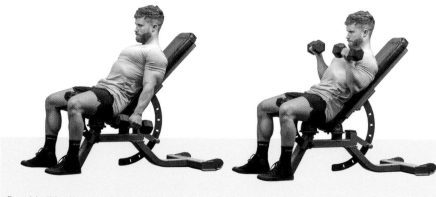

Dumbbell incline curl (side view)

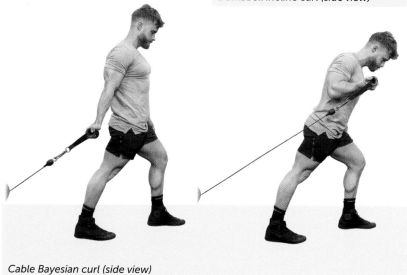

Cable Bayesian curl (side view)

Attach a D-shaped handle to the low cable pulley. Grab the handle with your back to the weight stack, take a few steps forward, and stand with your working arm slightly behind your torso and your opposite-side leg forward for stability. This puts your biceps in a deep stretch at the start of each rep. You can increase the stretch by setting the cable pulley higher, although you'll want to try it in the low position a few times before raising it.

A neutral hand position, with your palms facing each other, puts more emphasis on the brachialis, the short, thick muscle that sits between the biceps and the upper-arm bone. It also works the brachioradialis, the largest forearm muscle, in addition to the biceps.

Unlike other curl variations, the hammer curl works best when you take a firm grip. Wrap your thumb around the handle rather than letting it rest passively against the top head of the dumbbell.

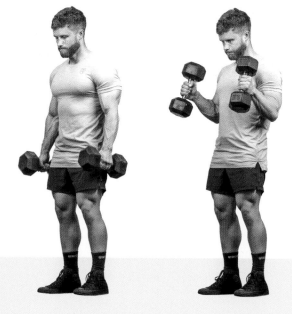

Dumbbell hammer curl (front view)

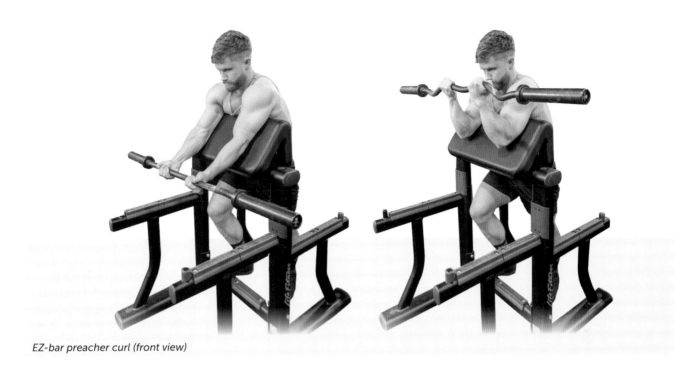

EZ-bar preacher curl (front view)

You can do preacher curls with a cambered bar, as shown, or with a straight bar, dumbbells, or a cable system. Another great option is the preacher curl machine, if your gym has one.

If your gym doesn't have a preacher curl bench, you can go old school and use the back of an incline bench. Keep your elbows pinned against the pad and make sure you get a full biceps stretch at the start of each rep.

TRICEPS EXERCISES

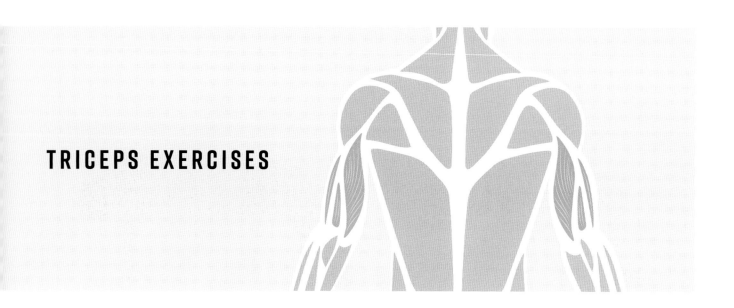

SKULL CRUSHER

PRIMARY MUSCLES TARGETED
Triceps

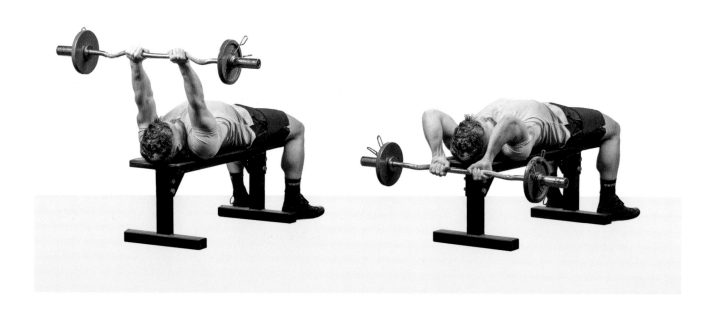

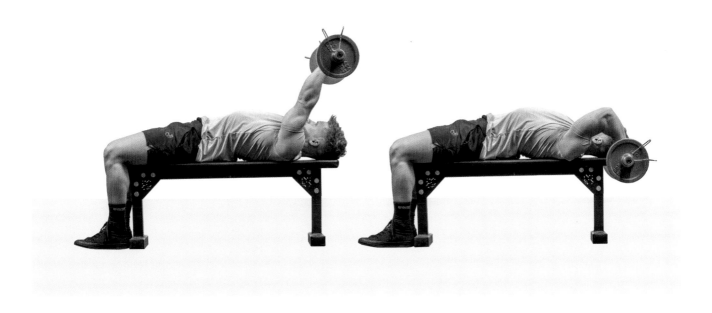

NOTE: *Despite the name, under no circumstances should you lower the weight to your forehead, much less make contact with it. It's safer to think of this exercise as a lying triceps extension. Your goal is to lower the weight behind your head and start the concentric phase with your triceps in a deep stretch.*

✓ Technique checklist

- Grab an EZ-curl bar with a shoulder-width grip and hold it on your lap or have a training partner hand you the weight while you're face-up on the bench.

- In one motion, lie back on the bench with your head at the end and the bar over your head with your arms straight. In this starting position, your arms are angled back toward your ears rather than perpendicular to the floor.

- Squeeze your shoulder blades back and down, as you would on a bench press.

- Bend your elbows and lower the weight slowly in an arc behind your head; go as low as you can without feeling discomfort in your elbows or moving your upper arms.

- Reverse the movement, squeezing your triceps at the top.

OVERHEAD TRICEPS EXTENSION

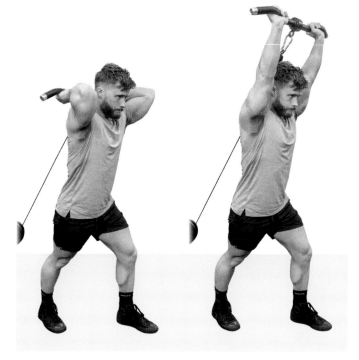

PRIMARY MUSCLES TARGETED
Triceps

✅ Technique checklist

- Set the cable pulley low with a straight or EZ-bar attachment.

- Grab the bar with an overhand grip and hold it behind your head as you stand with your back to the weight stack.

- Step into a staggered stance and lean forward slightly, with your elbows raised and in line with your head; make sure there's tension in the cable in this bottom position.

- Moving only at the elbows, press the bar directly overhead until your arms are straight.

- Reverse the movement under control, feeling a deep stretch in your triceps as you return to the starting position.

TRICEPS PRESSDOWN

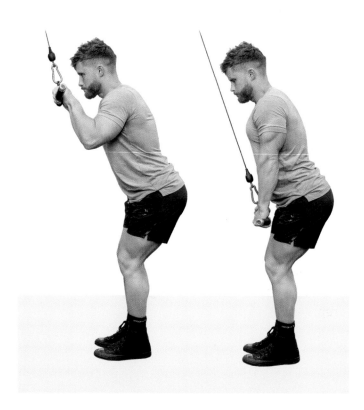

PRIMARY MUSCLES TARGETED
Triceps

✅ Technique checklist

- Set the cable pulley so the attachment (bar, rope, or whatever you prefer) hangs at or just above eye level.

- Grab the attachment with an overhand grip, step back, and set your feet between hip and shoulder width apart; lean forward slightly with your knees bent.

- Bring the attachment down to about chin level with your forearms touching your biceps and tension in the cable; this is your starting position.

- Press the weight down and slightly back toward your body, moving only at the elbows, until your arms are straight.

- Reverse the movement under control, keeping tension in your triceps all the way back to the starting position.

CABLE TRICEPS KICKBACK

PRIMARY MUSCLES TARGETED
Triceps

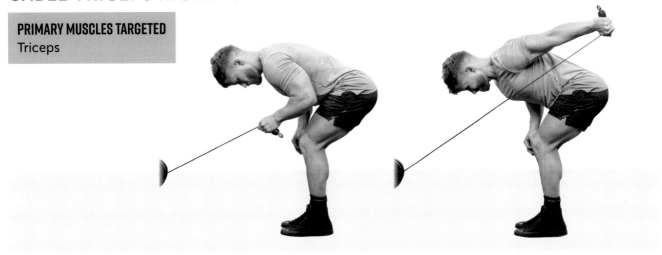

⊘ Technique checklist

- Set the cable pulley to its lowest position; you can attach a D-shaped handle or use the cable itself.

- Grab the handle, brace your nonworking hand against your knee, and lean over until your back is slightly above parallel to the ground.

- Moving only at the elbow, pull the cable down and back behind your torso.

- Pause at the end with your elbow fully locked and squeeze the muscle.

- Reverse the movement under control and come to a full stop before beginning the next rep.

NOTE: *In contrast to the pushdown, which you typically perform with both arms and relatively heavy weights, the kickback is more of a finesse movement. It's incredibly easy to cheat and use momentum to knock out reps, but it's also pointless. You want to do each rep slowly, with continuous tension on the triceps and a full contraction at the end.*

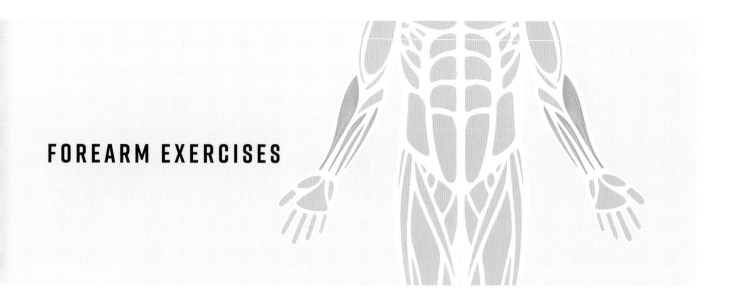

FOREARM EXERCISES

DUMBBELL WRIST CURL

PRIMARY MUSCLES TARGETED
Wrist flexors

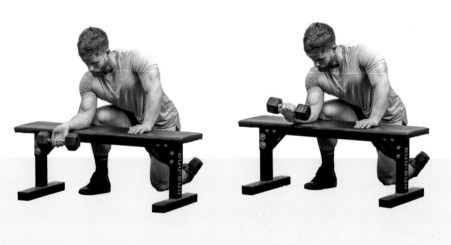

✓ Technique checklist

- With a dumbbell in your hand with your palm up, rest the back of your forearm against a flat bench so your wrist hangs over the edge.

- Bend your wrist down and let the dumbbell roll into your fingers; you should feel a nice stretch in your forearm muscles.

- Flex your wrist and close your fingers, curling the weight from below to above the bench.

- Reverse the movement under control and come to a full stop before beginning the next rep.

DUMBBELL WRIST EXTENSION

PRIMARY MUSCLES TARGETED
Wrist extensors

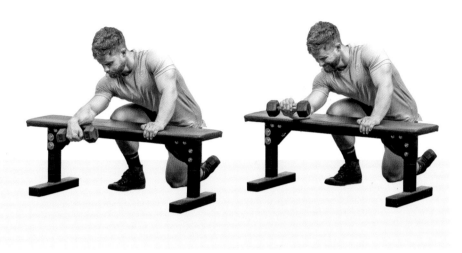

⊘ Technique checklist

- With a dumbbell in your hand with your palm down, rest the front of your forearm against a flat bench so your wrist hangs over the edge.

NOTE: *Most people find a false grip (without the thumb wrapped around the dumbbell) more comfortable.*

- Bend your wrist over the bench, feeling a stretch in the muscles on the back of your forearm.

- Extend your wrist, lifting the weight from below the bench to above it.

- Reverse the movement and lower the dumbbell under control to the starting position.

UPPER TRAP AND NECK EXERCISES

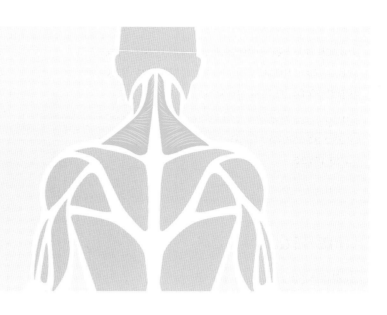

BARBELL SHRUG

PRIMARY MUSCLES TARGETED
Upper traps, levator scapulae

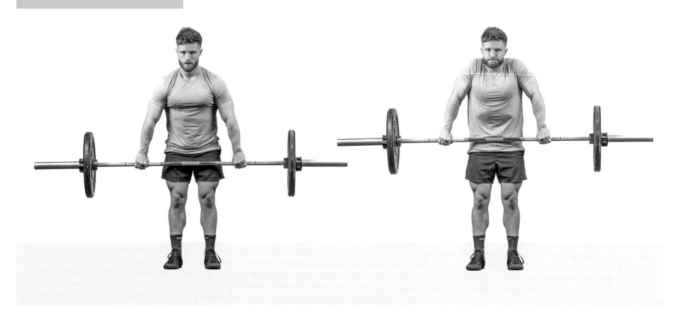

✓ Technique checklist

- Set up a barbell just above knee height. You might want to use a squat rack for this.

- Take a relatively wide overhand grip, approximately one-and-a-quarter to one-and-a-half times shoulder width.

NOTE: *As your upper-back strength improves and you work with increasingly heavy weights, your grip will become a limiting factor, and you'll need to use wrist straps.*

- Unrack the bar and take two or three steps back; you should feel a deep stretch in your upper traps in this starting position.

- Shrug your shoulders toward your ears; pause at the top with your upper traps fully contracted.

- Reverse the movement and pause one or two seconds in the starting position, feeling a deep stretch in your traps, and then start the next rep.

DUMBBELL SHRUG

PRIMARY MUSCLES TARGETED
Upper traps, levator scapulae

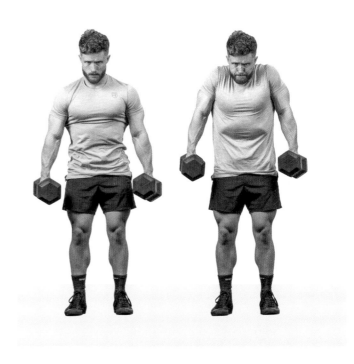

✅ Technique checklist

- Grab a pair of dumbbells and hold them at your side. As with the barbell version (page 134), your grip strength will eventually become a limiting factor, and you'll need to use wrist straps.

- Execution is the same as described for the barbell shrug; make sure you pause at the top to feel the contraction and pause again at the bottom to feel the stretch.

NOTE: *The following are two more shrug variations you can work into your program for variety. The technique is the same for both.*

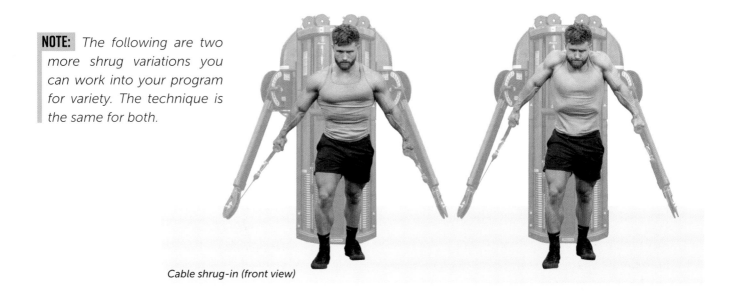

Cable shrug-in (front view)

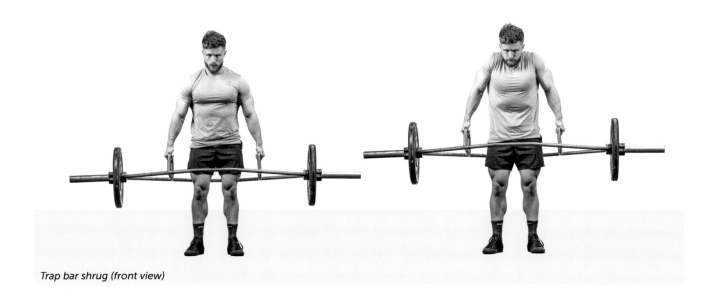

Trap bar shrug (front view)

PLATE-LOADED NECK CURL

PRIMARY MUSCLES TARGETED
Neck flexors (front and sides of the neck)

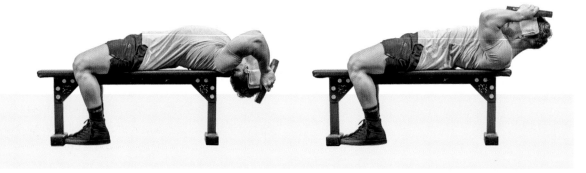

NOTE: *Training the neck muscles directly has obvious value in combat and contact sports, as well as some motor sports. Because it increases neck circumference, it's useful for lifters who are genetically small-framed and want to appear more muscular, especially in clothes.*

Personally, I've found that strengthening my neck helps reduce headaches and day-to-day neck pain. However, this exercise isn't popular in gyms today, which is why I consider it optional in most circumstances.

☑ Technique checklist

- Position yourself face up on a flat bench with your shoulders resting on the end of the bench and a towel on your forehead for protection.

- Hold a weight plate in both hands and position it on the towel.

- Tuck your shoulder blades in and down to create a slight arch in your upper back, as you would on a bench press; plant your feet firmly on the floor for balance.

- Slowly lower your head over the edge of the bench, feeling the stretch on the front of your neck. There's no need to go very deep at first; you can increase your ROM as you get more comfortable with the movement.

- Raise your head using the muscles on the front of your neck. Do not use your hands for assistance; their only role is holding the weight in place.

- Reverse the movement and continue with a smooth, consistent tempo; the amount of weight is far less important than having full control over it.

PLATE-LOADED NECK EXTENSION

PRIMARY MUSCLES TARGETED
Neck extensors (back of the neck), upper traps

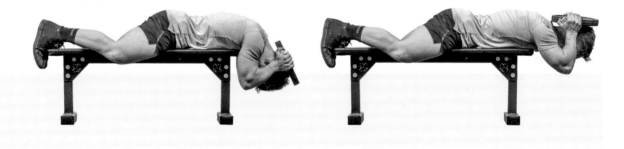

☑ Technique checklist

- Lie face down on a flat bench with your chest at the edge and your head and shoulders free to move; you'll need to hook your feet on the opposite end to avoid falling off.

- Place a towel on the back of your head for protection, set a weight plate on the towel, and hold the plate with both hands.

- Lower your head slowly, feeling a stretch on the back of your neck. There's no need to work through the full ROM right away; wait until you're comfortable with the exercise.

- Reverse the movement and continue with a smooth, consistent, controlled tempo.

HEAD HARNESS NECK EXTENSION

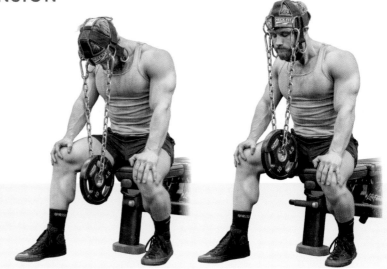

☑ Technique checklist

- Adjust the head harness so it's tightly secured.

- Loop a weight through the chain and attach it to the harness.

- Sit on a flat bench, brace your hands on your knees, and sit in a comfortable posture with your shoulders back.

- Lower your head slowly until you feel a stretch on the back of your neck.

- Raise your head until your neck is in or near a neutral position; you'll probably have to lean forward a bit to keep the weight plate from resting on your chest.

- Reverse the movement and continue with slow, smooth, controlled repetitions. You'll know you have it right if the chain and plate only move up and down; any other movement means you're not in full control.

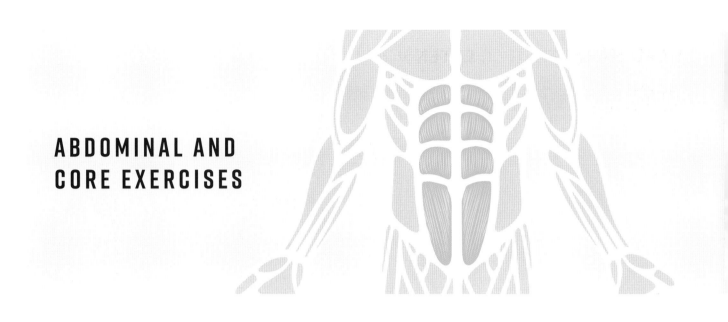

ABDOMINAL AND CORE EXERCISES

CABLE CRUNCH

PRIMARY MUSCLES TARGETED
Abs (rectus abdominis
and external obliques)

✓ Technique checklist

- Raise a cable pulley to a high position with a rope attached.

- Grab the ends of the rope, with your pinkies on the plastic ends, and kneel facing the weight stack.

- Start with your hands just above your head and tension in the cable.

- Pulling only with your abdominal muscles, crunch down until your elbows are near the floor and your upper back rounds forward.

- Feel the squeeze in your abs; then reverse the movement under control and begin the next rep.

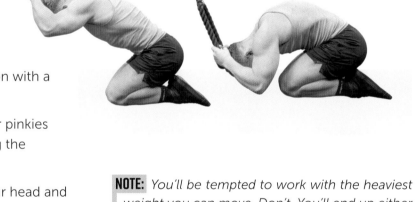

NOTE: *You'll be tempted to work with the heaviest weight you can move. Don't. You'll end up either raising and lowering your entire torso, which means you're using your hip flexors instead of the rectus abdominis and external obliques (aka spinal flexors) or yanking on the rope with your arms, which will activate your lats, among other muscles.*

PLATE-LOADED DECLINE SIT-UP

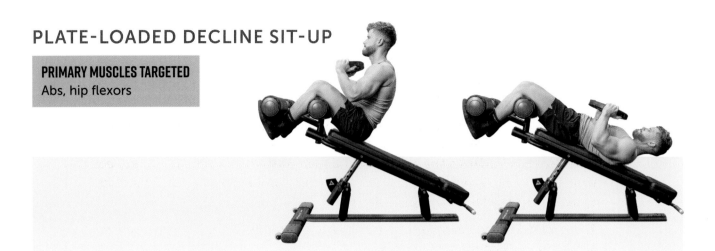

PRIMARY MUSCLES TARGETED
Abs, hip flexors

☑ Technique checklist

- Sit on a decline bench with your feet and ankles secured while holding a weight plate to your chest.

- Lower your torso under control until your back is flat on the bench.

- Curl your body up, initiating the movement with your hip flexors but completing it with your abs; crunch your chest toward your thighs at the end, feeling the squeeze throughout your core.

- Continue with strong but controlled repetitions; end the set if you start pulling with your legs or lifting your hips off the bench to generate momentum.

HANGING LEG RAISE

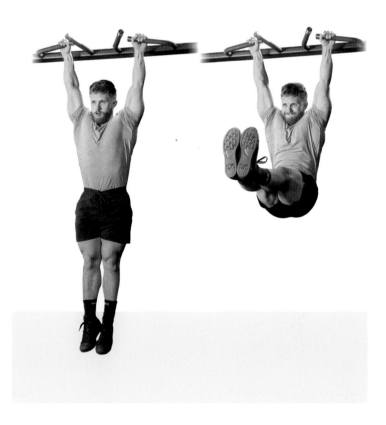

PRIMARY MUSCLES TARGETED
Abs and hip flexors

☑ Technique checklist

- Grab a pull-up bar in an overhand grip with your hands a comfortable distance apart.

- With your knees straight (or nearly straight), lift your legs out and up until your feet reach chest height.

- Lower your legs under control and come to a complete stop before starting the next rep. Although some swaying is inevitable as you learn the movement, your goal over time is to eliminate it entirely (or at least minimize it).

NOTE: *Your hip flexors do all the work at the beginning of the movement. It takes a lot of focus to train your abs to take over the second half of the ROM so you can finish with your pelvis tilted upward.*

You also want to avoid using your upper body for assistance. You'll feel some activation in your middle back as your shoulder blades move down and toward each other for stability. That's fine as long as you keep your arms straight. But if you feel your torso rising, especially if your elbows bend, you'll know your lats and other upper-body muscles are trying to take over.

This is obviously an advanced movement, and even some strong and experienced lifters never get comfortable with it.

However, most lifters can eventually master either the bent-knee variation of the hanging raise or leg raises in a Roman chair.

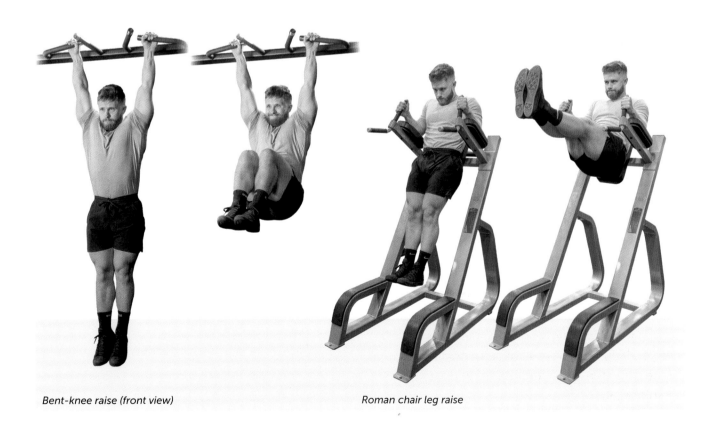

Bent-knee raise (front view)   Roman chair leg raise

PLANK

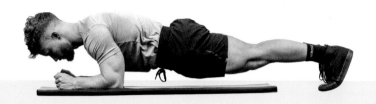

✓ Technique checklist

- Get into plank position with your arms shoulder width apart and your weight on your forearms and toes; use a mat to protect your elbows if you don't have a well-padded floor.

- Tighten your torso, core, glutes, and legs so your body forms a straight line from neck to ankles.

- Hold this position for a predetermined amount of time:

  - A beginner might hold for as little as 10 to 15 seconds at a time, doing sets of 3 to 4 holds with short breaks in between to relax and reset.

  - End the hold when you lose your initial posture—your glutes rise, your hips sink, your shoulder blades cave in, and so on.

  - Once you can do multiple 30-second holds, or a single plank for more than 60 seconds, you can try a more advanced variation, like the long-lever pelvic tilt plank (page 143).

LONG-LEVER PELVIC TILT (LLPT) PLANK

PRIMARY MUSCLES TARGETED
Abs, obliques, shoulder
stabilizers

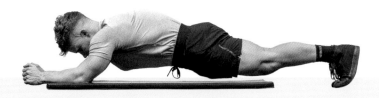

The LLPT plank has two important modifications from the standard plank:

- Your elbows are beneath your eyes rather than beneath your shoulders.

- Your pelvis is in a posterior tilt, which you achieve by contracting your glutes and activating your lower abs to pull the bottom of your pelvis forward. That pushes your upper pelvis up and back, flattening your lumbar spine.

NOTE: *At first, it's challenging enough to make these two modifications and hold for any amount of time. Working up to a 30-second hold is an accomplishment.*

STILL WITH ME?

Great!

That means you understand how to perform the fundamental exercises included in this chapter. And if you understand these, you'll be able to figure out the many, many variations available to you in any well-equipped gym.

The next chapter shifts attention from exercise technique to exercise selection. How do you decide which ones are best for you? Time to find out.

CHAPTER 5

EXERCISE SELECTION

WHAT ARE THE BEST EXERCISES?

With the two sides of the Muscle Ladder firmly in place and the first rung of technique secured, it's time to step onto the second rung, where you select the best exercises for building muscle. Exercise selection comes relatively early in the climb because the exercises you perform are the fundamental tools you use to skillfully craft new muscle tissue.

Think of it this way: If you want to sculpt a statue from a chunk of marble, one of the first things you'll want to know is which tools to buy. Future rungs of the ladder emphasize how often to do the chiseling, how much pressure you should apply to the marble, and so on, but those instructions aren't of much use unless you know what the *best* tools for the job are.

I should probably point out that although the sculpture analogy is a longtime bodybuilding favorite, it isn't perfect. Building muscle honestly isn't as intricate as sculpting a statue out of stone, and, unlike the art of sculpting, you can use a virtually endless number of tools to get the job done in the gym.

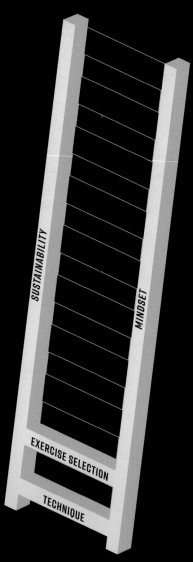

SUSTAINABILITY

MINDSET

EXERCISE SELECTION

TECHNIQUE

So I put exercise selection early in the ladder not because there are a small handful of must-do exercises that are far superior to the rest but because without knowing which exercises to emphasize, you won't know how to put the other training variables into practice.

As long as you're using good technique, training hard, and doing enough volume (enough total sets and reps), it doesn't actually matter much if you do a shoulder press with a barbell or with dumbbells or with a shoulder press machine. The specific choice of equipment is a relatively minor factor for muscle growth, and your muscles often won't know the difference.

Then why does exercise selection seem so much more complex than what I just described? In part, I think it's because denigrating certain exercises is so popular. A trainer can get lots of clicks and views by offering reasons why you

should *never* do Exercise A, followed by why you should do Exercise B instead.

I'm not a big fan of this approach. If you understand the principles of exercise selection, you should realize there are many ways to get the job done. Rather than thinking of a given exercise as "good" or "bad," it makes more sense to ask if an exercise is more or less appropriate for your body, your goals, your training history, and your strengths and weaknesses.

In this chapter, I cover all the information you need on how to select the best exercises for your goals and how they can be most effectively organized into a workout.

COMPOUND VERSUS ISOLATION EXERCISES

Let's start with some basic terminology to make sure we're on the same page. Throughout this chapter and the remainder of the book, I refer to two exercise classifications: compound exercises and isolation exercises.

Compound exercises target multiple joints and activate multiple muscles at once. The bench press, for example, is a compound exercise because it involves the shoulder joints and the elbow joints. Your pecs and front deltoids

contract to generate movement at the shoulder joints, and your triceps contract to generate movement at the elbows.

Isolation exercises, by contrast, require action at a single joint and aim to target a single muscle. For example, the biceps curl is an isolation exercise because it involves movement at the elbow joint when the biceps contract.

Then you have an exercise like the lat pulldown. The name suggests it's an isolation exercise, targeting the lats, and many people think of it as an isolation exercise because it's performed using a machine rather than free weights. Although it doesn't feel as rigorous as a squat, bench press, or deadlift, the lat pulldown is, in fact, a compound movement, and a fairly complex one at that. The movement begins with action in your mid-back muscles (the rhomboids and the middle and lower parts of your traps), which pull your shoulder blades down and together. Your lats also generate movement at the shoulder joints to pull your arms down. And your biceps act on the elbow joints to finish the movement.

That said, there is a practical difference between an exercise like the bench press and an exercise like the lat pulldown, apart from the muscles they target. The bench press is generally more strength-oriented, and the lat pulldown is generally more muscle-oriented. For this reason, it's sometimes helpful to divide compound exercises into two subcategories: primary and secondary movements. Isolation movements are tertiary exercises. (See Figure 5.1.)

Figure 5.1

Compound and isolation exercises

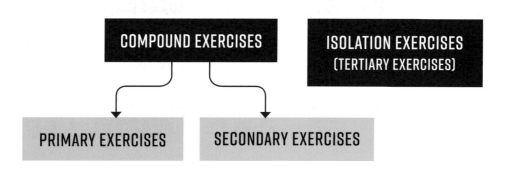

- *Primary exercises* are compound movements best trained with heavier weights, lower reps, and an emphasis on progressively building strength. My list of primary exercises is short: squat, bench press, deadlift, and overhead press. However, I can stretch the definition to include other compound movements you do with the goal of getting stronger. For example, if you're doing barbell rows with heavy loads

for 4 to 6 reps per set, you can consider them a primary exercise.

- *Secondary exercises* are compound movements that either involve less muscle mass or don't lend themselves as well to a focus on strength progression. Examples include lat pulldowns, cable rows, lunges, hip thrusts, and pull-ups. With these exercises, you often use higher reps and focus more on feeling the target muscles in action than you would with primary exercises.

- *Tertiary exercises* are isolation movements. They involve movement at one joint, targeting a single muscle or muscle group. Most of the time, you do higher reps with lighter loads.

There's a lot of chatter within the lifting community about the relative value of compound versus isolation exercises in stimulating muscle growth. Some argue that compound movements are superior because they activate more total muscle mass. Others argue that isolation exercises are better because they allow you to fully stimulate one muscle at a time.

But that's a false dichotomy. Training doesn't need to be either/or. A well-designed bodybuilding routine includes both compound and isolation movements rather than relying on one or the other. Each exercise category offers advantages and disadvantages that can make them more or less effective in different situations. Tables 5.1 and 5.2 outline some of the pros and cons of compound and isolation exercises.

Table 5.1: Compound Exercises Pros and Cons

Pros	Cons
Generally more time efficient because you activate a lot of muscle mass at once.	Because you activate a lot of muscle mass at once, you may not be able to achieve optimal activation in some of the smaller muscles that assist the larger ones.
Generally allow for the use of heavier loads, developing total-body strength faster.	Working with heavier loads creates more fatigue, which means you may need more time to recover.
Generally easier to track and assess strength gains, which can be highly motivating.	The stronger you get, the more time you'll need to warm up for your heaviest lifts, which can make workouts longer.
Technique, like strength, often carries over to other movements, making you a better all-around lifter.	You need more time and practice to become proficient in primary compound lifts.

Table 5.2: Isolation Exercises Pros and Cons

Pros	Cons
Generally better at targeting smaller muscles that may not be fully stimulated when they're assisting larger muscles on compound movements.	Training muscles one at a time can be less time efficient.
You can often train lagging muscle groups with higher volume and frequency because you need less time to recover.	It's more difficult to track progress because you might go weeks or even months at a time without any change in strength.
Technique is more easily mastered, making isolation exercises more accessible to new lifters.	Technique and strength in single-joint exercises have less carryover to other movements.
Reduced recovery demand allows you to train closer to failure, which is beneficial in some contexts.	May be worse at hitting certain smaller, stabilizing muscles that are easily reached with compound exercises.
You typically get a better "feel" for the target muscle working, which helps you develop a stronger mind-muscle connection.	If you like working with heavier weights on compound movements, you may not feel as motivated when you do isolation exercises.
You can use advanced training techniques like rest-pause or drop sets without the same recovery cost.	Some isolation exercises require equipment you may not have access to, like cable machines with a variety of handles.

As you can see, compound and isolation movements complement each other. Each has advantages that make up for the other category's disadvantages. An effective bodybuilding program includes both.

I cover how to implement compound and isolation movements in more detail throughout the chapter, but to get things started, here are a few general guidelines:

- If your goal is to maximize muscular development, you shouldn't use compound or isolation exercises exclusively. Use both.

- There's no precise ratio of compound to isolation movements that applies to every lifter. A good bodybuilding program will have a roughly even mix. In my own workouts, I have 50 to 70 percent compound exercises and 30 to 50 percent isolation exercises. You can tweak these ratios to suit your goals and preferences.

- Compound exercises usually work best early in a workout. There can be exceptions, of course, but most of the time, you want to do the most technically complex and physically demanding exercises when you're fresh and focused.

- Isolation exercises should be used to fill any gaps in your workout. Let's say it's leg day and you start your workout with barbell back squats (a compound exercise that primarily targets the quads and glutes). You'd be wise to also include hamstring curls and calf raises, which isolate muscles that won't be sufficiently activated by the primary movement.

THE BIG SIX

The Big Six are the most basic movements and form the foundation of all my training programs. I believe any complete training program should include at least one exercise from each of the six fundamental movement patterns. If you're a new lifter, I recommend learning the Big Six within your first few months of training. Table 5.3 on page 155 summarizes the Big Six.

SQUAT-TYPE MOVEMENT

As the name implies, squat-type movements feature joint actions similar to those of a squat. Those include knee extension (where the knees straighten) and hip extension (where the hips straighten).

All squat-type exercises involve the quadriceps (mainly responsible for straightening the knees), the glutes (mainly responsible for straightening the hips), and the adductors (the large muscles on the inside of the thigh that perform a crucial stabilizing role). See Figure 5.2 for the location of these muscles.

Examples of squat-type exercises include

- Barbell back squat (page 65)
- Barbell front squat (page 67)
- Goblet squat (page 69)
- Leg press (page 71)
- Lunge (pages 70–71)
- Step-up
- Bulgarian split squat
- Hack squat
- Machine squat

Figure 5.2

The main muscles targeted by squat-type movements

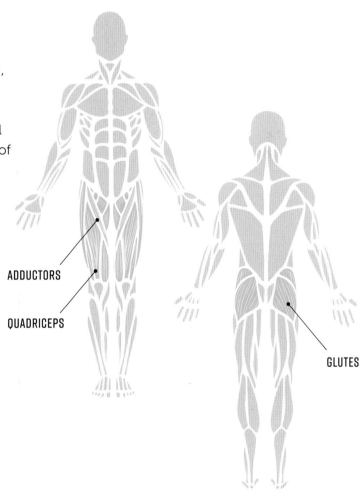

ADDUCTORS

QUADRICEPS

GLUTES

HIP HINGE

Hip-hinge movements involve bending and straightening at the hips. They typically begin with the torso bent forward, followed by hip extension, which brings your upper body back into alignment with your lower body. The glutes and hamstrings are the primary hip extensors, with your spinal erectors working hard in a stabilizing role. (See Figure 5.3 for the location of these muscles.) There's relatively little action at the knee joints.

Examples of hip-hinge exercises include

- Conventional deadlift (page 74)

- Sumo deadlift (page 77)

- Romanian deadlift (page 83)

- Good morning (page 84)

- 45-degree back extension (page 80)

- Reverse hyperextension

Figure 5.3

The main muscles targeted by hip-hinge movements

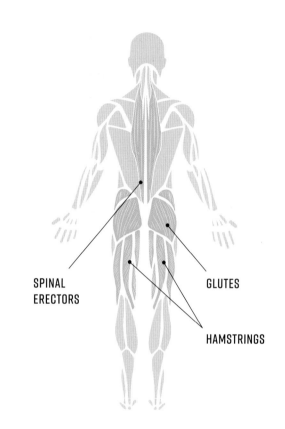

SPINAL ERECTORS

GLUTES

HAMSTRINGS

VERTICAL PUSH

Vertical pushing movements are most often referred to as overhead presses or shoulder presses. (You might also hear the term "military press," which, literally, would mean standing at attention with the heels together and toes out and lifting a barbell overhead.) Whatever you call the exercises, they mainly target the deltoids (see Figure 5.4). The front delts get the most work, followed by the side delts, triceps, and the clavicular head of the pecs, also known as the "upper chest."

Examples of vertical pushes include

- Barbell overhead press (aka OHP) (page 116)

- Seated barbell overhead press

- Dumbbell shoulder press (standing or seated)

- Machine shoulder press

- Vertical (aka inverted) push-up

Figure 5.4

The main muscles targeted by vertical push movements

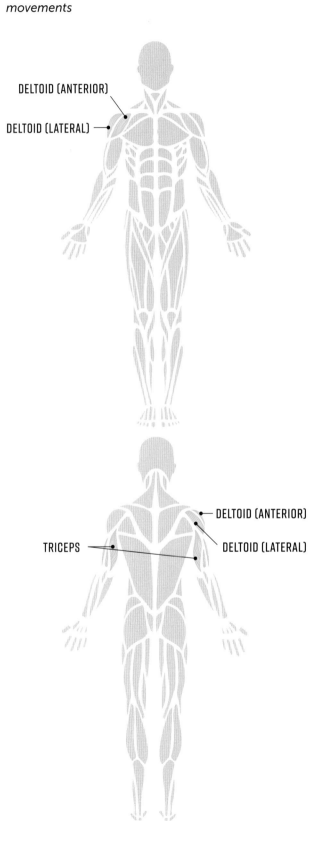

HORIZONTAL PUSH

Chest presses or bench presses are the most recognizable of the horizontal push exercises, but the category is actually broader than that. It includes any pushing movement in which the arms are either straight out in front of the torso (horizontal to the ground if you're standing up; perpendicular to the ground if you're lying on a flat bench) or diagonal to it. A flat bench press or traditional push-up mainly works the pecs, triceps, and front delts (see Figure 5.5). Incline variations put more emphasis on the upper chest, whereas decline presses and parallel-bar dips put more emphasis on the lower chest.

Examples of horizontal pushes include

- Barbell bench press (flat, incline, or decline) (pages 102, 107, and 108)

- Close- or wide-grip bench press (page 107)

- Dumbbell bench press (flat, incline, or decline) (pages 109–110)

- Parallel-bar dip (page 111)

- Push-up (traditional or with hands or feet elevated) (page 114)

- Machine chest press

Figure 5.5

The main muscles targeted by horizontal push movements

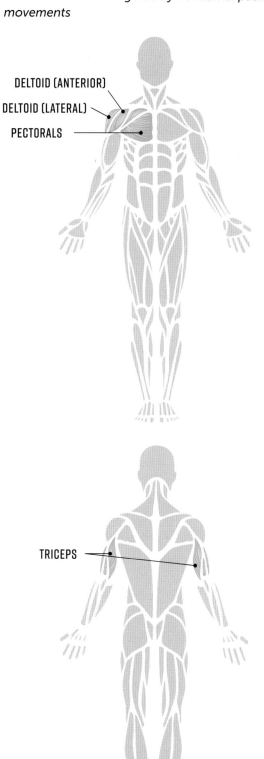

DELTOID (ANTERIOR)

DELTOID (LATERAL)

PECTORALS

TRICEPS

VERTICAL PULL

Vertical pulls are the mirror image of vertical pushes. Instead of straightening your arms overhead, you're pulling them down to your sides. The lats are the primary target, but vertical pulls activate a long list of other muscles too (see Figure 5.6): traps, teres major, rear delts, and almost everything that supports and stabilizes the shoulders, spine, and scapulae. And that's just in your back and shoulders. You also work your biceps and the gripping muscles in your hands and forearms. Even the pecs and triceps play a minor role.

Examples of vertical pulls include

- Pull-up (overhand grip) (page 92)

- Chin-up (underhand grip) (page 94)

- Lat pulldown (page 94)

- Machine pulldown

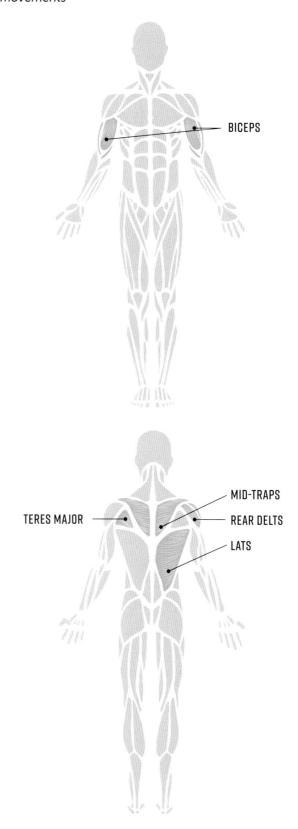

Figure 5.6

The main muscles targeted by vertical pull movements

BICEPS

MID-TRAPS

TERES MAJOR

REAR DELTS

LATS

HORIZONTAL PULL

Horizontal pulls use the same movement path as horizontal pushes, but the arms move in and toward the torso instead of out and away from it. The traps and lats are the primary targets of the movement, with help from the rear delts, biceps, and smaller muscles acting on the shoulders and middle back. See Figure 5.7 for the muscles affected by horizontal pulls.

Examples of horizontal pulls include

- Barbell or dumbbell row (pages 96 and 98)

- Cable row

- Machine row

- Chest-supported T-bar row (page 99)

- Pendlay row (page 97)

- Face pull

Figure 5.7

The main muscles targeted by horizontal pull movements

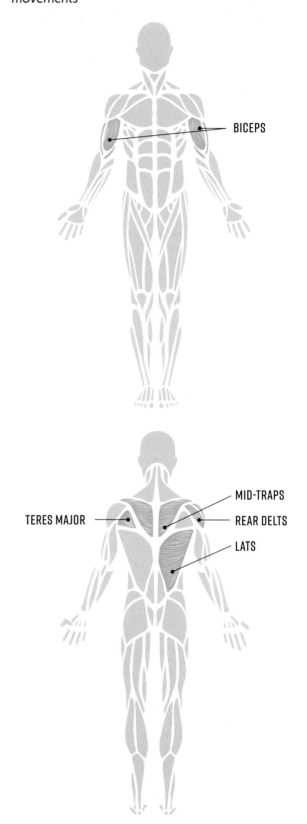

Table 5.3: The Big Six

Fundamental Movement Pattern	Exercise Examples		Main Muscles Targeted
Squat-type	Barbell back squat Barbell front squat Goblet squat Leg press	Lunge Step-up Bulgarian split squat Hack squat Machine squat	Quadriceps Glutes Adductors
Hip hinge	Conventional deadlift Sumo deadlift Romanian deadlift	Good morning 45-degree back extension Reverse hyperextension	Glutes Hamstrings Spinal erectors
Vertical push	Barbell overhead press (standing or seated) Dumbbell shoulder press (standing or seated)	Machine shoulder press Vertical/inverted push-up	Deltoids (anterior and lateral) Triceps Pectorals (clavicular head)
Horizontal push	Barbell bench press (flat, incline, or decline) Close- or wide-grip bench press Dumbbell bench press (flat, incline, or decline)	Parallel-bar dip Push-up (traditional, incline, or decline) Machine chest press	Pectorals Deltoids (anterior and lateral) Triceps
Vertical pull	Pull-up Chin-up	Lat pulldown Machine pulldown	Lats Teres major Trapezius (middle and lower) Biceps Forearms Deltoids (posterior)
Horizontal pull	Barbell or dumbbell row Cable row Machine row	Chest-supported T-bar row Pendlay row Face pull	Trapezius Lats Rhomboids Teres major Biceps and forearms Deltoids (posterior)

MUSCLE ISOLATION: BEYOND THE BIG SIX

With the Big Six movement patterns as the foundation of your program, you'll not only get bigger and stronger, but you'll also become more physically fit. More capable. More athletic. You can do more than you could before, both in and out of the gym. You'll feel the difference in every waking moment.

Although compound exercises work every major muscle group, some of those muscles won't be fully or optimally stimulated. Some won't develop in proportion to others. That's where isolation exercises come in. They fill in the gaps.

What does that mean? Let's take a look at each muscle group—what it does, and what it might require to reach its full potential for size and aesthetics.

SHOULDERS

The human ball-and-socket shoulder joint is unique in the animal kingdom. Some believe its structure (see Figure 5.8) and range of motion evolved for hunting—specifically, to throw a blunt or pointed object far enough and hard enough to take down something our ancestors couldn't outrun.[1]

Figure 5.8

The ball-and-socket shoulder joint

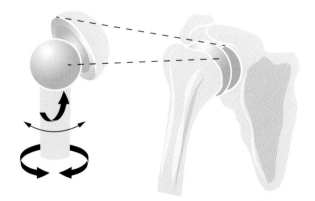

The deltoid muscle had to be strong and versatile enough to perform a variety of lifting and carrying functions without limiting the ability to throw. That's why you can lift your arm to the front, back, or side; rotate it in circles; or swing it back and forth. And it's why you can train your deltoids with so many different movements.

Anatomical data suggests the deltoid has seven distinct intramuscular segments (see Figure 5.9), and each segment performs a slightly different function.[2] If you only train your shoulders in one or two directions, you probably won't fully stimulate the muscle.

Figure 5.9

The seven intramuscular segments of the deltoid

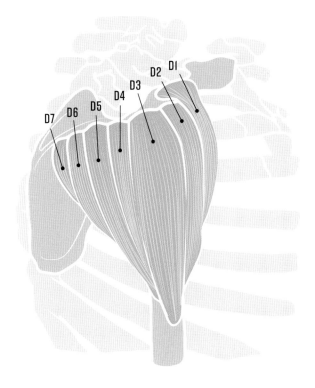

That said, for practical training purposes, it doesn't make much sense to target each of the seven segments. Instead, I'm focusing on the three you're already familiar with: anterior (front), lateral (side), and posterior (rear). You can think of the D1 and D2 segments in Figure 5.9 as the anterior deltoid, the large D3 segment as the lateral delt, and the smaller D4, D5, D6, and D7 segments as the posterior delt. Even with just three segments, there's still some overlap in function.

You can activate the front delts to a high degree on two Big Six movements: horizontal and vertical presses. Further isolating them is seldom necessary. In fact, bodybuilders frequently have the opposite problem: Their anterior delts are so big in comparison to the other two heads, they create an imbalanced, "front-heavy" appearance. Front raises and other isolation exercises for

the anterior delts are usually redundant. The side delts and rear delts are more important to isolate.

The side delts will be activated on horizontal and vertical presses, but to a lesser extent than the front delts. For example, one study from 2020 found that the bench press activated the front delts about four times more than the side delts.[3] A 2013 study found roughly twice as much activation in front delts compared to side delts with shoulder presses.[4] Both studies used EMG (electromyography) to measure muscle activation, which may or may not predict long-term muscle hypertrophy.[5] We don't yet know if higher activation means faster growth rates or if lower activation means slower growth rates. (The neurophysiology is complex and not worth getting into here.)

DELTOID ACTIVATION DURING BENCH PRESS[3]

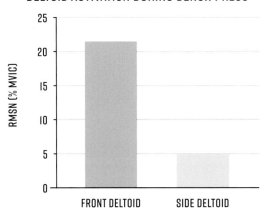

DELTOID ACTIVATION DURING SHOULDER PRESS[4]

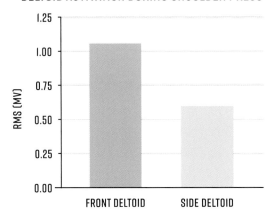

However, despite potential limitations of EMG data, well-understood biomechanics tells us that the front delts tend to take over on both vertical and horizontal presses. That's why I doubt that vertical and horizontal pressing alone will maximize lateral deltoid development. I recommend targeting them with at least one isolation exercise. That's especially true if you want to build broader shoulders and an aesthetic, tapered physique.

The lateral raise is the best exercise for isolating the side delts. You can do them with dumbbells, cables, or a lateral raise machine. All should yield similar results as long as you're pushing them hard and using good technique. Cable and machine lateral raises may have a slight benefit over dumbbells simply because they provide more tension when the delts are highly stretched, but that's hairsplitting that you don't need to worry about for now. I periodically include all three variations in my own training.

The rear delts, by contrast, are virtually silent on all horizontal and vertical presses, according to EMG activation data.[6] Again, this makes sense when you consider the biomechanics. They are, after all, on the rear aspect of the shoulder. They're poorly positioned for presses but ideally placed to assist with pulling movements. Almost any horizontal and vertical pulls will activate the rear delts to some degree.

However, for *optimal* rear delt activation, you have to go beyond pulldowns and rows, which are dominated by bigger, stronger muscles like the lats and traps. To be clear, your rear delts *will* grow if your routine contains only rows and pull-ups/pulldowns, but you likely won't see visually noticeable improvements to their development beyond the beginner-intermediate stage if you don't do rear delt isolation.

Including any of the following exercises will get the job done for the rear delts:

- Dumbbell or cable reverse fly (page 112)

- Reverse pec deck (page 122)

- Face pull (usually with a rope attachment)

- Band pull-apart

CHEST

The pectorals are divided into two heads: the relatively smaller clavicular head (the upper chest) and the much larger sternal head, which includes the middle and lower pecs.

Both heads are highly active in any horizontal press. The clavicular head also contributes to vertical pressing, especially if you perform it with a slight arch in your upper back (as you should). Thus, the pecs are one of the few muscles where isolation work isn't mandatory.

At some point, however, you may realize that you need more work for your chest to keep it growing. If you simply add more presses and dips, you may place undesired stress on your anterior delts or triceps. That's where isolation exercises can be useful. They give your pecs the volume they need to develop without imposing an unwanted recovery demand on other muscles.

These are the main exercises I recommend for chest isolation:

- Cable fly (page 113)

- Cable crossover

- Pec deck (page 114)

- Dumbbell fly (page 112)

BACK

I touched on the complexity of your back muscles earlier in the chapter, especially compared to the muscles on the front of your torso. You have dozens of muscles layered on top of each other. The largest of them, the lats, connect your upper arms to your middle and lower back. The second-largest, the trapezius, has multiple segments responsible for moving your shoulder blades up, in, and down. That's just the top layer of muscles. Beneath and between them are muscles that move and stabilize your neck, shoulders, and spine.

Despite all their unique anatomical features, most of these muscles are functionally complementary. You usually don't need to isolate them because they work together on the Big Six pulling exercises. Any well-executed row lights up virtually all of them: lats, traps, rhomboids, teres, and more. Vertical pulls crush almost anything that isn't fully stimulated by the horizontal pulls. Change the angle, apparatus, or attachment, and you'll hit even more.

Although you couldn't isolate most of those muscles even if you wanted to, there are two exceptions. The lats are a key muscle, along with the side delts, for developing an aesthetically desirable V-taper. Their main function is shoulder extension—driving the arms down—which you can come close to isolating with pullover variations. (The triceps and pecs will come in to help the lats out.)

Cable and machine pullovers (page 100) are my preferred options, since they provide consistent tension throughout the range of motion. Dumbbell and barbell pullovers are perfectly fine alternatives, though. Just keep in mind that you'll only have tension on your lats in the final part of the movement, when your arms are positioned behind your head. To get the most out of free-weight pullovers, I suggest staying in the bottom half of the movement, where your lats are most stretched.

Another exercise I like for the lats is the one-arm, half-kneeling lat pulldown. It's not technically an isolation movement because the biceps are involved in flexing the elbow. But it attacks the lats from a unique angle—one that minimizes assistance from other back muscles.

The upper traps are the other exception. They don't contribute a lot to horizontal pulls, and don't really do much at all on vertical pulls. They do have an important stabilizing role on some row variations, and they reach a reasonable level of activation on heavy deadlifts and loaded carries, where they contract isometrically to keep your shoulder joints from flying apart.

To fully develop the upper traps, you want to work them through an active range of motion. Here are some isolation exercises I recommend:

- Barbell shrug (page 134)

- Dumbbell shrug (seated/standing) (page 135)

- Trap bar shrug (page 136)

- Cable shrug-in (page 135)

BICEPS

For all of the attention the biceps get, they're a pretty simple muscle to train and grow. They're already activated to a significant degree by any horizontal and vertical pulls in your program. A 2015 study on novice lifters found that lat pulldowns were able to produce biceps hypertrophy similar to that from barbell biceps curls.[7] Although a later 2019 study found that dumbbell rows stimulated less than half as much growth as dumbbell curls, it still showed that vertical and horizontal pulls build the biceps (at least in new lifters).[8]

Despite the evidence from these two studies, my coaching experience with bodybuilders leads me to doubt that pulldowns and rows are enough to maximize biceps hypertrophy for very long. Once you gain basic lifting experience, and you get better at activating your back muscles on pulling exercises, you'll need to isolate your biceps if you want them to continue growing.

The biceps are an example of what's called a biarticular muscle, meaning it crosses both the elbow joint (where it bends the elbow) and the shoulder joint (where it assists the front delt in lifting the arm). Because of this, altering your arm position can provide a slightly different stimulus and possibly even target the short head (on the inside) versus the long head (on the outside) to different degrees.

A lot of the recommendations I see in this area are some combination of hype and mental gymnastics, in my opinion. Gymnastics can be fun, but in a book about training fundamentals, I think it's best if we keep our feet on the ground. The bottom line? Any biceps curl that feels like it's working the muscle and that allows you to get progressively stronger will do the job.

It also helps to rotate among exercises that put the arm in different positions. Here are some examples:

- Standing barbell/EZ-bar curl (upper arms aligned with your torso) (pages 124 and 125)

- Incline dumbbell curl (upper arm slightly behind your torso) (page 126)

- Bayesian single-arm cable curl (upper arm slightly behind your torso) (page 126)

- Preacher curl (upper arms in front of your torso) (page 127)

Two other muscles assist the biceps in flexing (bending) the elbow. The first is the brachialis,

a large, flat muscle positioned between the biceps and the upper-arm bone. The second is the brachioradialis, one of the most prominent forearm muscles. Both are more active when your wrist is in a neutral position (palm turned toward the torso) or pronated (palm turned toward the ground).

You can target these muscles with dumbbell hammer curls (page 126) or reverse curls (with your palms facing down). Keep in mind, these muscles may not need isolation work right away because you will hit them alongside your upper back any time you do vertical pulls and rows, especially when using a neutral or overhand grip.

TRICEPS

As the name implies, the triceps are made up of three heads: the long head, the medial head, and the lateral head. The long head is the biggest. It's closest to your torso and beefs up the back of the arm. Interestingly, it's another biarticular muscle, acting on both the elbow joint and the shoulder joint. That's why it's active in pullovers and, to a lesser degree, pull-ups. The medial head runs down the middle, and the lateral head sits on the outside, where it combines with the long head to give the triceps their iconic horseshoe shape.

Any horizontal and vertical pressing in your program hits the triceps, especially if you use a close grip. But for full and proportional development, you need isolation exercises, which allow you to emphasize different heads of the triceps with different arm positions.

The medial and lateral heads aren't affected much by your arm's position. They should activate similarly whether the arm is overhead or by your side. But the long head will be activated differently depending on how you position your arm. When your arm is overhead, the long head of your triceps works in a deeper stretch. And when your arm is by your side (like in a pressdown) or behind your torso (like in a kickback) the long head gets a stronger peak contraction.

To be clear, you don't need to include every type of isolation movement in every program. Beginners may not need *any* triceps isolation work to make progress, as long as the program has enough pressing.

That usually changes when you reach the intermediate to advanced stage, though. At that point, it makes sense to include at least one overhead triceps variation, especially because new research suggests that those exercises are superior to pressdowns for stimulating triceps growth.[9] (That's probably because the long head seems to grow better when it's highly stretched.) For the most proportional development, I suggest including exercises with each of the three arm positions. You still want to emphasize the overhead position, but don't skip on the other two entirely.

FOREARMS

The forearms include layers of muscles with names few of us can remember without checking an anatomy chart. But for our purposes, I'm dividing them into two basic functional categories: the wrist flexors on the inside of the forearm and the wrist extensors on the outside.

You activate the flexors on any exercise that requires gripping. That's a long list: deadlifts, vertical pulls, horizontal pulls, curls, loaded carries. Really, any time you pick up a weight, you work those muscles.

Your extensors include the brachioradialis, which, as I mentioned earlier, is active in most compound pulling exercises as well as in hammer and reverse-grip curls.

Despite this crossover with so many common exercises, some trainees may find that they still want to develop their forearms more with isolation. In this case, here are some great isolation exercises for the forearm flexors:

- Dumbbell wrist curls (page 132)

- Plate pinches

- Barbell iso-holds

- Hand gripper

To work the forearm extensors, in addition to the brachioradialis-targeting exercises I already mentioned, you can use

- Dumbbell wrist extension (page 133)

- Wrist roller

NECK

While forearm training is still quite popular, neck training is largely neglected. Most lifters assume their necks will grow just fine with heavy compound lifts. While that rings true for the forearms, research shows that the neck muscles get bigger and stronger in response to isolation exercises.

In a classic 1997 neck-training study, researchers found that significant hypertrophy of the neck muscles occurred only when an exercise targeting them directly was added to a workout that already included deadlifts, shrugs, and pulls from the mid-thigh.[10]

Isolation exercises for the neck offer benefits beyond hypertrophy. They also can reduce headaches and improve safety in contact sports. Here are some exercises I recommend:

- Plate-loaded neck curl (page 136)

- Plate-loaded neck extension (page 137)

- Head harness neck extension (page 138)

- Head harness neck curl

QUADS

The quadriceps, true to their name, have four distinct muscle heads. Three of them—vastus medialis, vastus lateralis, and vastus intermedius—are responsible for one thing: extending (straightening) the knee. A 2016 study suggests there may be a fourth knee extensor, the tensor vastus intermedius, which means the quads may actually be quints.[11] I only mention it because I'm amazed that, after hundreds of years of anatomical research, a muscle could go unnoticed until the second decade of the twenty-first century.

The fourth quadriceps muscle, the rectus femoris, performs two actions: It assists the other quad heads in extending the knee and also acts as a hip flexor—lifting your leg out to the front. Because it's a biarticular muscle, it warrants some special training considerations, which I'll discuss in a moment.

Before I get to isolation exercises for the quads, I want to emphasize that squat-type exercises harness most of their growth potential. Include one or two from the Big Six in each program and you're covered. You can see for yourself if you go to a powerlifting meet or watch Olympic weightlifting on TV. Look at the size of the competitors' quads. That's all from squats and other squat-type movements.

Even so, quad isolation sometimes makes sense for bodybuilders for two main reasons:

- Squat-type movements hit dozens of muscles in addition to the quads. The harder you train, the more recovery those muscles require. In the barbell back squat, for example, you get high activation in the glutes, adductors, and spinal erectors. The calves and hamstrings play important stabilizing roles. If you need additional work for your quads, you may not want to impose that much fatigue on all those other muscles.

- Because the rectus femoris head of the quads is biarticular, its muscle length doesn't change much throughout the squat. It lengthens at the hip as it simultaneously shortens at the knee; as such, it can't reach the high levels of tension that the other heads can.

That's where leg extensions (page 73) come in. Setting the seat back at a larger angle will take the hips out of flexion and allow that tricky rectus femoris head to get more involved. Usually, tilting the seat back by 20 to 45 degrees is enough to get the job done.

You may wonder about the safety of leg extensions. In my view, there's been a lot of unjustified fear mongering about injury risk. Recent research refutes the idea of leg extensions causing knee damage.[12] I'm not saying there's *no* risk. There's some risk with virtually any exercise you perform with enough intensity to drive new growth. I'll discuss this in more detail later in the chapter. For now, I'll just say this: If you experience knee pain while doing leg extensions, adjust the apparatus to see if you can find a more comfortable position. If that doesn't work, it may not be a good exercise for you.

The sissy squat is another option for emphasizing your quads. Unlike the traditional squat, where your knees and hips flex and extend, you maintain a fixed hip position throughout the sissy squat. All the movement occurs at the knee and ankle joints. It isn't technically an isolation exercise because more than one joint is involved. But when you try it, you'll find it hits your quads like nothing you've experienced before, and it targets the rectus femoris more effectively than other squat variations.

Reverse Nordics are another fun exercise I've been including more lately. These are a great option for people without access to a leg extension machine and actually get the quads into a deeper stretch than most leg extension machines will. Don't knock them until you try them!

HAMSTRINGS

The hamstrings include three muscles: the semimembranosus, semitendinosus, and biceps femoris. The biceps femoris is further subdivided into short and long heads, each of which has important training implications.

The hamstrings are yet another example of a biarticular muscle, with actions at both the knee and hip joints. You already know about the hamstrings' role in hip-hinge movements, where they work with the glutes to straighten the hips when they're bent forward. Exercises in the Big Six—deadlift variations, good mornings, back extensions—cover that function and work the hamstrings well.

But nothing in the Big Six addresses the other function: bending the knee. If you don't target knee flexion with an isolation exercise, you're missing an opportunity to fully develop the hammies. That's because one part of the hamstrings, the short head of the biceps femoris,

doesn't act on the hip joint, which means it isn't activated by hip-extension movements. At all. For this reason, the hamstrings are one of the few muscle groups where isolation is nearly mandatory.

The solution is easy enough, though: Do some kind of leg curl. Here are some variations I recommend:

- Seated leg curl (page 87)

- Lying leg curl (page 86)

- Glute-ham raise (page 88)

- Nordic ham curl (page 89)

Nordic ham curls and glute-ham raises are great options for those who don't have access to leg curl machines. Neither, however, is a pure isolation exercise. You perform both exercises with your hips straight, which requires an intense isometric contraction from your glutes and low back. They're also extremely challenging. Even advanced trainees will struggle with them.

Leg curls are a different story. They're accessible to lifters at all levels. If you have multiple options at your gym, the seated version may be the best choice. A 2021 study found that seated leg curls produced greater hypertrophy than lying leg curls after twelve weeks of training.[13] I don't consider a single study to be the final word, but if you're trying to decide which variation to start with, the study works well enough as a tiebreaker. Even so, it's a good idea to use different variations. I suspect the differences between these machines won't matter much in the long run.

GLUTES

The hips are ball-and-socket joints, like the shoulders. Also like the shoulders, the hips move in multiple directions and allow a massive range of functions. Many of them are powered primarily by the glutes.

You're already familiar with one of those functions, hip extension, which you perform in both hip-hinge and squat-type movements. The glutes also help lift the leg out to the side (hip abduction), rotate the leg outward (hip external rotation), kick the leg behind the body, and even rotate the pelvis (a move exercise scientists refer to as "twerking").

The glutes include three muscles: The gluteus maximus is the most famous and both the biggest and strongest of the glute muscles. The gluteus medius, a much smaller muscle, is positioned on the side of your hips, directly below your obliques. The even smaller gluteus minimus sits directly beneath the medius. These three muscles have fibers running in many different directions that can be targeted with different movement patterns.

Despite the muscles' complexity, the Big Six exercises are really all you *need* to develop your glutes, at least in your first few years of training. Simply including a squat-type movement and a hip-hinge movement (like a deadlift or good morning) is enough for most people to make some serious glute gains for years.

That said, the smaller gluteus medius and minimus muscles are better trained through hip abduction (moving your leg out to the side). So one priority in terms of glute isolation is including hip abduction movements, such as these:

- Machine hip abduction (page 81)

- Cable hip abduction (page 81)

At this point, you may be wondering why I haven't mentioned hip thrusts. In just a few years, they've gone from an exercise you never saw in a gym to one you see every day. They're especially popular among female lifters, for good reason.

The Big Six movements train your glutes primarily in the stretched position (at the bottom), with much less activation in the contracted position (at the top). Think about a barbell squat: How much work are your glutes doing when you're just standing there in the starting position? They certainly have a stabilizing role for your hips and lower back, which is important. You'd never want to relax your glutes completely when there's a heavy weight on your shoulders. But the real tension comes at the bottom of a squat and through the midrange of the lift. It tapers off after that.

The same is true for hip-hinge movements— high activation in the stretched position, low activation in the contracted position. That's not necessarily a bad thing. In fact, accumulating evidence suggests that loading muscles while they're highly stretched is great for muscle growth.[14]

Still, given the size and complexity of the glutes, it makes sense to include an exercise that overloads the contracted position. Plus, research has shown that the glutes fire hardest when you're at or near full hip extension.[15] These movements are all good choices:

- Hip thrust (page 79)

- Glute bridge

- Single-leg hip thrust

I don't want to overhype the importance of overloading the glutes in both stretched and contracted positions. I know athletes who've built incredible glutes without doing any hip thrusts or glute bridges. Many people, me included, find the setup tedious and time-consuming. That's why they've never been an integral part of my programming. In fact, as I write this, I'm realizing that I haven't done a hip thrust or a glute bridge in many months. I've gotten all the glute stimulus I need from Big Six exercises combined with some hip abduction. When I do feel like I need to add some glute-stabilization work, I add single-leg hip thrusts with light loads, which are easy to set up.

I say that knowing some people see a better payoff from hip thrusts or bridges than I do. You don't really know until you try them.

Finally, sometimes trainees require more glute volume than the Big 6, hip abductions, and hip thrusts can provide. In this case, further isolation can be beneficial, especially if you have big glutes goals and as you enter into the intermediate-advanced stage. In this case, you can add the following exercises to accumulate additional glute volume and stimulate the glutes via slightly different loading parameters:

• Glute kickbacks

• Lateral banded walks

CALVES

The calves are so notoriously hard to grow that some fitness leaders I know have made it a part of their branding strategy to actively promote their paltry calf development. COME ON. Growing the calves is not *that* complicated. You just can't expect them to grow as fast as other muscles, most of the time.

One reason could be a relatively low density of androgen receptors. These are the places where hormones like testosterone can bind to tissues and promote muscle growth. With

fewer receptors, you might expect the calves to be slightly more "stubborn" than other muscle groups.

There's also the challenge of genetics. You can't change your bone structure or where your calves insert on your lower leg. Some people have high-inserting calves that can make the lower leg appear smaller compared to people with low-inserting calves, even when there may not be any actual difference in muscle mass.

Figure 5.10

Comparing low calf insertions and high calf insertions

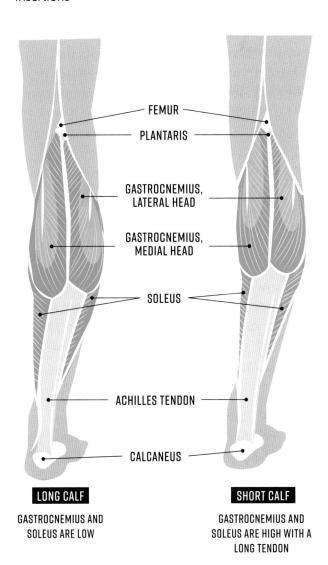

Regardless of your genetics, the only way to get bigger calves is to train them thoroughly and consistently. Let's start with some basic anatomy.

What we call the calves are technically known as the triceps surae muscle group (not to be confused with the triceps brachii of the upper arm) that is made up of two main muscles: the gastrocnemius (gastroc for short) and the soleus. Both of these muscles plantarflex the ankle (point the toes down) but the gastroc also flexes (bends) the knee.

Most compound lower-body exercises work the calves to some degree. Squats, for example, require a lot of movement in the ankle joint and the calves are largely responsible for creating that movement. Leg curls also activate the gastroc, which assists the hamstrings in curling the leg.

And, of course, everyday movements like walking and climbing stairs produce some degree of tension in the lower legs. But only those with truly blessed calf genetics can maximize their development without hitting them directly with isolation exercises. Here are the main isolation exercises I recommend:

- Standing calf raise (page 90)

- Leg press calf press

- Seated calf raise (page 91)

You perform the first two with your legs straight. They both hit every part of the calf. The seated calf raise, however, uses a bent knee, which slightly shifts the emphasis to the soleus, the flat muscle underneath the gastroc. The soleus, interestingly, has a higher ratio of slow-twitch type I muscle fibers than any other muscle in the human body. Type I fibers are more fatigue resistant than type II fibers, which produce strength and power in short bursts. It makes

sense that a calf muscle would be dominated by endurance-oriented fibers. That's why we can take thousands of steps a day and still recover in time to take thousands more the next day.

Most of us assume that a muscle with more type I fibers should be trained with higher reps. The evidence is conflicting, but I recommend doing seated calf raises with 10 to 20 reps per set rather than 6 to 12 reps for straight-leg calf raises.

ABS/CORE

For training purposes, I like to split the "core" into two categories of muscles. There is the "six-pack" itself, formally known as the rectus abdominis, and then there is all the stuff that surrounds the six-pack, mainly the transverse abdominis and obliques. Let's start with the six-pack.

A popular misconception among strength coaches is that heavy compound exercises like squats and deadlifts work the core muscles hard enough to render any direct ab work unnecessary. But EMG data shows the opposite: The rectus abdominis is actually barely active on squats and deadlifts, which makes sense when you consider the biomechanics of those lifts.[16]

When you do a squat or deadlift, you maintain a neutral spine—at least, it shouldn't bend much while you perform these lifts. However, the rectus abdominis's main purpose is to bend the spine forward, like you would do in a crunch exercise. These actions are opposites of one another. Therefore, to target the abs effectively, you should do exercises in which you bend your spine against some sort of load.

You can do that from two different directions. You can crunch your upper torso down toward your legs, and you can raise your legs up toward your torso. The first puts slightly more emphasis on the upper abs, whereas the second is more of a challenge for the lower abs. For proportional development, I recommend doing one of each.

These movements target the upper abs:

- Weighted cable crunch (page 139)

- Plate-loaded decline sit-up (page 140)

These movements put slightly more emphasis on the lower abs:

- Hanging leg raise (page 140)

- Reverse crunch

Two more points about core training:

Some early research suggested that repetitively flexing the spine is inherently risky. Although there's still some debate (and probably always will be), the older studies were well-intentioned but overcautious and not based on human models. Today, most experts recognize that these abdominal exercises are safe and effective as long as total load and volume are managed properly.

It's also worth noting that the appearance of the core muscles is largely determined by genetics and diet. Yes, the muscles will get bigger with resistance training, like any of the muscles we've discussed. But the shape of the muscles is whatever your genes say it's going to be. Some of us will have a photogenically symmetrical six-pack. Others will look more like an earthquake zone, with blocks of muscle on one side of your linea alba (the strip of connective tissue that runs down the middle) higher than the blocks on the other side. This asymmetry is entirely genetic and can't be modified with training. Similarly, some of us have what looks more like a four-pack, whereas others somehow end up with what looks like an eight-pack when they're completely shredded.

Genetics also affect where your abs are positioned on your abdomen. Some folks will have a visible six-pack when they're relatively lean but not close to shredded. I'm the opposite: My abs sit relatively deep in my midsection. They don't pop out much, even when my body fat is very low.

Now we come to diet. I like to say that abs are built in the gym and revealed in the kitchen. Unless and until you have sufficiently low body fat, you may not be able to see your abs, even if they're relatively well developed.

For men, the six-pack generally becomes blurry but visible at around 20 percent body fat and becomes sharp and defined at around 10 percent. For women, it becomes blurry but visible at around 28 percent and sharp and defined at around 18 percent.

The trick is to reach that low body-fat percentage while maintaining the muscle you worked so hard to build. That requires a sustained caloric deficit, one that's large enough to force your body to use fat for energy but not so large that you lose muscle along with the fat. You also need enough energy to continue training and enough protein to maintain muscle and recover from your workouts.

I'll cover nutrition in more detail in Chapter 14.

EXERCISE VARIATION

Research shows that muscles develop best when you train them with a variety of exercises, instead of using just one exercise for each muscle.

A well-known 2014 study from Fonseca and colleagues compared muscle growth in subjects doing one exercise for their quads (squats) to subjects doing the same amount of work spread across four exercises (squats, leg presses, lunges, and deadlifts).[17] After twelve weeks of training, the increase in quad size was similar in both groups. But the subjects who did four exercises had more proportional gains across all four heads of the quads, while their counterparts who did squats exclusively had significant hypertrophy in just two of the four heads.

It's reasonable to draw two inferences: First, total training volume is likely more important for overall muscle growth than exercise variety. Second, the exercises you do will determine exactly where the growth occurs. A variety of exercises should lead to more evenly distributed growth across all parts of the muscle you're training.

A follow-up study in 2021 showed similar results. This time, the researchers had their volunteers do a total-body program, instead of focusing on just one set of muscles.[18] One group did the exact same exercises every workout. The other did a different exercise for each muscle group on each training day. For example, the no-variety group did bench presses for their chest every workout, and the other group did bench press on Monday, incline bench press on Wednesday, and decline bench press on Friday. *Note:* The volume of work was the same for both groups, regardless of which exercises they used. Table 5.4 shows a more detailed look at the study's training protocol.

The program lasted nine weeks, which means the volunteers did twenty-seven total workouts. The researchers took before and after measurements for each participant at twelve muscular sites. Once again, overall muscle growth was similar in both groups, but only the group that did a variety of exercises showed significant growth at all twelve sites. The no-variety group had growth in ten of the twelve.

Table 5.4: No-Variety Versus Varied Programs from de Vasconcelos Costa et al. (2021)

	Monday	Wednesday	Friday
No variety group	Bench press	Bench press	Bench press
	Lat pulldown (front)	Lat pulldown (front)	Lat pulldown (front)
	Arm curl	Arm curl	Arm curl
	Triceps extension	Triceps extension	Triceps extension
	Leg press	Leg press	Leg press
	Lying leg curl	Lying leg curl	Lying leg curl
Variety group	Bench press	Incline bench press	Decline bench press
	Lat pulldown (front)	Lat pulldown (neck)	Lat pulldown (narrow grip)
	Arm curl	Preacher curl	Incline curl
	Triceps extension	Cable seated triceps extension	Cable triceps kickback
	Leg press	Half squat	Machine hack squat
	Lying leg curl	Seated leg curl	Seated single-leg curl

This suggests, once again, that the best way to achieve full and proportional development is by including a variety of exercises for each muscle group in your program. Different exercises activate different fibers in different muscle regions in different ways. The differences may be small, especially at first, but over time, the effects should be both visible and measurable.

However, as with most good things, too much variety can impede your progress in multiple ways. Remember the first rung of the Muscle Ladder: technique. Learning the basic movement patterns takes time and practice. If you're switching exercises up too much, you won't get enough consistent practice with each to master your form. Excessive variety also makes it more difficult to track progress. How do you know if you're getting stronger if you're constantly and haphazardly switching exercises?

(Yes, I know some people have branded it as "muscle confusion." Keep reading to see why it doesn't actually work the way its advocates suggest.)

There is, of course, a sweet spot for exercise variation. In the 2021 study I just described, the training program had lots of variety from day to day, but the participants did the same exercises from week to week. That kind of consistency from week to week allows you to measure your progress on each individual exercise. If there had been a third group that randomly switched exercises from week to week, I suspect their gains would have been significantly worse. Controlled and consistent variety is good. Haphazard variety isn't.

To summarize this section: Pick a handful of exercises that fit your goals and stick to them for a while. Get better at those movements and watch your strength improve over time. There's no reason to change exercises if you're still making progress, especially if you're a new lifter. After a few months, when your progress slows or you feel like your workouts are getting stale, swap out a few of the stale exercises to keep your training novel and interesting. But don't swap out all of them. I'll show you a precise method for rotating exercises later in the book.

FREE WEIGHTS VERSUS MACHINES

Debates about the value of free weights versus machines have gone on for decades.

Free weights, of course, are "free" in the sense that they're not attached to any other piece of equipment. That includes dumbbells, barbells, kettlebells, and that big stone in the corner of your gym. Resistance comes from both the load and gravity.

Machines create resistance in a number of ways. The most common are selectorized machines, where you choose how much you want to lift by inserting a pin into a weight stack. Most of the machine exercises I've mentioned in this chapter, from lat pulldowns to pec deck flies, are performed on this type of machine, with resistance provided by a combination of weight plates and pulleys or levers. Others use bands or pneumatic pressure to create resistance. And on some, like the leg press and Smith machine, you load them with the same plates you'd put on a barbell.

The most commonly noted difference is that free weights allow unrestricted movement, whereas many machines lock you into a specific trajectory. For example, you can do almost anything with a dumbbell: curl it, press it, pull it, squat while holding it, and more. But, a leg extension machine is meant to do one thing: leg extensions.

Within some circles, there's no question that free weights are superior for developing strength and muscle mass. And if your goal is to be a competitive strength athlete, they're mostly right. There's no Olympic medal for the leg press or pec deck. But if your goal is to build your best physique, you won't find much evidence that one is better than the other.

For example, two papers published in 2020 compared free weights to machines.[19] Both studies showed similar increases in muscle mass. That doesn't mean there are no differences between the two. Each has its pros and cons, which you need to keep in mind when creating a training program. Tables 5.5 and 5.6 highlight these differences.

Table 5.5: Free-Weight Exercises

Pros	Cons
You activate more muscle mass. Free-weight exercises typically require more balance and coordination, which means higher activation of smaller stabilizing muscles.	**Technique can be harder to learn.** The learning curve can be discouraging for some new lifters, especially those who work out at home or who don't have access to a qualified coach at their gym.
They offer more versatility. Dumbbells give you nearly countless options for every movement pattern and muscle group.	**The setup is more time-consuming.** To get set up for barbell exercises, you need a bar, plates, collars, and a bench, power rack, or floor space.
Equipment is less expensive. You can equip a home gym with a barbell and dumbbells for less money than you might pay in membership fees at a higher-end health club.	**You need more time to warm up.** At home or in a gym, you need to invest more time and effort in getting your body ready for heavy compound exercises. That means either longer workouts or less time for accessory movements.
They're more accessible. No matter where you work out, a 40-pound dumbbell is a 40-pound dumbbell. But 40 pounds on a machine in one gym might feel heavier or lighter than 40 pounds on a similar machine in a different gym.	**The resistance curve isn't always ideal.** Many free-weight exercises don't offer continuous resistance throughout the range of motion. For example, a standing dumbbell curl provides zero tension on the biceps when they are stretched (at the bottom) and maximum tension when the elbow is at 90 degrees. Many machines and cables, by contrast, offer continuous resistance.

Table 5.6: Machine-Based Exercises

Pros	Cons
Technique can be easier to learn. Because there's less of a learning curve, machines can be less intimidating to new lifters.	**You may activate smaller stabilizing muscles less.** Machines with a fixed movement path require less balance and coordination, which means there's often less activation of stabilizers.
Setup is easy and fast. Machines are usually ready to go—adjust the seat, select a weight, and start lifting.	**Some machines can be confusing to figure out.** Some newer machines require multiple adjustments and have several moving parts. Even experienced lifters can struggle to set up the machine.
It takes less time to warm up. Because machines require less stability and coordination, you can lift safely with just one or two warm-up sets.	**Machines are less predictable.** Forty pounds on one machine might feel very different from 40 pounds on another machine, even though both machines are designed for the same exercise. Even the same machine might be calibrated differently in different gyms.
Some machines offer better muscle isolation. The upside of activating fewer stabilizers is more direct work for the targeted muscles.	**You can't always find your favorite machines.** Because commercial-grade machines are expensive, gyms have to choose the ones that fit their budget as well as their space. If you have to change gyms, you may not find one with the machines you liked at your last gym.
The resistance curve is often superior. Many machines offer more continuous resistance through the full range of motion.	**Machines are less versatile.** Most machines have one function: one exercise, one movement path. You can't always progress to a more challenging variation of the same exercise or movement pattern. (Cable machines are a notable exception in that they can be used to do a wide range of effective exercises.)

As you can see, free weights and machines are equally viable options in a well-designed training program. In my own bodybuilding programs, I generally use a 50-50 mix of free-weight and machine exercises. The exact ratio depends on the situation. When there's a clear advantage to using one over the other, that's what I'll choose.

Sometimes there really isn't a choice. If you work out at home, for example, you're most likely not going to fill your limited space with a bunch of machines. You'll probably choose equipment that gives you the most options. You can hit all the primary movement patterns with a barbell, bench, power rack, and set of dumbbells. I'd also want an adjustable cable machine in my home gym. It doesn't take up a lot of space and gives you a ton of options.

Conversely, if you have access to a commercial gym but limited time to train, you might want to use machines instead of free weights. That way you gain efficiency without sacrificing results.

EXERCISES TO AVOID

Just about any exercise can be a bad idea for some lifters in some situations. Some may actually be a bad idea for most people most of the time.

I'll use one of my least favorite modalities as an example: unstable-surface training. Maybe exercises on a stability ball or foam pad makes sense for competitive athletes where balance is important for their sport or in certain rehab contexts. But when your goal is to build muscle, it doesn't make sense to use an unstable surface over standing, sitting, or lying on something solid. When your body is unstable, you reduce tension on the targeted muscles without gaining any benefits in return.

The most obvious exercises to avoid are those that cause pain or discomfort. Behind-the-neck presses and behind-the-neck pulldowns, for example, cause shoulder pain in some lifters without offering any obvious advantage over the conventional versions of those exercises. I think they're worth skipping for most lifters.

A lot depends on the individual. The most productive exercise for one lifter might cause shoulder, back, or knee pain in another. The depth and orientation of your hip sockets can affect your range of motion on squat-type movements. The shape of your shoulder bones can impact which pressing exercises feel the best for you.

But your individual response to an exercise might be clouded by something called the nocebo effect. It's the inverse of the placebo effect, which you're probably familiar with. The classic example is when you feel relief from a headache, even though the pill you took was a placebo, with no active ingredients. The headache stops simply because you expect it to.

In a training context, you might experience a placebo effect from a supplement that purports to increase strength or give you more energy. You get those benefits because you believe you'll get them.

The nocebo effect, on the other hand, can create unwarranted fear of exercises that typically work well. Consider upright rows. In my experience, they are very effective for building the traps and side delts when performed correctly, as shown here:

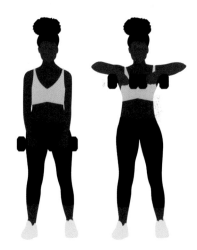

However, upright rows are a popular choice on lists of exercises you should avoid. If you feel discomfort while doing them, is it because they actually caused that discomfort or because you expected them to? Did you wince during leg extensions because you anticipated pain, or because your knees really aren't comfortable with the movement? And was the pain or discomfort unusual, or was it something you'd barely notice when doing exercises that aren't routinely vilified?

For this reason, I am wary of using pain as a reliable criterion for guiding exercise selection. Still, the reality is that some movements do give certain people issues more than others, and if there is a substitute that provides you the same benefits with a higher level of comfort, I see no reason not to go with the more comfortable variation.

You may also wonder if you should continue with exercises you just don't "feel." To be sure, some of the most effective movements don't lend themselves to a strong mind-muscle connection. Squats are a good example. You won't feel your quads working the way you do on leg extensions, but that doesn't mean you aren't working those muscles. You definitely are!

Your feel for an exercise matters most when you get beyond the Big Six. If you're deciding between two comparable exercises, the one that feels better to you is almost always the better choice. My gym, for example, has a Hammer Strength chest press machine that absolutely lights my pecs up. I can feel my chest working from the start of the first rep to the completion of the last one. But when I do the same basic movement on the Smith machine, I just don't feel my pecs working as well. My decision of which machine to use is easy.

Staying outside the Big Six, I generally recommend avoiding exercises you don't enjoy. For me, it's the barbell hip thrust. The time needed to set everything up, the pain of the barbell on my hips (even when I use a pad or reposition the barbell), and the general lack of mind-muscle connection led me to conclude it isn't a great exercise for me. The decision to axe the barbell hip thrust from my program was made even easier by having so many good alternatives. (The dumbbell single-leg hip thrust is one I particularly like.)

But even within the Big Six, there are no "must-do" exercises for hypertrophy. With so many options in each category, you should be able to find exercises you enjoy—or at least don't hate.

"Don't do exercises you hate" sums up this section pretty well. It covers exercises that don't suit your goals or cause discomfort. It could apply to exercises you can't get a feel for. And it certainly includes exercises you actively dislike. Separately and together, they make training untenable in the long term. (Refer to Chapters 2 and 3 for more information about sustainability and mindset.)

OPTIMIZING EXERCISES

Beyond the general guideline of picking from the Big Six movements and filling in the gaps with ancillary exercises, there are a few other exercise selection principles I use to guide more experienced trainees toward optimal gains. As you gain lifting experience, you'll soon realize that certain exercises seem to work better for you than others. That's usually because they tick the following three boxes:

- High tension

- Feels good

- Simple to overload

If an exercise ticks all three boxes, it's most likely an optimal exercise for you. Let me briefly explain what they each mean.

High-tension exercises force your muscles to work hard against resistance. This means that you should feel like your muscles are stretching and pulling *against something*. For example, a stability ball squat will severely limit tension on your quads because the lack of stability disperses tension across the body. As such, a hack squat would be a much more optimal choice for quad growth.

An exercise feels good if it doesn't cause you pain and it has a smooth resistance profile. Giving you a good pump and a strong mind-muscle connection wouldn't hurt either. For example, I find my shoulders get a bit cranky if I do weighted dips too often. I also don't feel them in my pecs all that well, regardless of how I modify the technique. I still think they're an amazing chest builder for a majority of lifters, but, based on my experience, they're probably

not optimal for me. I find I can get a similar stretch with a dumbbell chest press, and I can adjust my elbow path so it feels good on my shoulders. So even though I still include both periodically, the dumbbells do a better job at ticking the "feels good" box, and I tend to go for it more often these days.

An exercise is simple to overload if you can easily add weight or reps from week to week. This is crucial for ensuring continued progress over time. For example, as you gain strength, a goblet squat becomes difficult to overload because the dumbbells simply don't go heavy enough. A 100-pound squat would be considered beginner-level strength for most lifters. Yet most gyms' dumbbell racks stop at 100 pounds. So with the goblet squat, you'll end up being limited by how much weight you can hold in your hands rather than how much load your quads can actually handle. A barbell squat or leg press would be a more optimal option as you gain experience because you can repeatedly add a little weight or an extra rep.

EXERCISE ORDER AND WEAK POINT PRIORITIZATION

How you organize exercises within a training session makes a difference. Research shows enhanced performance in exercises you do earlier in a workout, when you're fresh and fully energized.[20]

That's why, most of the time, you should begin your sessions with compound exercises—those that require the most effort and work the most muscle mass. Placing these more complex movements near the beginning of a workout, when you are less fatigued, allows them to be completed with more focus and overload. Also, since many lifters measure strength gains on these compound movements, performing isolation exercises that target smaller muscles first can muddy progress.

Additionally, if you're trying to emphasize a weak muscle or lagging body part, you should target it earlier in your session. For example, if your chest is a weak point and you have a goal of increasing your bench press, it makes obvious sense to place your bench press first in your workout. However, if you train chest and triceps on the same day and your triceps are a weak point, you should still hit bench press first and then move on to your triceps isolation work. You can emphasize triceps on the bench press by taking a closer grip, but in most instances, you should perform compound exercises first.

It's also worth mentioning that the effect of exercise order isn't so huge that exercises can't be shuffled around within reason. For example, lately I've been kicking off my leg days with hamstring curls before hitting my squat-type exercise for the day. I find the hamstring curls get my knees nice and warmed up for the heavy squats to follow without significantly reducing my strength performance. So, while there are exceptions, putting your compounds earlier rather than later in the session is a good rule of thumb.

It's also inevitable that muscles on one side of your body will be a little bigger or stronger than the other, especially when first starting out. We all have asymmetries that, although not inherently bad for health or performance, you may want to correct for aesthetic purposes. In this case, the best solution is to simply prioritize the weak point by hitting it first. For example, my right biceps is smaller than my left biceps. To help even them out, I'll simply start with my right side when doing single-arm biceps curls. I'll push my weaker arm hard and then match the reps with my stronger arm. This way, my weaker side will set the pace and get a slightly better growth stimulus. This can help even things out over time.

You can also organize your training split so you hit your weak points after a rest day. By giving those muscles more time to recover, you ensure they're primed for maximum performance. I'll revisit this in Chapters 9 and 13 when I talk about training splits and periodization, respectively. For now, in the next chapter, let's get into how hard you should train to build muscle and gain strength.

CHAPTER 6

EFFORT

AM I TRAINING HARD ENOUGH?

No matter how much you optimize all the other variables, what you do won't matter if you don't push yourself hard enough. You need effort to maximize the benefits of technique and exercise selection, the first two rungs on the Muscle Ladder. And effort determines how much you get out of the next seven rungs.

Here's what I mean: The next time you're in the gym, look around at your fellow lifters. How many of them do you think are training hard enough to build muscle?

In 2017, a research team in Brazil conducted an ingenious experiment to assess the training effort of typical gym-goers.[1] They recruited 160 healthy men with at least six months of weight-training experience and gave them a simple task: Select a weight they would normally use on the bench press for a set of 10. But instead of stopping at 10 reps, do as many as possible.

Try to guess how many reps participants managed to get on average. Eleven? That would mean they were leaving one rep in the tank. Twelve? Fourteen?

Nope.

Participants got a staggering 16 reps with their usual 10-rep weight on average. And it gets worse: Zero percent of them (not a single one of the 160 subjects) got fewer than 10 reps. In a group of 160 lifters, none overestimated their abilities.

You can see the full breakdown in Table 6.1. What I found most astounding was that 26 percent of the participants got at least 19 reps. That suggests they would leave half their potential reps in the tank on a typical set in a typical workout.

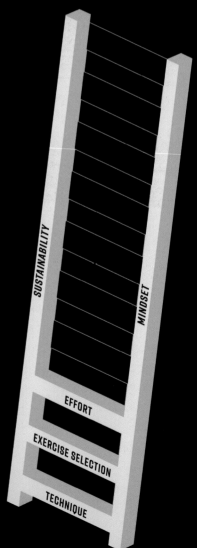

Table 6.1: Distribution of Reps Achieved by Participants from Barbosa-Netto et al. (2017)

Number of Reps Achieved with Typical 10-Rep Weight	Percent of Participants
<10 reps	0%
10 to 12 reps	22%
13 to 15 reps	31%
16 to 18 reps	21%
19 and up	26%

I wish I could say this study was an outlier, but it's not. Most lifters—newbies and experienced trainees alike—stop sets long before they've pushed themselves hard enough to force their muscles to adapt. Put another way, most lifters *under*train. In my view, this is the single most important reason why so many lifters stop making progress after their first year or two in the weight room and why so few reach their true muscular potential.

WHAT MAKES MUSCLES GROW?

To understand why it's so important to train hard, it helps to understand something far more fundamental: what makes muscle tissue grow in the first place.

For a long time, we thought growth was primarily driven by muscle damage. Resistance training creates small tears within muscle fibers. Those fibers then get bigger and stronger during post-training recovery, as long as you give them enough time and provide the right nutrients. This is the "no pain, no gain" theory of bodybuilding, and many people still think it accurately describes how muscles grow.

Research, however, tells a different story.[2] We now know there isn't a strong link between muscle *damage* and muscle *growth*. On the contrary, excessive damage can *impede* growth because the body prioritizes tissue repair. That leaves fewer resources for tissue growth.

Figure 6.1 shows how this works during a theoretical training program.

Figure 6.1
Repair-oriented versus hypertrophy-oriented training[3]

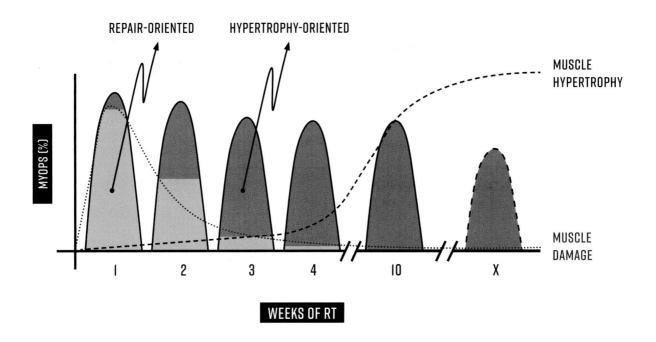

As you can see, the first few workouts create a lot of muscle damage. That's because you're doing things your muscles aren't prepared for—new exercises, heavier loads, higher volume, and so on. Repairing that damage is an obvious priority. But as your muscles grow accustomed to the new challenges, the workouts create less damage, and your body can direct its resources to muscle growth.

Here's another myth many bodybuilders believe: You need a skin-tearing pump to make your muscles grow. Contrary to the "no pain, no gain" theory, a pump is something you can see. Your muscles get bigger as they fill with blood. Who doesn't love being swole? And even if the swelling is temporary, why wouldn't the metabolic disruption caused by that surge of nutrient-rich blood be the thing driving new muscle growth?

Alas, the latest evidence tells us it doesn't quite work that way either.[4] The metabolic stress from a pump most likely plays a minor role in hypertrophy. I don't knock the idea of chasing pumps. I enjoy them as much as anyone. But I also realize they aren't the main thing driving muscle growth.

So what is most important? Mechanical tension. Almost all muscle growth results from your muscles straining against resistance.

Think of your biceps. The muscle originates on the inside of your shoulder blade and ends on one of your forearm bones just below the elbow. The role of the biceps, as you know, is to bend the elbow. When you do that with a dumbbell in your hand, the biceps pulls and stretches. Molecules within the muscle called mechanosensors respond to that tension by triggering a complex set of neural and hormonal signals, resulting in new muscle tissue (see Figure 6.2).[5]

The details don't really matter (assuming your career doesn't require you to understand them). What does matter is that you need to train hard to get the process started.

Figure 6.2

Neural and hormonal signals that trigger muscle growth

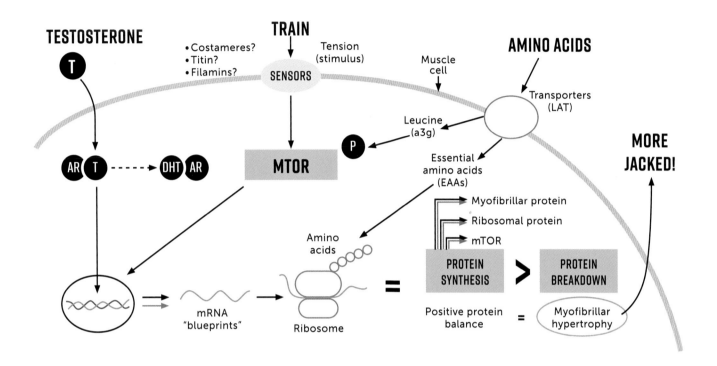

Let's return to our favorite muscle. Imagine you're doing biceps curls. You pick a light weight that you could probably curl for 20 reps if you *really* had to. But let's say you take that same light weight and do only 10 reps instead of an all-out 20. At around rep 6, you start to feel the blood pooling in the muscle. At rep 8, you start to feel a mild burning sensation. At rep 10, your arms are starting to feel uncomfortable, so you terminate the set and put the weight down. This is a common way to train, but unfortunately, it does almost nothing for muscle growth. That's because, despite the pump and the mild burn, not enough muscle fibers are being challenged to reach high levels of *tension.*

On the other hand, imagine that you curl the same dumbbell, but instead of stopping at rep 10, you keep pushing. You go beyond the pump and the burning sensation until you get to the point where you physically cannot complete

another rep. (Sometimes trainers come up with psychotic examples to encourage this level of effort, such as, "Do as many reps as you can and if you stop short, you die.") In this case, your biceps must activate all (or nearly all) of its individual muscle fibers to keep the weight moving. This time, you get all the way to rep 20. You go for rep 21 but fail to complete a full range of motion. By doing so, you elicit a very high level of tension in the muscle. This is building muscle.

Before I go on, I want to clarify that this "do-or-die" style of lifting isn't how I suggest you train—at least not all of the time. It definitely isn't the way I train on every set.

I just described an example of taking a set to absolute muscular failure. A cross-section of bodybuilders believe their muscles will never reach their maximum potential without that level of effort, but it's by no means unanimous within bodybuilding circles. Nor is it a mainstream view among exercise scientists and high-level practitioners.

Most coaches who follow the science recognize the need to push sets *close* to muscular failure to maximize your gains, but very few say you need to go all the way there. It's fine for the more sadomasochistic bodybuilders. It's just not something I encourage you to do.

But what is the difference between reaching failure and just getting close to it? It's time to be a little more precise.

HOW DO YOU DEFINE "FAILURE"?

According to researchers James Fisher and James Steele, muscular failure occurs when, "despite attempting to do so, they cannot complete the concentric portion of their current repetition without significant deviation from the prescribed form of the exercise."[6]

Put simply, you don't stop when it gets uncomfortably difficult. You keep going until your muscles cannot produce enough force to complete another rep without bizarre, acrobatic contortions (aka "cheating").

Some coaches disagree about how much cheating is allowed when getting to failure. Are you allowed to use some swinging at the hips to curl the weight up—even just a little? Or do you count failure at the first sign of shifting posture? These disputes have led coaches to come up with two categories of failure:

- *Absolute failure* is when you just can't move the weight, even if you change your form or get other muscles involved. To return to the set of biceps curls from the previous example, let's say your strength is nearly depleted after rep 16. So, to complete rep 17, you generate some momentum by bending and straightening your knees. You do that on rep 18, but now you also rise on your toes. You start rep 19 with a hip swing. And to complete the twentieth and final rep, you start with a hip swing but finish with a back bend that looks like you're doing the limbo at a wedding reception.

- *Technical failure* is what I described for rep 16: You can't do another rep *with good form*. You've gone beyond that point when you have to cheat to complete a repetition.

To be clear, it's quite hard to reach technical failure. Most recreational lifters, most of the time, don't get there. But it's important to get there at least sometimes, so you know what it feels like. It gives you a dependable metric to track over time. If you can get two extra reps before hitting technical failure on a given exercise with a given weight, you've gotten stronger. But if you have to cheat to get those reps, you probably haven't.

I should note that I'm not on board with a super-strict definition of technical failure. Small changes in form are acceptable and inevitable, especially on free weight exercises. Humans aren't robots. Even experienced lifters deviate from textbook form as fatigue sets in. The more experienced you are, the more you understand which deviations are acceptable in pursuit of muscle activation and which give you a false sense of progress.

As the researchers phrased it, the key is to stop before you commit a "significant deviation" from proper technique. If you stop when you detect the *slightest* change in form, you risk terminating the set before the target muscles have reached the level of fatigue required to stimulate new growth.

Keep in mind that technique comes before effort on the Muscle Ladder. Most of the time, you should prioritize good form. The less experience you have in the weight room, the more you need to focus on both learning and practicing proper technique. Don't deviate until you understand what you're deviating from.

As you gain confidence in your ability to do the exercises correctly, you'll notice times when form and effort are at odds with each other. That's when you can experiment with the outer edges of proper technique. Look for small adjustments that allow one or two or three more high-quality reps, but don't go so far that you set off the lunk alarm.

Another key point: Technical failure can look different on machines versus free-weight exercises. Because your body is usually locked into position on a machine, it's easier to maintain consistent form all the way to muscular failure.

Some researchers have investigated failure in terms of rep speed rather than small shifts in technique. It's an interesting idea because we've all experienced it. The more fatigue you feel, the slower the reps become. It's what we mean when we talk about "grinding" out those last few reps when it feels like some crazy physicist has found a way to increase the force of gravity.

One study found that rep speed slowed down by 30 percent halfway through sets of bench presses.[7] When the participants reached their last possible rep, the weight moved about 80 percent slower.

Some coaches, especially in powerlifting circles, now use high-tech rep-speed trackers to measure changes throughout a set. That gives the coach an objective way to measure how close a lifter is to failure and use that data to decide how hard they should push for the rest of the workout.

I highlight this research not because I think anyone reading *The Muscle Ladder* needs to time their reps. I just want you to be aware that your lifting velocity will decline as your muscles fatigue. If your reps aren't getting slower, you're most likely not close to failure, no matter how you define it.

SO HOW HARD SHOULD YOU PUSH IT, EXACTLY?

Some bodybuilders, as I mentioned, insist that taking every set to failure is crucial to their success. They use phrases like "the muscle only knows failure," implying that the only good set is an all-out set. It doesn't take much digging to see it isn't true. It's been debunked in both research and practice.

In research, a 2021 review showed that lifters can achieve statistically similar increases in muscle size regardless of whether they train to failure or merely close to failure.[8] A litany of other studies shows the same thing.[9] You need to train hard. You need to be close to failure. But reaching failure isn't always necessary.

The best study I've seen illustrating this was conducted in 2024 by a team of researchers in Australia.[10] They had eighteen resistance-trained subjects train one leg to failure, while the other leg did the same number of sets but left one or two reps in the tank. So one leg was going to failure, the other leg was stopping one or two reps shy. Everything else in the study was kept as controlled as possible, so the only difference was failure versus not failure. What did they find after eight weeks of training? No difference. This, combined with other studies showing similar results strongly suggest that leaving one or two reps in the tank is most likely equally effective as training all the way to failure for muscle growth.

As for practice, I recently analyzed the training footage of some of the most successful bodybuilders across several decades. It's quite clear that many of the best all-time bodybuilders often didn't push sets all the way to failure. There are a few notable exceptions, including six-time Mr. Olympia Dorian Yates, who was notorious for consistently pushing himself to gut-wrenching failure (and beyond). But in my detailed digging, it became clear that the best bodybuilders in the world were able to build mounds of muscle with both failure and nonfailure approaches to training.

Nearly without exception, folks who advocate for pushing all sets to failure also endorse shorter workouts with fewer total sets. They recognize that you can't have it both ways. If you're going to push each set as hard as possible, you simply can't do as many sets. And if you're going to push each set less hard, you need to do more sets to compensate. I believe this is the correct way to think about it.

Let's return to the research for a moment:

A 2017 study by Morán-Navarro and colleagues showed that pushing sets to failure causes more fatigue, which seems obvious if you've ever done it.[11] Less obvious are the consequences of training to that level of fatigue. In this study, the researchers looked at creatine kinase, an enzyme often used as a proxy for muscle damage. Creatine kinase levels were significantly above baseline in the failure group forty-eight hours post-exercise, which wasn't the case in the nonfailure group.

A workout that causes so much fatigue and muscle damage will be much harder to recover from. That's true in any athletic endeavor, whether training or competing. Every body has a tolerance threshold, beyond which it begins to break down.

Bodybuilding is no different. If your program is based on failure training, you have to give your muscles more time to recover between workouts, which means less total work. That might be the optimal approach for someone with limited time to train. Pushing every set to failure means shorter, more efficient workouts. You're getting the best possible results per unit of time.

But is the most *efficient* training system also the most *effective* way to maximize muscle growth? I doubt it.

We have piles of research showing a clear relationship between volume—the total number of sets you do for any given muscle group—and hypertrophy. I'll explain this in more detail in the next chapter. For now, I'll just note that, on average, more volume leads to more muscle growth, at least up to a point.

The data in Figure 6.3 is taken from a meta-analysis led by James Krieger.[12] As you can see, eleven of the fifteen studies included in the study favored higher volumes, as does the average overall effect. I think this result is intuitive for most lifters. If you do more work, you'll build bigger muscles. (I'll discuss the point of diminishing returns in the next chapter.)

Figure 6.3

Studies investigating the effect of volume on muscle growth

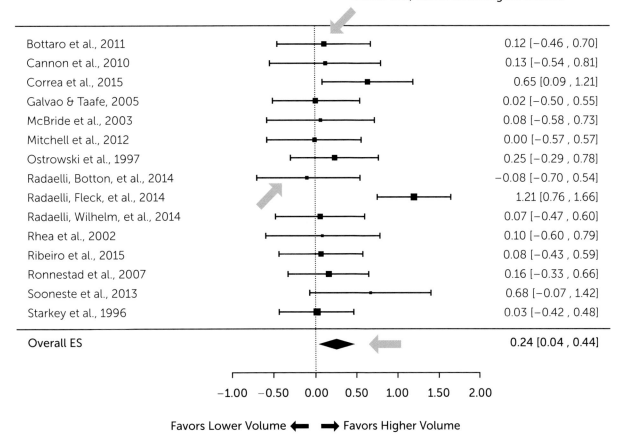

11 of the 15 studies are clearly to the right of the center line, which favors higher volume

Bottaro et al., 2011	0.12 [−0.46 , 0.70]
Cannon et al., 2010	0.13 [−0.54 , 0.81]
Correa et al., 2015	0.65 [0.09 , 1.21]
Galvao & Taafe, 2005	0.02 [−0.50 , 0.55]
McBride et al., 2003	0.08 [−0.58 , 0.73]
Mitchell et al., 2012	0.00 [−0.57 , 0.57]
Ostrowski et al., 1997	0.25 [−0.29 , 0.78]
Radaelli, Botton, et al., 2014	−0.08 [−0.70 , 0.54]
Radaelli, Fleck, et al., 2014	1.21 [0.76 , 1.66]
Radaelli, Wilhelm, et al., 2014	0.07 [−0.47 , 0.60]
Rhea et al., 2002	0.10 [−0.60 , 0.79]
Ribeiro et al., 2015	0.08 [−0.43 , 0.59]
Ronnestad et al., 2007	0.16 [−0.33 , 0.66]
Sooneste et al., 2013	0.68 [−0.07 , 1.42]
Starkey et al., 1996	0.03 [−0.42 , 0.48]
Overall ES	0.24 [0.04 , 0.44]

−1.00 −0.50 0.00 0.50 1.00 1.50 2.00

Favors Lower Volume ⬅ ➡ Favors Higher Volume

Now, if you can get a similar hypertrophic stimulus without training to failure, and you can do a higher volume of training by not training to failure, and higher volume gives you a greater hypertrophic stimulus, doesn't that seem like an obvious argument for not taking every set of every workout to failure?

Let's be clear about what I'm *not* saying: I'm not saying you should *never* take a set to failure.

To the contrary, I think research tells us we need to train *close* to failure to maximize the hypertrophic response. You can't know when you're close to failure unless you sometimes push a set as hard as you can.

To do that, you need an accurate way to plan for and manage your proximity to failure.

RIR AND RPE

Managing your proximity to failure allows you to accomplish your three key objectives:

- You provide enough tension to your muscles to stimulate growth.

- You perform a sufficient volume of training to maximize hypertrophy.

- You do both of those things without compromising recovery.

There are two pretty good ways to do it: RIR and RPE.

REPS IN RESERVE (RIR)

Imagine doing a set of biceps curls with a mob boss standing next to you. When you think you've finished the set, he pulls out his pistol, points it at your head, and says, "One more rep." You do the rep, and he says it again. And again. And again. Finally, with your life literally on the line, you just can't crank out another one.

Rest in peace, and may your memory be a blessing.

Had you lived, you would know what it feels like to hit zero reps in reserve with that specific weight on that specific exercise. If the last rep you performed was the fourteenth, you had one rep in reserve (RIR) at rep 13, two RIR at rep 12, and so on. Before the gangster intervened, you were going to stop the set after 10 reps, when you had four RIR.

How many reps you can leave in the tank and still optimize muscle growth isn't perfectly clear. Is it zero to three RIR? Zero to four? Zero to five? I doubt if it's even possible to answer the question definitively. There are simply too many variables to consider: what exercise you're doing, how heavy the weight is, how explosively you're moving the weight, how many sets and reps you're going to do, and so on.

For our purposes, I'm going with zero to three RIR as the "anabolic sweet spot" where most of your training should occur. If you regularly leave more than three reps in the tank, you probably aren't generating enough tension in the muscle to maximize the hypertrophic response.

Some of you reading this may think that standard is too lenient and that I'm encouraging some cautious lifters to stop their sets too soon and they'll end up with mediocre results. I doubt that for two reasons. First, for some lifters, three RIR may be closer to failure than they would typically train. Second, it's not at all clear that three RIR isn't hard enough to maximize gains. At least one study showed that training with five to ten RIR gained as much muscle as training within a few reps shy of failure![13]

I'm not recommending five to ten RIR. Zero to three RIR, like I said, should produce enough tension to work well for most lifters in most circumstances. If you feel you aren't working hard unless you finish your sets with zero to two RIR, great. You're within the range I recommend. If you don't like training that close to failure, you're fine with two to three RIR. You're also ahead of the majority of your fellow gym-goers. (Remember the 2017 Barbosa-Netto study I mentioned earlier, in which just 41 percent of participants trained at zero to four RIR.[14] And 23 percent stopped their sets with 10 or more reps in the tank.)

As a final note, I want to highlight that throughout this section, I've been using terms like "optimize" and "maximize" hypertrophy. This distinction is extremely important. Even if you are training further from failure, let's say four to six RIR, there is still evidence to support that you will make *some* gains, just not *optimal* gains. However, just like with where the cutoff is for optimal gains, it's still not quite clear how far from failure you can train and still see some gains. For beginners, my guess would be six to eight RIR; for more experienced lifters, I think this would likely be closer to four to six RIR.

RATING OF PERCEIVED EXERTION (RPE)

RPE was originally developed in the 1970s as a way for endurance athletes to gauge how hard they were training. The 6 to 20 RPE scale was based on percentages of the athlete's maximum heart rate. So someone doing extremely light cardio, with their heart rate at 60 beats per minute (bpm), might be at RPE 6—the bottom of the scale. If they started moving faster and their heart reached 120 bpm, they might be at RPE 12.

Lifters picked up on RPE in the early 2000s. But because the heart-rate-calibrated 6 to 20 scale didn't make much sense for resistance training, researchers used a modified scale that goes from 1 to 10. One means no effort at all and 10 is the equivalent of that gangster's gun to your head.

I like to use an RIR-based RPE, which you can see in Table 6.2.

Table 6.2: Interpreting the RPE Scale[15]

RPE Score	RIR/Description
10	Maximal effort
9.5	No RIR but could increase load
9	1RIR
8.5	Definitely 1, maybe 2RIR
8	2RIR
7.5	Definitely 2, maybe 3RIR
7	3RIR
5 to 6	4 to 6RIR
3 to 4	Light effort
1 to 2	Little to no effort

The system is about as simple as it gets. An RPE of 10 means gun-to-the-head, no-freakin'-way, zero RIR. RPE 9 means one RIR, and so on. The final meaningful RPE is 5, which suggests five in the tank. That's fine for a warm-up, but probably not where you want to be for most of your actual training sets. At least not if your goal is to maximize muscle gain. Once you get to the bottom of the RPE scale, you may as well be using Grandma's neoprene-covered "hand weights."

It's easy to figure out what RPE 10 feels like. Just push until you can't do another rep. But to stop at a specific point below your max effort? How do you know what an RPE of 8 or 9 feels like, and how do you tell the difference between them?

For that, you *really* need to know your own body, which only comes with experience. Discipline also helps.

A common critique of RPE is that it's too subjective and therefore not accurate enough to be useful. RPE is certainly subjective—you're estimating how many reps you *feel like* you have left. But that doesn't mean it can't be accurate or

useful. It's a tool that, like any other, works better with practice.

The following strategies can help you fine-tune your accuracy in estimating RPE:

- **Get more experience with lifting.** Serious lifting, over time, teaches you what hard work feels like. If you focus on how your body performs with different degrees of exertion and levels of fatigue, you'll develop an intuitive sense of how close you are to failure.

- **Become "comfortable" with what failure feels like.** Failure is an uncomfortable sensation, so many lifters shy away from it. But you won't know what RPE 10 feels like until you get there. And if you never get to 10, you can't possibly estimate what it feels like to reach RPE 9 or 8 or 7.

There are several practical ways to implement failure training. You might take the final set of one or two exercises per workout all the way to zero RIR. After a couple of weeks, take those sets to RPE 9 (one RIR). Or you can run a short training block (two to four weeks should be plenty) where you do fewer sets of each exercise, but take every set to failure.

- **Use anchoring sets.** This tactic works well with either of the previous suggestions. When you plan to take a set all the way to failure, use the final reps to guess how close you are to that point. For example, call out when you think you're at an RPE of 8 but then keep pushing all the way to RPE 10. See how close you were with your guess. You can try anchoring sets once every few weeks or months to see if your estimates are getting more accurate as you gain experience.

- **Record your sets.** You may be surprised by what your video shows compared to how you felt when you performed the sets. Maybe you thought you were close to failure—RPE 8 or 9. But when you run the video, you see your rep speed didn't change much, and there's nothing in your face to suggest you were working especially hard. In this case, the video gives you more objective feedback than your body provided.

- **Get feedback from a coach or training partner.** I had the opportunity to train with Eric Helms, one of the world's leading experts on RPE, when we were both speaking at a fitness conference in Australia. Eric did his doctoral dissertation on RPE and has continued to perform valuable research with bodybuilders and powerlifters. During my sets, I would tell him what I thought my RPE was, and he would either agree or disagree. I then used his feedback to adjust my effort up or down. Even though it was humbling at times, having a second pair of eyeballs on my training gave me a wealth of useful information and insights.

Here are my recommendations for how to incorporate RPE and RIR in your training:

- For muscle growth, most sets should be taken to an RPE between 7 (three RIR) and 10 (zero RIR).

  - Recall that heavier compound exercises like squats, presses, and deadlifts are the primary exercises. These are notable exceptions where I'd suggest staying slightly further from failure. On these more fatiguing movements, aim for an RPE of 6 to 8 most of the time. For hypertrophy, there's no obvious benefit to going any closer to failure, but there's plenty of risk.

    - This means that if you are doing 3 sets of a primary exercise at a fixed weight, you might target RPE 6 on the first set, RPE 7 on the second, and RPE 8 on the third.

    - Occasionally pushing sets to an RPE of 9 or 10 can have merit on heavier compound exercises, especially as a means of anchoring what an RPE of 6 to 8 should feel like. However, they should be done sparingly (generally not more than once every few months) due to their larger impact on fatigue and recovery.

  - Secondary exercises are compound exercises best trained with more moderate weights (lat pulldowns, cable rows, lunges, hip thrusts, pull-ups, etc.). On these exercises, I suggest aiming for an RPE of 8 to 10.

    So let's say you're doing 3 sets with the same weight on lat pulldowns. You could take the first set to RPE 8, the second set to RPE 9, and push the last set all the way to failure. It's normal for your RPE rating to increase from set to set as fatigue accumulates, which is why I prefer to think of RPE as a fuzzy range rather than a strict target.

- On isolation exercises like biceps curls, triceps pressdowns, and lateral raises, I advise shooting for an RPE of 9 to 10 most of the time. The injury risk is minimal, and fatigue is less likely to have a negative impact on your training overall.

  - So if you're doing three sets with the same weight on isolation exercises, you could take the first set to RPE 9, the second set to RPE 9, and push the last set all the way to failure.

  - For any body part, I recommend waiting until the final set before going beast mode with RPE 10. Going to failure too early or too often limits your volume and load, which means less benefit despite the higher effort.

- For strength gain, there's more room to be flexible with RPE. In general, bigger muscles tend to be stronger, and stronger muscles tend to be bigger. But *maximal* strength, unlike hypertrophy, develops through neuromuscular adaptations and skill acquisition. That's why you can build strength at lower RPEs.

  - For heavier compound exercises like squats, presses, and deadlifts, you can use a wide range of RPEs in training:

    - RPEs of 4 to 6 can be useful for practicing your technique and accumulating volume.

    - RPEs of 6 to 8 should be the norm for most of your strength-focused training volume.

    - RPEs of 8 to 10 should be reserved for testing your maximum strength (although it's okay to grind out those final reps just for the sake of grinding every now and then).

- When you're doing isolation and assistance exercises with lighter weights, my recommendations are similar to those for hypertrophy training: RPEs of 7 to 10.

Now that we're clear about the importance of effort and how to measure it objectively, it's time for the next step in our Muscle Ladder: making sure your effort leads to progress.

CHAPTER 7

PROGRESSIVE OVERLOAD

AM I ACTUALLY PROGRESSING?

The technical definition of progressive overload is a "gradual increase in the amount of stress placed on the body from exercise."[1]

The concept is simple enough: For the most part, each of us has already adapted to the stresses we routinely put on our bodies. Without additional stress, our bodies have no reason to get bigger and stronger. If you want your body to make further adaptations—that is, to get bigger and stronger than you are now—you have to give your body new challenges. That's the "overload."

But you have to be smart about it. The overload should be strategic, systematic, and, most important of all, incremental. Too much overload, applied too soon or too haphazardly, will waste time and energy at best. At worst, it can increase risk of injury. That's why it needs to be "progressive."

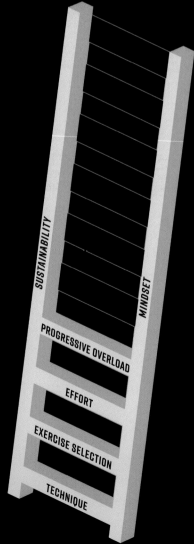

SUSTAINABILITY

MINDSET

PROGRESSIVE OVERLOAD

EFFORT

EXERCISE SELECTION

TECHNIQUE

Recall what I discussed in Chapter 6: To build muscle, you need high levels of mechanical tension, which requires pushing sets reasonably close to failure. That will be extremely challenging at first. But as your body adapts by getting stronger, you need to increase the challenge.

Here's an example: Let's say, in the first week of your program, you do 8 reps of biceps curls with 50 pounds. It's *really* hard. You barely squeeze out the eighth rep with good form. Just for fun, you decide to go for a ninth rep but can't get the weight up. You hit failure, reaching an RPE of 10, with zero reps in reserve. (If you don't know what I mean by RPE and RIR, go back and read Chapter 6.)

In week two, 8 reps with 50 pounds feels a little easier. You still stop at 8 reps, but you probably could've gotten 9 or 10 this time. By week three, you feel like you could do 10 or 11. If you continue with this pattern, using the same weight for the same reps, your biceps will get a lot better at doing curls. But the tension on the muscles will diminish to the point that you're barely stimulating a growth response.

That, in essence, is why so many lifters start spinning their wheels after a year or two of training. As a beginner, basically any lifting you do will elicit a growth response. But as you gain strength, the workouts that caused newbie gains are no longer getting the muscles close enough to failure to keep the gains coming. Instead of becoming an advanced lifter, you become a lifetime intermediate.

The problem is easily solved: Increase the reps or increase the load so you're once again training sufficiently close to failure.

Before I dig into specific ways to do that, I need to make a technical distinction between *progressive overload* and a *progression scheme. Overload,* as I said, refers to gradually increasing the stress you impose on your body through training. You accomplish that by using a *progression scheme* (a plan for adding weight, reps, sets or some combination, that aims toward overload).

The reason I highlight this distinction is that trainees sometimes become so fixated on a specific progression *scheme* that they forget that the entire point of the scheme is to aim at progressive *overload.* In other words, just because you're adding weight to your lifts doesn't necessarily mean you are progressively overloading. If the weight is too easy to present a disruptive stress to your system, you aren't progressively overloading. This is why the effort rung comes before the progressive overload rung. Even if you're following a progression scheme to a tee, if it isn't at an appropriate, challenging effort level then you aren't actually achieving progressive overload.

A FAREWELL TO MUSCLE CONFUSION

"Muscle confusion" is the antithesis of progressive overload. Equating the two is like comparing a local jam band to a professional orchestra.

The idea behind muscle confusion, as you may know, is that muscles grow in response to unpredictable challenges. High reps one week, low reps the next. Barbells today, dumbbells tomorrow. Squats here, leg presses there.

But there's an obvious problem. Muscles don't actually experience confusion. They can't predict what you're going to throw at them because muscles don't make predictions. Muscles adapt to stimuli. If the stimulus is prolonged, repetitive movement, the muscles adapt by developing more endurance. If the stimulus is a high degree of mechanical tension, the muscles adapt by getting bigger and stronger.

To be fair, plenty of bodybuilders have made progress by using muscle confusion. But that's because they trained so hard for so long that they were able to generate enough tension almost by accident. But in general, because the muscle confusion approach is random, the results will be random as well. And this is why, for every bodybuilder who has had success with muscle confusion, there's a swath of people spinning their wheels in the gym, mindlessly hopping from exercise to exercise.

MUSCLE GROWTH AND STRENGTH

Up to this point, I've talked a lot about muscles getting "bigger and stronger." Now it's time to explore the relationship between muscle growth and strength gains.

The most obvious way to apply progressive tension to your muscles is to use heavier weights. Increased strength is the most obvious result of working with heavier weights. It's natural to assume that you need to get stronger to get bigger or that strength drives muscle growth. If that were true then the best bodybuilders would all train with super heavy weights and super low reps.

But that is *not* the way bodybuilders typically train.

To be sure, the vast majority of successful natural bodybuilders are also extremely strong. That's not a coincidence. There's a powerful

relationship between strength and size, and getting stronger is a great way to know if you're applying sufficient tension to your muscles.

But getting stronger isn't the only way to get bigger, as you'll see.

GENERAL APPROACHES TO PROGRESSIVE OVERLOAD

Most people familiar with progressive overload think it simply means "adding weight to the bar," but that is just one of nine ways of applying the principle. One overload strategy isn't necessarily better than the others. You can choose different strategies in different contexts. All of them lead to an increased challenge to the muscle and better growth over time.

STRATEGY 1: INCREASING LOAD (LINEAR PROGRESSION)

Increasing load is the most common and intuitive approach to progressive overload. It's the first one I recommend for most beginners, and in some contexts, it's the most important.

This example (shown in the graph in Figure 7.1) involves doing the barbell back squat with the same sets and reps while incrementally adding a minimal amount (5 pounds) to the load.

Barbell back squat

Week 1: 3 sets × 6 reps × 135 lb
Week 2: 3 sets × 6 reps × 140 lb
Week 3: 3 sets × 6 reps × 145 lb
Week 4: 3 sets × 6 reps × 150 lb

Figure 7.1

Increasing load

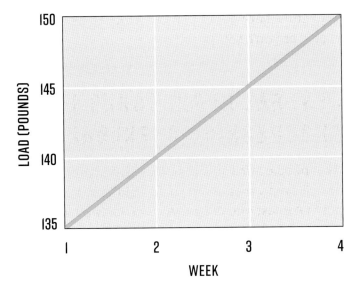

You can see why it's called linear progression. You're progressing one variable by a fixed amount while leaving everything else the same. If you could do that for fifty-two consecutive weeks, you'd be squatting 395 pounds for 6 reps after a year of training. Of course, this isn't possible for many people and certainly can't happen forever. If everyone could add 5 pounds to the bar every workout, we all would be squatting 1,000 pounds by year 4. Which, yes, is absurd. I only know of five people on the planet who can squat that amount of weight.

The more realistic scenario is that you start with a moderately challenging weight. After increasing the load in a linear fashion for several weeks or months, you can no longer complete all 6 reps in all 3 sets.

At that point, you have a couple of options:

- Add weight every second or third workout.

- Increase the weight by smaller increments, using micro or fractional weight plates.

The first option is simple enough. You let your body tell you when it needs a new challenge.

The second option, which only applies to barbell exercises, is a little trickier. Most gyms have plates ranging from 45 pounds (20 kg) to 2.5 pounds (1.25 kg). That's fine when your goal is to add 5 pounds per week. Slap an extra 2.5-pound plate to each end of the bar, and you're there. If you want to increase the weight in smaller increments, you need micro or fractional plates, which come in sizes as small as a quarter pound. Although some niche strength gyms have micro plates available, you'll probably need to buy your own set online and bring them with you to the gym.

I honestly don't recommend micro plates very often, and I don't use them myself. Unless you're a competitive powerlifter aiming for a specific record, I don't think it's all that useful to micromanage your progression by adding fewer than 5 pounds at a time. The fractional plates can be sometimes helpful when you feel like you can add a bit of weight but not a full 5 pounds, but since there are eight other ways to apply progressive overload, fixating on micro-loading feels a bit fussy for my taste.

A QUICK NOTE ABOUT PROGRESSION EXPECTATIONS

You are not a robot. You know that, of course. You may have even said as much to a boss or coworker or family member who seemed confused about your personal or professional bandwidth. But in the gym, you probably expect robotic consistency in your training. You think your strength and energy level should be exactly the same every time you train.

However, your body doesn't work like that. It's normal to experience fluctuations in your performance, for any number of reasons—

stressors in your personal and professional life, the quality and quantity of your sleep, your nutrition and hydration status. You might be coming down with an illness and have no idea anything's wrong until you run out of gas halfway through a workout. Any of those things can affect your strength.

There will be days when your body is at odds with your progression scheme. Your plan might call for you to increase your loads this week, but your muscles can't even handle the weights you worked with last week.

Conversely, you might feel so good that everything you lift feels lighter than it should, even if it's heavier than any weight you've used on that exercise in that rep range. But just when you think this is your new normal, your strength fluctuates in the opposite direction.

Or perhaps you've hit a plateau after several months of steady, dependable gains. It happens to everyone. Maybe micro plates can help you continue moving forward, at least on barbell exercises. But you can't do that with dumbbells, which are rarely available in increments smaller than 5 pounds. If you're doing a bilateral exercise, you can only move up 10 pounds at a time.

A cable machine might have 5- or even 2.5-pound plates you can add to the stack, but other types of machines might not offer any flexibility at all.

That's when you need to look at other ways to apply progressive overload.

STRATEGY 2: INCREASING REPS AT THE SAME LOAD

Eventually, everyone gets to a point where they can't add more weight and still complete all their reps. That's when you shift your progression strategy from adding more weight to doing more reps with the same weight.

I'll stick with the barbell back squat example. Let's say, thanks to linear progression (Strategy 1), you worked your way up to squatting 185 pounds for 6 reps. That's awesome! What's not awesome: When you tried 190 pounds, you could only get 5 reps.

Assuming you weren't just having a bad day, it's probably time to consider a new overload strategy. Now, instead of increasing the weight while keeping a fixed rep target, you keep the weight fixed and increase reps:

Barbell back squat
Week 1: 3 sets × 6 reps × 185 lb
Week 2: 3 sets × 7 reps × 185 lb
Week 3: 3 sets × 8 reps × 185 lb
Week 4: 3 sets × 9 reps × 185 lb

Rep overload is a great tool, but it often has an even shorter shelf life than linear overload with weight. If you committed to adding even just 1 rep each week, you'd be doing sets of 20 after a few months and sets of 100 reps after a few years. This isn't realistic.

In fact, even the preceding squat example would be a stretch for most lifters. Adding reps to already challenging loads can get real tough, real quick. If the reps become too challenging, you don't need to add reps to every set, every week. Instead of adding a rep to all three sets, you could instead commit to adding just one rep to one of the three sets. This way, you give yourself more time to build from 3 sets of 6 reps to 3 sets of 9 reps.

Still, even if you drag the progression calendar out, you'll still eventually hit a wall with rep overload on its own. For that reason, I think the best way to use rep overload is in tandem with another type of progression, as I describe in the next section.

STRATEGY 3: DOUBLE PROGRESSION

In double progression, you're working with two variables—reps and load—instead of one or the other. This is the way most coaches implement progressive overload, and it's an intuitive one for most lifters.

Note that the following example starts with a lighter weight than you maxed out on in the previous example, and you're working with a range of 6 to 8 reps:

Barbell back squat
Week 1: 3 sets × 6 reps × 175 lb
Week 2: 3 sets × 7 reps × 175 lb
Week 3: 3 sets × 8 reps × 175 lb
Week 4: 3 sets × 6 reps × 180 lb
Week 5: 3 sets × 7 reps × 180 lb
Week 6: 3 sets × 8 reps × 180 lb
Week 7: 3 sets × 6 reps × 185 lb
Week 8: 3 sets × 7 reps × 185 lb
Week 9: 3 sets × 8 reps × 185 lb
Week 10: 3 sets × 6 reps × 190 lb
Week 11: 3 sets × 7 reps × 190 lb
Week 12: 3 sets × 8 reps × 190 lb
Week 13: 3 sets × 6 reps × 195 lb
Week 14: 3 sets × 7 reps × 195 lb
Week 15: 3 sets × 8 reps × 195 lb
Week 16: 3 sets × 6 reps × 200 lb

As you can see, the general pattern is to add one rep each week until you hit the top end of the rep range (in this case, 8 reps). At that point, you add some weight and return to the low end of the rep range (in this case, 6 reps).

In the preceding example, you don't reach your current 6-rep max of 185 pounds until Week 7. But you're hardly wasting time by working at a submaximal level in those first seven weeks. You're taking a running start. That's how you can blow past your previous stopping point in the next seven weeks. By the end you're working with 200 pounds—an 8 percent increase in your 6-rep strength.

Here's an example of double progression on the bench press, using a lower rep range:

Bench press
Week 1: 3 sets × 4 reps × 135 lb
Week 2: 3 sets × 5 reps × 135 lb
Week 3: 3 sets × 6 reps × 135 lb
Week 4: 3 sets × 4 reps × 140 lb
Week 5: 3 sets × 5 reps × 140 lb
Week 6: 3 sets × 6 reps × 140 lb

And here's an example of double progression on an isolation exercise, using a higher rep range:

Triceps pressdown
Week 1: 3 sets × 10 reps × 50 lb
Week 2: 3 sets × 11 reps × 50 lb
Week 3: 3 sets × 12 reps × 50 lb
Week 4: 3 sets × 10 reps × 55 lb
Week 5: 3 sets × 11 reps × 55 lb
Week 6: 3 sets × 12 reps × 55 lb

The progression from 50 to 55 pounds is nominally small. But it's still a 10 percent increase. Fortunately, gyms typically have 2.5-pound add-on plates for cable machines, which in this example would be a more manageable 5 percent increase.

Progressive overload gets more complicated when you're working with dumbbells on an isolation exercise. Let's say you're doing lateral raises. You start with 10 pounds, work your way up to a dozen reps, and then increase the weight to 15 pounds. (This example assumes your gym doesn't have 12.5-pound dumbbells—or 17.5 or 22.5, etc.) Again, you work your way up to 12 reps, and you think you're ready for 20 pounds. But you can't even get 8 reps, and the 7 reps you do complete feel ... different. You feel more stress in your shoulder joints and less activation in your deltoids.

It's only 5 pounds per arm, but it's also a 33 percent increase. That's a lot of extra weight!

In cases like these, your best tactic is a wider rep range, which allows you to continue with rep overload longer than you would in the previous examples:

Dumbbell lateral raise
Week 1: 3 sets × 10 reps × 15 lb
Week 2: 3 sets × 11 reps × 15 lb
Week 3: 3 sets × 12 reps × 15 lb
Week 4: 3 sets × 13 reps × 15 lb
Week 5: 3 sets × 14 reps × 15 lb
Week 6: 3 sets × 15 reps × 15 lb
Week 7: 3 sets × 10 reps* × 20 lb
Week 8: 3 sets × 11 reps × 20 lb

*You might even start at 8 reps, which you couldn't manage at the beginning of this sequence. That widens the rep range even more—from 8 to 15 reps.

Another thing to keep in mind: Your rep counts won't always be as neat and tidy as they appear in the examples. And that's okay! For one thing, you may not be able to reach the exact same rep count for all three sets on any given day. The next page shows a real-life example from one of my old training logs.

As you can see, my progression worked, even though I didn't hit the exact same rep count on every set. But I did manage to stay within the target rep range and do at least 10 per set—even when I moved up to 20-pound dumbbells in week 16.

But what if I hadn't been able to hit that rep count with the heavier weights? What if I only got 7? Clearly, that would mean the weight is still too heavy. At that point, I could drop the weight back to 15 pounds and widen the rep range (up to 20 reps, for example), or try a different overload strategy (such as those I describe later in this chapter).

It's also worth mentioning that many coaches schedule deloads every four to eight weeks within these progression schemes. I'll cover deloading in more detail in Chapter 13, but for now, I'll just say that deloading is simple during a double progression. For one week, return to the bottom of your rep range. Depending on the exercise and how fatigued you're feeling, you may need to reduce the load as well. The next week, pick up the progression where you left off before the deload.

Week	Exercise	Rep Range	Set 1	Set 2	Set 3	Notes
Week 1	Dumbbell lateral raise	10 to 15	15 lb × 10 reps	15 lb × 10 reps	15 lb × 10 reps	I started at the bottom of the 10- to 15-rep range with 3 sets of 10 reps.
Week 2	Dumbbell lateral raise	10 to 15	15 lb × 11 reps	15 lb × 11 reps	15 lb × 11 reps	I was able to add 1 rep to all 3 sets.
Week 3	Dumbbell lateral raise	10 to 15	15 lb × 12 reps	15 lb × 12 reps	15 lb × 10 reps	Due to fatigue, I could only add a rep to sets 1 and 2. For set 3, I got just 10 reps.
Week 4	Dumbbell lateral raise	10 to 15	15 lb × 12 reps	15 lb × 12 reps	15 lb × 11 reps	This time I was able to add 1 rep to set 3 but stayed at 12 reps for sets 1 and 2.
Week 5	Dumbbell lateral raise	10 to 15	15 lb × 12 reps	15 lb × 12 reps	15 lb × 12 reps	This time I got 12 reps on all 3 sets! Next week, I'll aim to increase the reps to 13.
Week 6	Dumbbell lateral raise	10 to 15	15 lb × 13 reps	15 lb × 12 reps	15 lb × 11 reps	Because 13 reps was challenging on the first set, I got only 12 and 11 reps for sets 2 and 3.
Week 7	Dumbbell lateral raise	10 to 15	15 lb × 13 reps	15 lb × 13 reps	15 lb × 12 reps	This week I was able to add 1 rep to sets 2 and 3.
Week 8	Dumbbell lateral raise	10 to 15	15 lb × 13 reps	15 lb × 13 reps	15 lb × 13 reps	This time I got 13 reps on all 3 sets! Next week, I'll aim to increase the reps to 14.
Several more weeks passed. Each week, I gradually added reps within the 10- to 15-rep range until I was able to complete 15 reps for all 3 sets at the same weight.						
Week 15	Dumbbell lateral raise	10 to 15	15 lb × 15 reps	15 lb × 15 reps	15 lb × 15 reps	After 15 weeks, I went from doing 3 sets of 10 to doing 3 sets of 15 at 15 pounds. Next week, I'll aim to increase the weight to 20 pounds.
Week 16	Dumbbell lateral raise	10 to 15	20 lb × 10 reps	20 lb × 10 reps	20 lb × 10 reps	This week, I increased the weight to 20-pound dumbbells and dropped the reps all the way back to 10.

STRATEGY 4: ADDING SETS

Continuing with the lateral raise example, let's say you built up to 3 sets of 12 reps with 20-pound dumbbells. But now you're stuck: Heavier weights feel like they're hitting your joints more than your muscles, and your technique quickly breaks down with higher reps.

The solution is simple, if not easy: Add another set, using the same weight and rep range. In the short term, it's a great way to give your targeted muscles more work with minimal risk. But it does have downsides.

The first and most obvious downside is the impracticality of adding volume. Going from 2 to 3 sets is a natural progression. Going from 3 to 4 sets is a viable way to get through a plateau. But going from 4 to 5 or 5 to 6? That's usually a nonstarter, especially when you're talking about an isolation exercise. It's just not a good use of your time.

The second downside is diminishing returns. At some point, more sets don't lead to bigger gains and might actually be counterproductive. (I'll discuss "junk volume" in the next chapter.)

The third and more subtle downside is that additional sets tend to dilute your focus and energy. When I'm doing 3 sets of any given exercise, I can focus on getting the most out of each one. But what if I'm doing 6 sets? Do I really push myself as hard on each one?

Finally, the fourth and even more subtle downside is the fatigue factor. Think of it as a math problem: In a double progression, most of the time, you're adding 1 rep per set per week. If you're doing 3 sets, you're adding 3 reps. And when you increase the weight, you reduce reps to the bottom of the range. But when you add a set, that's 8 to 15 more reps you're adding! Do that for multiple exercises, and you've significantly increased your workout

volume. You not only need more time to *do* the workouts, you may need more time to *recover* from them.

So while adding a set *can* be a viable overload strategy, you should use it sparingly. It's most effective when you apply it to a specific exercise after progress has stalled with the other methods.

One way to get around the issues I just described is to use sets as part of a double progression. In this example, you're adding sets with a fixed number of repetitions, rather than adding reps with a fixed number of sets:

Seated leg curl
Week 1: 2 sets × 8 reps × 100 lb
Week 2: 3 sets × 8 reps × 100 lb
Week 3: 4 sets × 8 reps × 100 lb
Week 4: 2 sets × 8 reps × 110 lb
Week 5: 3 sets × 8 reps × 110 lb
Week 6: 4 sets × 8 reps × 110 lb
Week 7: 2 sets × 8 reps × 120 lb

The range is two to four sets. Your goal is to use the increased volume to achieve the second part of your double progression: increased load. Each time you add weight, you decrease sets to the bottom of your set range.

Once again, I should emphasize that while increasing sets can be a powerful stimulus for sparking new growth and busting a plateau, it can also quickly increase recovery demand. For this reason, set overload requires closer monitoring than the other overloading methods I've covered. When adding sets, keep a close eye on your recovery by making sure you're not seeing a sudden and otherwise unexplained drop in strength or excessive exhaustion both in and out of the gym. If you're experiencing dwindling strength and feelings of constant exhaustion, you may need to return to a fixed number of sets (one you can recover from) and consider using another progression strategy.

STRATEGY 5: OVERLOADING VIA TECHNIQUE

All the methods I've described so far assume consistent technique. The reality, though, is that an experienced lifter can manipulate their technique to increase tension or muscle activation.

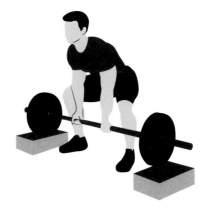

One way is to slow down the negative (eccentric) phase of the lift. So instead of lowering the weight at your normal pace (about one to two seconds), you take two to three seconds. That increases the muscles' time under tension, making the set more fatiguing without adding reps or load. Even if you slow down the negative on only the final two reps of each set, it still presents a new challenge to your muscles.

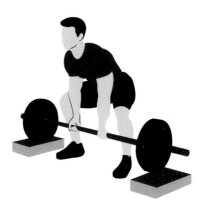

Another way to overload via technique is to pause at the moment when the muscle is in its deepest stretch. On a calf raise, for example, you could pause at the bottom and intentionally feel a more intense stretch. Again, even if you only do it for the last few reps, you'll feel the difference in activation.

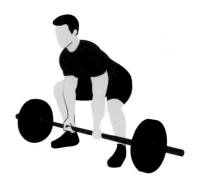

You can also expand the range of motion. You can gradually increase your squat depth, for example, if your mobility allows it. Or you can use a higher platform for step-ups. If you deadlift off blocks (or from the supports of a power rack), you can progressively decrease the height of the blocks until you're pulling from the floor.

STRATEGY 6: OVERLOADING VIA VELOCITY

Research shows that using explosive force on the positive (concentric) phase of a compound lift can activate larger, higher-threshold muscle fibers. That should help with your goal of creating an overloading stimulus. Let's use the barbell bench press as an example.

Last week, you lifted 225 pounds for 4 reps. You weren't lifting deliberately fast or slow; you were completely focused on moving the weight without thinking about how fast you were moving it. But what if you tried to push the bar off your chest as fast as possible? What if you pressed like your goal was to launch the bar into the ceiling (without actually letting it leave your hands)?

Of course, this method of lifting isn't suitable for all exercises. Generally, you don't want to lift explosively on isolation exercises or most machines—a smoother cadence on the positive and negative is usually better for these movements. Bench and overhead presses lend themselves well to explosive lifts, as do pull-ups, chin-ups, and rows. Just make sure you still control the negative.

STRATEGY 7: OVERLOADING VIA MIND-MUSCLE CONNECTION

As you recall from Chapter 4, you create a mind-muscle connection when you focus on the muscle you're training. Studies have shown it not only increases muscle activation at the moment, it leads to bigger muscles over the long term.[2] It's also one of the more "instinctive" training variables, and one that improves with time and training experience.

However, it's easy to overstate its importance. For example, if you can't feel your pectoral muscles working on a bench press, does that mean they aren't being activated? Of course not. A chest press involves a joint action called horizontal shoulder adduction—pushing your upper arms toward the midline of your torso. The pecs are driving that movement. They're activated even if your mind can't connect with them.

Additionally, the mind-muscle connection can be a distraction in some circumstances. For example, if you're doing relatively low reps (eight or fewer) with relatively heavy weights, you want an external focus on how your body is moving rather than an internal focus on specific muscles. That's especially true with compound exercises like squats and deadlifts.

The best application of the mind-muscle connection is on isolation exercises or when doing higher-rep sets of select compound exercises, as shown in Table 7.1.

Table 7.1: Exercises That Benefit from Mind-Muscle Connection

Exercise	Muscle	Mind-Muscle Connection Cues
Biceps curl	Biceps	"Squeeze your biceps to move the weight."
Cable crunch	Abs	"Crunch your abs together."
Cable pec fly	Pecs	"Squeeze the middle of your pecs together at the top."
Lat pulldown	Lats	"Feel your lats pulling apart on the negative."
Lateral raise	Side deltoids	"Think about the middle of your shoulder as you lift."
Leg curl (lying or seated)	Hamstrings	"Squeeze and stretch your hamstrings like an accordion."
Leg extension	Quadriceps	"Squeeze your quads to move the weight."
Overhead triceps extension	Triceps	"Feel your triceps pulling apart on the negative."
Shrugs	Traps	"Feel your traps squeeze at the top and stretch at the bottom."

STRATEGY 8: OVERLOADING VIA SHORTER REST PERIODS

The shorter your rest periods between sets, the less time your muscles have to recover. That leads to higher cumulative fatigue, which—in theory—forces your muscles to work harder.

I say "in theory" because reducing rest periods is usually a bigger challenge for your cardiovascular system than your muscles. Oftentimes, people find shorter rest periods more difficult, not because their muscles are achieving higher tension but because they're struggling to catch their breath. While this is good for overall conditioning, it can be suboptimal for muscle growth and strength gain.

For example, a 2015 study showed that three minutes of rest between sets resulted in greater hypertrophy than one minute of rest, and a 2017 meta-analysis found that more than one minute of rest was better for muscle growth than less than one minute of rest.[3]

With that said, shorter, faster workouts are sometimes a necessity when you have limited time to train. By progressively reducing your rest periods, you can do more exercises and complete more total sets. You not only improve your conditioning, but you exploit that improved conditioning by getting more work done in the same amount of time. I do count that as a form of progressive overload, even if it may not be suitable for everyone's goals.

I also might recommend shorter rest periods when muscular endurance is at least as important as muscle size. That's often the case for military and law-enforcement personnel. Same with someone who's interested in CrossFit, adventure racing, or any other activity that challenges both endurance and strength.

But for lifters chasing maximum muscle growth, I think it makes more sense to separate hypertrophy work from conditioning work. You want to maximize tension when you're training for hypertrophy, and that's best accomplished with longer rest periods and more complete recovery between sets. And when you're training for muscular endurance or cardiovascular fitness (both of which are worthwhile goals), do what works best in those areas. I'll revisit the topic of rest periods in Chapter 11.

STRATEGY 9: EXTENDING SETS BEYOND FAILURE

Advanced intensity techniques like drop sets, iso-holds, myoreps, forced reps, static holds, and partial reps help you push a set past failure and increase stress on the target muscle.

I call them "advanced" techniques for a reason: They're best used by advanced trainees who are close to their muscular potential and have already gotten what they can from more conventional progression schemes and overload strategies.

For someone who's not advanced, the soreness and fatigue can be so extreme they impair future workouts. I'm not saying your muscles will fall off your bones if you're in your first year of lifting and you occasionally experiment with drop sets or add a partial rep to the end of a set. I just don't think they should be a regular part of your training until you actually need them.

When's that? Usually not in your first year or two of training. Not before you've made substantial gains in size and strength. And not before you've employed most of the previously described overload methods.

That's when it's useful to test your limits and get a sense of what it means to go beyond failure. You'll find a deep dive into this masochistic toolbox in Chapter 12.

ROTATING EXERCISES

If you take away one message from this chapter, I hope it's this: On any given exercise, each progressive overload strategy has a natural lifespan. It works until it doesn't. At some point, you can't lift heavier weights, add sets or reps, make the lifts any slower or faster, or push your mind any further into the muscle.

That's when it's time to start over. Pick a new exercise for the same muscles and begin the process again. You're not actually abandoning the original exercise. You might even keep it in your program (more on that in a moment), or at least plan to come back to it later. But you'll focus most of your attention and energy on the new exercise and the many ways to make progress with it.

I'll revisit the idea of rotating exercises in Chapter 13, when I discuss periodization. For now, I'll leave you with these guidelines:

- Once you select an exercise, you want to train with it for at least a month.

- If you're new to serious training, you want to stick to the same exercises for at least your first three to six months. Improve your technique and use linear progressions for as long as they continue working, which might be a year or more. Your body will thank you later for mastering the fundamentals first.

- Intermediate lifters progress more slowly and encounter plateaus more frequently. That's the "penalty" for getting closer to your genetic potential. At this stage, it makes sense to rotate exercises every two to six months.

- At any level, you don't want to switch things up too much. I know it's tempting to try the flashy new exercise you just discovered on social media. I also know the value of adding a little adventure to your workouts. Just remember that the spice is not the meal.

- I use the same movement patterns in every program I design. You'll always see squat-type movements, hip hinges, presses, and rows. But I rotate variations throughout the year—flat and incline bench press, back and front squat, dumbbell and machine shoulder press, etc. I alternate secondary and tertiary exercises more frequently.

Throughout this chapter, I've talked about how to make progress on specific exercises. Sometimes progress requires higher volume—adding reps and/or sets. But how much volume is enough? How much is too much? That's the next rung on the Muscle Ladder and the topic of Chapter 8.

CHAPTER 8

VOLUME

HOW MUCH WORK SHOULD I DO?

Now that we're halfway up the ladder, let's stop momentarily to catch our breath. (Metaphorically speaking—if you're actually out of breath, you may need a bit more cardio in your program.)

So far, we've gone from technique on the first rung to exercise selection, effort, and progressive overload. The fifth rung, volume, is something I've touched on a few times already, especially in the previous chapter. Now it's time to explain what it is and why it matters.

Simply put, volume is the amount of work you do. It seems straightforward, but it's been the source of sometimes heated debates in bodybuilding and exercise science circles.

Some bodybuilders hearken back to the '90s era of low-volume, high-intensity training (HIT) popularized by Dorian Yates and Mike Mentzer. Advocates for this approach say the goal isn't to do more work; it's to do better work. Quality over quantity. Put absolutely everything you have into one or two sets of each exercise. Then get out of the gym, feed your muscles, and watch them grow.

Despite HIT's rugged appeal, most bodybuilders train with higher volume. Yes, the quality of your work clearly matters, but quantity matters too, as shown by bodybuilding greats like Arnold Schwarzenegger, Ronnie Coleman, and Jay Cutler. All of them used enormous workloads in their training.

But let's not pretend we can settle the volume debate with dueling anecdotes. We can draw inspiration from the bodybuilding legends, but we can't pretend we'll get the same results from their training programs. Even if we could somehow replicate their genetics, there's no way to match all the other variables, including their specific drug regimen.

We can, however, do something much better: look at the scientific literature and expert consensus.

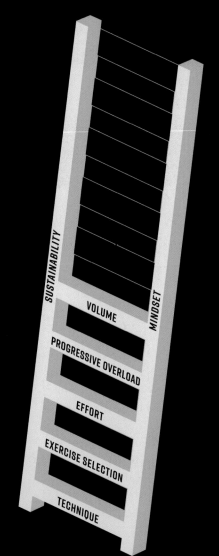

WHAT IS TRAINING VOLUME?

We can talk about the volume of water in a glass any number of ways—liters, fluid ounces, half empty, or half full—but we're still talking about the same thing: the amount of water in that glass.

Music volume can be described with a scale of very soft (pianissimo) to very loud (fortissimo), or we can get a precise measurement in decibels. Alternatively, we can wait for a neighbor to tell us when it's too loud.

So, when we talk about the training volume, it's no surprise we have multiple ways to do it. Historically, it was common to quantify either *rep volume* or *volume load*.

Rep volume is simple arithmetic: the number of reps you do in a workout. If you did 3 sets of 8 shoulder presses, your volume for that exercise was 24 reps. If you also did 3 sets of 12 cable lateral raises, your rep load for shoulders was 60 reps—24 shoulder presses and 36 lateral raises. You can look at those numbers over time to see how your rep volume matches your results.

Rep volume has been used in research to compare and contrast different levels of training volume. For example, a 2007 review by Wernbom and colleagues suggested there was a plateau in muscle growth after 40 to 70 total reps per muscle per workout.[1]

But it doesn't take much thought to find a glaring issue with rep volume as a primary tracking metric. It doesn't account for load, as if there's no difference between heavy and light reps or easy and hard reps.

That's why coaches and researchers turned to volume load to quantify total work. The math is still simple enough:

Volume load = sets × reps × load

Using this metric for the previous example, it looks like this:

Dumbbell shoulder press:
3 sets × 8 reps × 50 lb = 1,200 lb of volume

Cable lateral raise:
3 sets × 12 reps × 20 lb = 720 lb of volume

Combining the two shoulder exercises is a total volume load of 1,920 pounds.

That's somewhat better than rep load (on top of how cool it is to realize you lifted close to a ton), but volume load still has some issues. The most obvious is that you're combining loads from two very different types of resistance. With dumbbells, your muscles are moving weights against the force of gravity. But with a cable exercise, you have any number of pulleys between your muscles and the weight you've selected. Every type of machine is different, and even the same machine can offer more or less resistance, depending on its calibration and how worn the cable is. Twenty pounds on one machine might be harder to move than 30 pounds on another.

Another problem: High-rep sets massively inflate your volume load, just as they do your rep load. Because reps are being multiplied by the sets in both calculations, high-rep sets lead to gigantic volumes that don't reflect the actual high-tension work each muscle is performing all that well.

Because of these practical concerns, both rep volume and volume load have fallen out of favor in bodybuilding circles. Most coaches and experts these days choose a much easier approach requiring minimal math: counting the number of *hard sets*, sometimes called *set volume.*

Today, most people use "set volume" and "volume" interchangeably. Both mean the number of hard sets you do. I'm a huge fan of this approach because it makes training volume easy to monitor and modify. Just count how many hard sets you did.

If you think it might be *too* simple, consider this:

The latest research shows that you can build muscle with pretty much any rep range, as long as you meet two conditions: You're lifting at least approximately 30 percent of your one-rep max on that exercise, and you push yourself close to technical failure—the last rep you can do with good technique.

Practically speaking, I think that gives you a rep range from 5 to at least 30 when you're training for hypertrophy. Any hard set within that range counts toward your training volume.

WHAT IS A HARD SET, EXACTLY?

Put another way, how close to failure do you have to go for it to count as a "hard" set? Here's where it gets a little fuzzy. It depends to some extent on the exercise and your target reps.

Let's say you're doing a set of 10 reps on squats, and you take it to an RPE of 5 or 6. (Revisit page 187 in Chapter 6 if you need a refresher on RPE.) Even though you're leaving four or five reps in the tank, that will feel hard. Moderate- to high-rep squats are just difficult to do.

Conversely, 10 dumbbell lateral raises taken to an RPE of 5 or 6 won't feel hard at all. It's basically a warm-up set.

So, when you're trying to decide what counts as a hard set, consider these guidelines:

- For primary exercises (squats, presses, deadlifts, etc.), any set taken to RPE 6 or higher usually counts as a hard set.

- For secondary and tertiary exercises (lat pulldowns, lateral raises, etc.), any set taken to RPE 7 or higher usually counts as a hard set.

I say "usually" because a hard set needs to *feel* hard. More often than not, it's one you began with the *intention* of doing a hard set.

Some coaches call that a *working set* to distinguish it from a *warm-up set*. The terms pretty much explain themselves. A warm-up set gets your muscles ready for high-effort, high-tension working sets. Working sets count toward training volume. Warm-up sets don't.

For the rest of this chapter, if I mention "volume," I mean "set volume." And when I use "set," it implies "hard set" or, if you prefer, "working set."

WHY IS VOLUME SO IMPORTANT?

A large and growing body of research focuses on the link between volume and hypertrophy. It's generally understood that there is an inverted U-shaped relationship between training volume and muscle growth, as illustrated in Figure 8.1.

Figure 8.1

Relationship between muscle growth and training volume

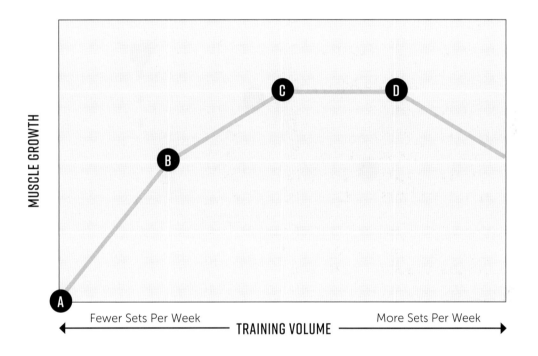

As you can see, if you're an average lifter, higher volume substantially increases muscle growth as you go from point A to point B. Almost any lifter closer to point A benefits from doing more sets and moving closer to point B. As you move from point B to point C, there's still a positive relationship between volume and hypertrophy, but you start to see diminishing returns. That is, each additional set contributes less to muscle growth.

Beyond point C, additional sets offer little, if any, hypertrophic benefit. Once you factor in

the recovery cost, they probably aren't worth it for most trainees in most circumstances. If you keep adding sets beyond point C, you eventually reach point D, where your volume is so high that it interferes with muscle growth.

To be clear, those additional sets don't result in muscle loss, but they overwhelm your body's ability to recover, resulting in fewer or slower gains than you could've made with lower volume and more complete recovery.

HOW MUCH VOLUME SHOULD I DO?

In Figure 8.2, I've added some numbers to the graph from Figure 8.1. Each number represents sets per week for an individual muscle group or body part.

Figure 8.2

How increasing training volume affects muscle growth

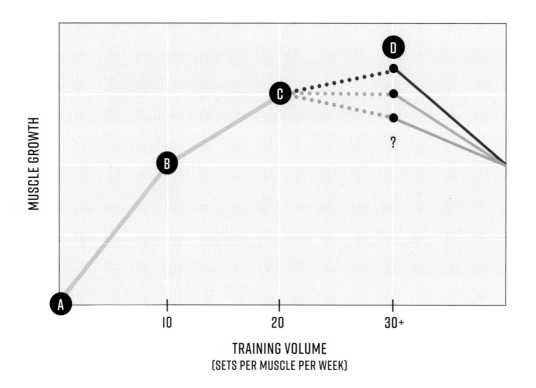

As you can see, for any given muscle group, every additional set from point A (zero sets per week) to point B (10 sets per week) should impact your gains. That's why I recommend a ballpark minimum of 10 sets per week for most muscle groups.

This is supported by a 2017 meta-analysis from Schoenfeld, Ogborn, and Krieger, which indicated a dose-response relationship between volume and hypertrophy when going from <5 to 5–9 to 10+ sets per muscle group per week.[2]

However, the curve begins to flatten as you move from 10 to 20 sets per muscle per week.[3] There's a smaller return on your investment with each additional set. The less advanced you are, the more you'll get from the lower end of that range. The more experience you have and the closer to your genetic potential, the more you need to push your volume toward the top of the range to see progress.

What happens when you do more than 20 sets?

Figure 8.2 shows three dashed lines between 20 (point C) and 30 sets (point D). Each represents a different possible outcome based on a lifter's training experience and genetic tolerance for volume.

Some elite lifters, represented by the red dashed line, continue making marginal gains as they increase volume. It's pretty rare, in my experience, for someone to do more than 20 truly hard sets per week and still benefit. Even then, they wouldn't be doing such gigantic volume for every body part. For example, some advanced female bikini competitors will do more than 20 sets a week for their glutes but do less volume for their quads and upper body.

The green dashed line—a plateau, essentially—shows what I would expect for an intermediate to advanced trainee. For most people in this category, going beyond 20 sets per muscle per week simply wastes time and energy.

The gray dashed line represents a beginner or someone with a lower tolerance for volume. In this case, the rate of progress turns negative when volume increases beyond 20 sets.

If we venture beyond point D and do more than 30 sets per week, most of us begin to see a drop-off in muscle growth. Although some new evidence suggests that single body parts might be able to handle very high volumes one at a time, it seems implausible to suggest that we

could do such high volumes for all body parts at once.[4] We simply don't have enough research to predict how steep the drop-off would be.

Here's what I recommend, based on the research we have:

Beginner: Aim for roughly 10 sets per muscle per week for optimal gains. If you're more concerned with time efficiency, even 1 to 5 sets per muscle per week is enough to get you some gains for a while.

Intermediate: Aim for 10 to 20 sets per muscle per week for optimal gains, depending on the body part you're training. (You'll find the details in Table 8.1.) Once again, you can still make *some* gains with less volume, but 4 to 8 sets per muscle per week is most likely your new minimum for making noticeable progress.

Advanced: Aim for 10 to 20 sets for most body parts for optimal gains. For stubborn body parts or muscles that seem to recover better than others, you can experiment with volumes beyond 20 sets per week. I have yet to recommend more than 30 sets per week for any trainee, regardless of body part. Doing so would almost certainly be counterproductive. You can most likely still maintain your gains by doing 4 to 8 sets per muscle per week, as long as you push those sets hard.

ADJUSTING VOLUME ACCORDING TO BODY PART

Spend enough time in the gym, and you start to see a divergence in how your muscles respond to volume. I can hit my shoulders and back with almost anything, and they'll rarely feel sore or even especially fatigued. But when I work my hamstrings, even moderate volume will haunt me for days. Your experience, however, might be completely different.

Keep that in mind as you look at Table 8.1. My body-part-specific volume recommendations are estimates of what works best for the average trainee in each category, but nobody is truly "average." Your limb lengths, training experience, injuries, and personal preferences can all affect how different muscles respond.

Table 8.1: Sets per Week per Body Part for Optimal Gains

Muscle	Beginner	Intermediate	Advanced
Abs	3 to 10	6 to 10	6 to 15
Back	10	10 to 20	10 to 30
Biceps*	3 to 6	6 to 10	8 to 20+
Calves	3 to 10	6 to 10	6 to 15
Chest	8 to 10	8 to 15	10 to 20
Forearms**	0 to 6	3 to 8	3 to 10
Glutes	10	10 to 20	10 to 30
Hamstrings	6 to 10	8 to 12	8 to 15
Neck***	0 to 6	3 to 10	3 to 10
Quads	8 to 10	10 to 15	10 to 20
Shoulders	10	10 to 20	10 to 25
Triceps*	3 to 6	6 to 10	8 to 20+
Upper traps	0 to 6	3 to 10	3 to 10

*Applies to isolation exercises only
**Includes both flexion (wrist curls) and extension (reverse wrist curls) exercises
***Refers to neck flexion (head forward) and neck extension (head back) exercises separately

Muscles that typically benefit from the highest volumes include back, glutes, shoulders, and quads. The back includes a mix of large and small muscles. The glutes, shoulders, and quads are single muscles with multiple subdivisions. You can optimize their development with 10 to 20 sets per week without compromising recovery. Some highly advanced trainees can benefit from more than 20 sets per week for a limited time. Very few can sustain that much volume over the long term.

The chest, another relatively large muscle with multiple subdivisions, seems to do best with slightly less volume than the four I just described.

The hamstrings are in a category of their own. Although they're a large, multijoint muscle, they typically respond better to lower volumes. I find most people have recovery issues if they exceed 12 to 15 sets per week. Why? I think it's because we tend to train them at long lengths, where they're most susceptible to muscle damage.

The biceps and triceps are also unique. If you're a beginner, your arms don't need a lot of isolation work to grow. The triceps work as assistance muscles on chest and shoulder presses, while the biceps assist on pulls and rows.

The opposite is generally true for advanced lifters. Even the heaviest pulls and presses barely move the needle for your biceps and triceps. It takes a higher volume of isolation work to get through that plateau and induce new growth in your arms.

Since this is a common area of confusion, I should note that in Table 8.1, I'm counting only sets of isolation exercises toward biceps and triceps volume. Of course, all presses hit your triceps indirectly, and all pulls and rows hit your biceps indirectly. But I find when

people ask, "How many sets of biceps should I do?" they're usually thinking of curls. So my recommendations in the table account for that.

You may also be surprised at the low recommended volume of direct abdominal work. A little volume goes a long way for beginners, whereas more experienced lifters generally need more to make progress. Keep in mind that even the highest volume of ab training won't guarantee visible abs if you carry a lot of fat around your waist. Conversely, someone who's extremely lean may rock a photo-ready six-pack with hardly any crunches or leg raises, thanks to the indirect stimulation the core receives from exercises that require a braced midsection.

The calves receive a lot of indirect stimulation from common lower-body exercises. As I mentioned in Chapter 5, the gastrocnemius assists the hamstrings on leg curls. They also play a stabilizing role in squats, deadlifts, and step-ups. That's in addition to all the real-life work they get if you spend a lot of time on your feet, especially if you carry loads up and down stairs, do construction or landscaping work, or walk on sand or other soft surfaces.

It's worth mentioning, however, that a lot of lifters struggle to build their calves. If you're one of them, and you've been training them long enough to know the difference between a "stubborn" body part and one that's simply underworked, you may want to experiment with high-volume calf training.

My recommendation for the forearms is to start at zero sets because you work them on every exercise that requires a strong grip. At the top of the list are deadlifts, rows, biceps curls, pull-ups, and chin-ups. You're also working them whenever you pick up dumbbells from the rack and carry them back to your bench or pick them up off the floor and return them to the rack.

Given all that incidental work and the sometimes heavy loads associated with it, direct forearm work is rarely truly required, especially for new lifters. Your forearms will grow in proportion to the muscles they assist. More advanced trainees, of course, may decide they need direct forearm work.

I also start at zero sets for the upper traps and neck muscles, mainly because, in my experience, those muscles tend to be a low priority for most trainees. The upper traps get some indirect work from deadlifts, lateral raises, and rows. But if you want to maximize their development, you need to train them directly with shrugs (an isolation exercise) or upright rows (a compound exercise that hits the upper traps along with the middle and rear deltoids).

Finally, if you're interested in building your neck muscles for functional or aesthetic reasons, I recommend at least three sets of neck flexion (head forward) and three sets of neck extension (head back) per week. More advanced lifters may need up to 10 sets per week of each movement to maximize development.

As a final note on Table 8.1, I want to emphasize that these volumes are intended for those seeking *optimal* gains. If you are not concerned with maximizing your development and instead are looking to build muscle in a time-efficient manner, you could cut the numbers roughly in half and still make respectable progress as long as you're pushing hard.

INDIVIDUALIZING VOLUME

A 2022 study from a team of Brazilian sport scientists represented a major leap forward in our understanding of individualizing training volume.[5] The researchers had participants train each leg with a different protocol for eight weeks. They did 22 sets per week with one leg. With the other, they added 20 percent to what they reported as their typical volume for their quads.

Ten of the study's 16 participants had more quadriceps growth in the leg that did the individualized protocol. Two had better results in the leg that did 22 sets, and the other four had similar growth in both legs.

You can act on this information immediately. If your progress has slowed or stopped altogether, consider increasing the volume of several key exercises by 20 percent. Chances are you'll see new growth without overwhelming your ability to recover.

This strategy, of course, has a practical limit. As I noted in Chapter 7, you can't increase volume every time you reach a plateau. Your workouts would eventually last all day. I recommend this instead: Find your volume sweet spot and stay there until your progress stalls. For most lifters, "just right" volume is around 10 to 20 sets per body part per week. But it's a little less for some people (perhaps 6 to 10 sets). For a rare few, especially the most advanced trainees, it's more (15 to 25 sets).

If your suggested volume sweet spot results in a plateau after several months of training, try adding about 20 percent to your current baseline. If that's obviously too much—you lose strength or feel chronically banged up—dial it back below your previous baseline. If you start making progress with lower volume, consider that your sweet spot.

Conversely, if you make progress with higher volume and have no problems with recovery,

that's your sweet spot. Stay there as long as you continue making progress. Once things truly stall, consider another slight increase in volume.

I've summarized the process of assessing progress and plateaus with the flow chart in Figure 8.3.

Figure 8.3

How to deal with stalled progress

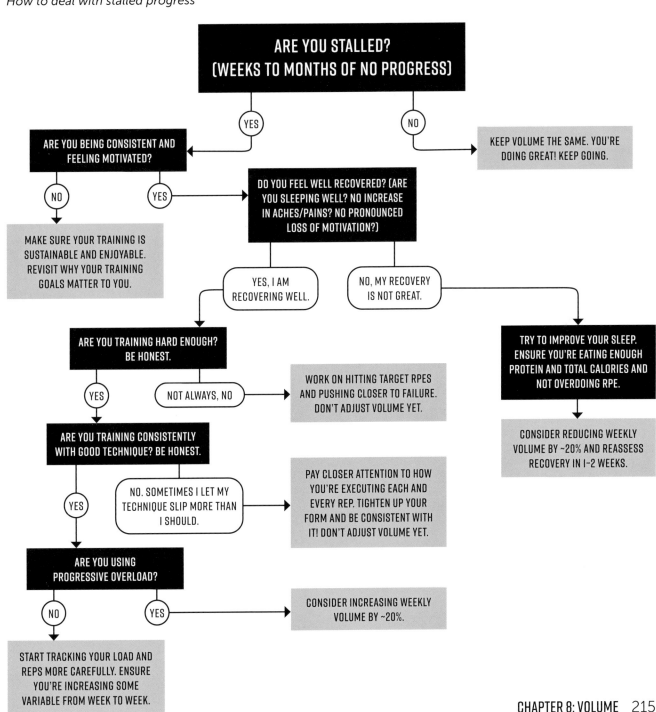

INCORPORATING VOLUME CYCLING AND SPECIALIZATION PHASES

Let's return to the time problem. Few of you reading this are professional bodybuilders. You have jobs, families, and any number of real-life responsibilities and interests. As passionate as you are about your workouts, there's only so much time and energy you can set aside for them.

To be sure, many trainees can add 20 percent more volume without losing their job or jeopardizing a relationship. And most lifters can make better use of their time in the gym through efficiency and effort. But some, especially the truly advanced, have reached their limit. If you're one of them, you know you can't train longer, harder, or smarter. Your only choice is to try something different.

That's when you can try volume cycling and specialization phases.

Volume cycling is when you increase volume for a limited time (usually four to eight weeks) with the goal of forcing new muscle growth. Because size is easier to maintain than build, you can return to your normal volume after your high-volume period without losing your new gains. After four to eight weeks to fully recover, you can try another higher-volume cycle.

I should note that volume cycling is an idea that makes sense in theory and, at least anecdotally, in practice among high-level natural bodybuilders. Still, we don't yet have enough research to say it's evidence-based.

Specialization phases are similar to higher-volume cycles. Instead of adding sets across your entire program, you increase volume by 20 to 40 percent for just one or two body parts at a time.

Let's say you want to build your chest even more than you already have across years of hard training. (Again, this assumes you're an advanced trainee.) Instead of doing your customary 12 sets per week, you do 15 to 17 sets per week during your specialization phase.

As a rule, the more you boost volume, the shorter the specialization phase should be. It can be as brief as four weeks for a 40 percent increase in weekly sets or as long as 12 weeks for a smaller bump. If you choose, you can then begin a new specialization phase for another muscle.

WHAT ABOUT MINIMALIST TRAINING?

So far in this chapter, I've mainly focused on volume in the context of maximizing muscle growth, even if squeezing out those gains requires more time in the gym and a bigger investment of both physical and cognitive energy. However, that's not a universal approach to training.

Many lifters, including some of you, would be perfectly satisfied with slower progress and less-than-maximal gains if it meant spending less time in the gym and having more energy for other interests and obligations. I respect that,

and I have great news for anyone who feels that way: The minimum volume required to build muscle is actually quite low.

A 2017 meta-analysis found that study participants who did just 1 to 4 sets per week built nearly two-thirds as much muscle as participants who did 10 or more sets per week, as shown in Figure 8.4.[6] That finding, however, comes with a caveat: Thirteen of the 15 studies included in the review used untrained participants.

Figure 8.4

Comparing the relative amount of hypertrophy from 1 to 4 sets and 5 to 9 sets per week to 10 or more sets per week

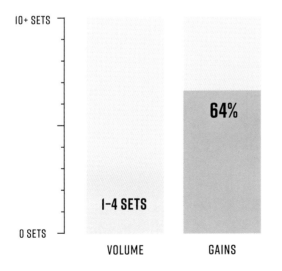
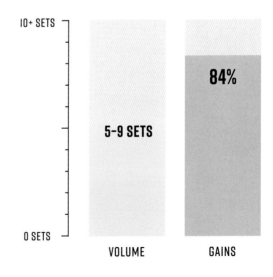

The two studies that used trained volunteers offer more equivocal findings. A 2002 study found no difference in hypertrophy between participants who did 1 or 3 sets of each exercise.[7] But I should note that the training program—three workouts a week for three weeks—was designed primarily for strength development. As you'd expect, the lifters who did more sets gained more strength.

The other study on trained subjects was from 1997 and found that participants who did low (3 sets per muscle group per week), moderate (6 sets), or high (12 sets) volume made similar gains in muscle, strength, and power during a ten-week program.[8] The gains were slightly better among those who did higher volume, but the differences didn't reach statistical significance.

Remember that I'm talking about *average* gains in all these studies. That means some individual participants made bigger gains than the composite results show, whereas some did worse.

It's also worth keeping in mind that participants in strength-training studies, more often than not, are pushed *hard*. Really hard. They usually hit technical failure on every set, and the research team adjusts their loads from workout to workout (and sometimes set to set) to make sure they're always within the study's parameters. RPE 9 is the *minimum* in many of these studies. Look around your gym and count the number of people who appear to be training with that kind of effort. You probably won't run out of fingers.

But while all-out effort is unusual for typical lifters in a typical workout, it's imperative for anyone who wants to maximize their gains with minimal volume. Each set takes on far more importance than it would in a higher-volume program.

UNDERSTANDING HOW VOLUME, EFFORT, AND FREQUENCY ARE INEXTRICABLY LINKED

So far, I've mostly talked about each rung of the Muscle Ladder as a stand-alone subject, but the higher you go, the harder it is to consider any of it in isolation. Effort (the third rung), volume (the fifth rung), and frequency (the sixth rung, which I cover in the next chapter) aren't independent variables. How you deploy each one depends on what you're doing with the others.

In this chapter, for example, I've offered ballpark estimates of the ideal volume for each muscle. But if you do most of your sets at RPE 4 or 5, forget maximizing your gains with 10 to 20 sets. Fifty sets might not be enough.

On the other hand, if you're consistently training with blood-vessel-bursting intensity, and your easiest sets are still at an RPE of 9 or more, my generic volume recommendations may be too much. Your best gains might come with a slightly lower volume.

Volume and effort, in other words, are two sides of an equation. When you push forward with one, you often need to pull back on the other.

That brings us to the next intermediating variable: frequency. The way you distribute your volume can have a big effect on your effort.

That's the subject of Chapter 9.

CHAPTER 9

TRAINING SPLITS & TRAINING FREQUENCY

HOW OFTEN SHOULD I LIFT?

Every day, in just about any gym, you'll hear this question: "What are you training today?" The usual responses are chest, back, or (if they seem particularly smug) legs.

The question assumes the other person is doing a training split. Their answer hints at what kind of split they use.

For example, if they reply with one or two specific muscles, you know they're doing a body-part split and primarily interested in hypertrophy. If they say "bench" (or "squat" or "deadlift"), you know they're a powerlifter. If they reply with a technical description of movement patterns ("hip-dominant," "vertical push-pull"), they're doing a functional routine to improve strength and performance.

BODY-PART SPLITS

A lifter new to training splits will often start by working a single body part each day. It might look something like this:

Monday	Chest
Tuesday	Back
Wednesday	Legs
Thursday	Shoulders
Friday	Arms & abs
Saturday	Rest
Sunday	Rest

This is a basic *body-part split.* Some would tauntingly call it a "bro split." A coach might describe it as a one-time-per-week training frequency because you focus on each body part just once, even though you're in the gym five days. The general idea is that the best way to build a muscle is to utterly destroy it on its dedicated training day and then give it a full week off to recover and grow before you destroy it again.

You can probably see some of the limitations of this approach.

First, most muscles don't need a full week to recover. They typically repair themselves and recover their strength in three to five days. As for muscle growth, research shows that post-workout muscle protein synthesis remains elevated for forty-eight to seventy-two hours in novice lifters.[1] For experienced trainees, it's more like twenty-four hours.

So waiting seven days between training sessions for any given body part is not only unnecessary but it's probably counterproductive. The data implies you could get faster results by hitting individual muscles more often.

However, I don't want to overstate this point. It's not clear that short-term post-workout protein synthesis is the best marker of long-term muscle growth. Some evidence shows that once-a-week training for a given muscle can be just as effective as more frequent workouts, especially for less experienced lifters.[2]

The second and more damning limitation of the basic body-part split is that it's a less-than-ideal way to distribute volume throughout the week. The more experienced you are, the bigger a problem it becomes.

Remember what I said in Chapter 8: For new lifters, 10 sets per week is a good volume target for the major muscle groups. But the longer you train, the more volume you need to make progress. Ten to 20 sets per week is usually the sweet spot for intermediate to advanced lifters (with a few exceptions for smaller muscles). Elite lifters may require 20 to 30 sets per week to see progress in certain muscles. It would be extremely difficult to squeeze that kind of volume into a single training session.

To illustrate what I mean, let's consider what Back Day—Tuesday in our sample body-part split—might look like for a beginner, intermediate, and advanced lifter.

Beginner

Goal: 10 sets per week (back volume only)

> Lat pulldown: 3 sets × 10 reps
> Barbell row: 3 sets × 8 reps
> Cable pullover: 2 sets × 15 reps
> Rope face pull: 2 sets × 15 reps

Total sets: 10

This is a pretty solid back workout. It shouldn't take too much time or leave you feeling absolutely destroyed by the end of the session.

Intermediate

Goal: 10 to 20 sets per week (back volume only)

Lat pulldown: 4 sets × 10 to 12 reps
Barbell row: 4 sets × 8 to 10 reps
Cable pullover: 4 sets × 15 to 20 reps
Rope face pull: 3 sets × 15 to 20 reps

Total sets: 15

As you can see, I chose 15 sets—the middle of the range—for this back workout. It's still a reasonable volume for a single training session, although your muscles will probably feel smoked by the time you get to the face pulls. Assuming all sets are hard, you'd expect technique to suffer by the final rows and pullovers. Bottom line: This is a lot to handle in a single workout.

Advanced

Goal: 15 to 30 sets per week (back volume only)

Lat pulldown: 5 sets × 10 to 12 reps
Barbell row: 5 sets × 8 to 10 reps
Cable pullover: 5 sets × 15 to 20 reps
Rope face pull: 5 sets × 15 to 20 reps
Seated cable row: 5 sets × 12 to 15 reps

Total sets: 25

Even for an advanced trainee, 25 sets is a *massive* amount of volume for a single workout. Performance will inevitably decline as it drags on. By the time you get near the end, you will find it nearly impossible to maintain a high level of effort. This means much of your training session will probably fall into the "junk volume"

category—wasted sets that contribute little (or maybe nothing) to your development.

Your goal, no matter your training split, is *effective* volume—doing each set with appropriate effort to ensure it effectively stimulates muscle growth.

Thus, a body-part split can work well enough when you're a new lifter. (Although it's not necessarily the best choice, as you'll see.) But the more experience you have and the more volume you need to make progress, the less effective it is to cram all of it into a single training session.

Let's consider some alternatives.

UPPER/LOWER SPLITS

If I had to recommend just one training split for anyone interested in building muscle and strength, it'd probably be this one. I like it for three reasons:

First, you're more likely to develop proportionally by balancing upper- and lower-body training. Second, training each major muscle group twice weekly makes your volume more sensibly distributed. Third, you can easily customize your workouts to accommodate a changing schedule.

FOUR-DAY-PER-WEEK UPPER/LOWER SPLIT

Monday	Upper body 1
Tuesday	Lower body 1
Wednesday	Rest
Thursday	Upper body 2
Friday	Lower body 2
Saturday	Rest
Sunday	Rest

You can see that you train your entire upper body on Monday and Thursday and your entire lower body on Tuesday and Friday. Let's revisit how the weekly distribution of back training might look for beginner and intermediate lifters using this upper/lower split.

Beginner

Goal: 10 sets per week (back volume only)

Split: 5 sets on Monday, 5 sets on Thursday

> Monday:
>   Lat pulldown: 3 sets × 10 reps
>   Rope face pull: 2 sets × 15 reps
>
> Thursday:
>   Barbell row: 3 sets × 8 reps
>   Cable pullover: 2 sets × 15 reps

Intermediate

Goal: 15 sets per week (back volume only)

Split: 8 sets on Monday, 7 sets on Thursday

> Monday:
>   Lat pulldown: 4 sets × 10 to 12 reps
>   Rope face pull: 4 sets × 15 to 20 reps
>
> Thursday:
>   Barbell row: 4 sets × 8 to 10 reps
>   Cable pullover: 3 sets × 15 to 20 reps

SIX-DAY-PER-WEEK UPPER/LOWER SPLIT

Monday	Upper body 1
Tuesday	Lower body 1
Wednesday	Upper body 2
Thursday	Lower body 2
Friday	Upper body 3
Saturday	Lower body 3
Sunday	Rest

Four workouts a week might not be enough for an advanced lifter doing 20-plus sets for some major muscle groups. That's when a six-day upper/lower split can be helpful. Even though you have just one rest day, you still give your upper- and lower-body muscles forty-eight to seventy-two hours to recover before working them again. And by distributing your volume across three workouts instead of two, you're not committing crimes against any single muscle group in any given workout.

Advanced

Goal: 25 sets per week (back volume only)

Split: 9 sets on Monday, 8 sets on Wednesday, 8 sets on Friday

Monday:

Pull-up: 3 sets × 6 to 8 reps
Seated cable row: 3 sets × 12 to 15 reps
Rope face pull: 3 sets × 15 to 20 reps

Wednesday:

Barbell row: 4 sets × 8 to 10 reps
Lat pulldown: 4 sets × 10 to 12 reps

Friday:

Single-arm pulldown: 4 sets × 12 to 15 reps
Cable pullover: 4 sets × 12 to 15 reps

STRENGTH VERSUS HYPERTROPHY EMPHASIS

Another way to use an upper/lower split is to target different types of adaptations in different workouts. So, if you're training four times a week, you could focus on strength development in two of those workouts, doing lower-rep sets with heavier weights. You could do higher-rep sets with moderate weights in the other two workouts. That would allow you to reach a deeper level of fatigue and, in the process, develop more muscular endurance.

Both styles of training contribute to hypertrophy, of course. But they do more than that. In addition to building muscle, the strength days will help you get stronger, and the hypertrophy days will improve your muscular endurance. Working with heavier loads improves bone density and increases the tensile strength in your connective tissues, providing a more solid base for additional muscle mass. Working with higher reps also improves muscular endurance, giving you a cardiometabolic base for longer, more productive workouts.

Here's how it would look:

Upper-body workout 1: Strength-focused (low-moderate reps and heavier weights)

Lower-body workout 1: Strength-focused (low-moderate reps and heavier weights)

Upper-body workout 2: Endurance-focused (moderate-high reps and lighter weights)

Lower-body workout 2: Endurance-focused (moderate-high reps and lighter weights)

In exercise science, this would be described as daily undulating periodization (DUP), a topic I'll cover in more detail in Chapter 13.

FULL-BODY SPLITS

Like upper/lower splits, full-body splits can be appropriate for any level of lifter and are easily modifiable as your weekly volume needs change. Full-body routines can take many different forms, as shown in Figure 9.1.

Figure 9.1

Example schedule for full-body splits

	1X/WEEK	2X/WEEK	3X/WEEK	4X/WEEK	5X/WEEK
Monday	Rest	Full body 1	Full body 1	Full body 1	Full body 1
Tuesday	Rest	Rest	Rest	Full body 2	Full body 2
Wednesday	Rest	Rest	Full body 2	Rest	Full body 3
Thursday	Rest	Full body 2	Rest	Full body 3	Full body 4
Friday	Rest	Rest	Full body 3	Full body 4	Full body 5
Saturday	Rest	Rest	Rest	Rest	Rest
Sunday	Full body	Rest	Rest	Rest	Rest

→ **MORE ADVANCED** →

At the minimalist end of the spectrum is one full-body workout per week. It might be the only option for someone whose weekday schedule is so jam-packed they can only work out on Saturday or Sunday. I assume that describes very few readers of *The Muscle Ladder*.

Practically speaking, the lowest frequency I normally prescribe is two full-body workouts per week. It's a viable option for beginners or early intermediates who don't require a lot of volume to make progress. It might also be the best option for someone who's so busy they can't get to the gym more often.

However, if the schedule isn't an issue, most beginners will do very well with three full-body workouts a week. That schedule can also be ideal for an older lifter who may need more recovery time between workouts.

More experienced lifters with higher volume requirements can do four or even five full-body workouts weekly. That means working each major muscle group at least three times a week, which moves you into a new category: *high-frequency training*.

HIGH-FREQUENCY, FULL-BODY TRAINING

Over the past few years, high-frequency training has become a contentious topic within the science-based lifting community. Proponents say it stimulates new growth in advanced trainees. Critics say there's no difference between high- and low-frequency training *as long as volume is the same.* That was the conclusion of a 2019 meta-analysis, which analyzed the results of 25 studies and found no impact of training frequency on hypertrophy.[3]

To be clear, this debate applies *only* to experienced, intermediate-to-advanced lifters. If you're one of them, high-frequency, full-body training can offer a viable structure to hit the volume you need to make progress.

Let's say the target volume for your chest is 15 sets per week. On a body-part split, your once-weekly chest workout might look something like this:

Chest day
Bench press: 3 sets × 6 to 8 reps
Incline dumbbell press: 3 sets × 8 to 10 reps
Weighted dip: 3 sets × 10 to 12 reps
Cable crossover: 3 sets × 12 to 15 reps
Pec deck: 3 sets × 15 to 20 reps

That's a lot for one day. But here's what it could look like if you spread that same volume across five full-body workouts:

Full body 1
Bench press: 3 sets × 6 to 8 reps

Full body 2
Incline dumbbell press: 3 sets × 8 to 10 reps

Full body 3
Cable crossover: 3 sets × 12 to 15 reps

Full body 4
Weighted dip: 3 sets × 10 to 12 reps

Full body 5
Pec deck: 3 sets × 15 to 20 reps

As you can see, on a high-frequency, full-body split, you do just one chest exercise daily. That allows you to do higher-quality work because built-up fatigue won't affect your performance.

Look at full-body 3, for example. Your entire chest component is 3 sets of cable crossovers. Even if you do those crossovers toward the end of the workout—following squats, deadlifts, chin-ups, or whatever else—you'll still be able to do them with more intensity than if they followed 6 sets of barbell and dumbbell presses and 3 sets of weighted dips.

I say all this while acknowledging that the evidence supporting high-frequency training is both scant and equivocal. I've had success with it, and many of my clients and followers have come to love it. If nothing else, it's a novel way to train and a great way to keep your program fresh and interesting.

But I don't want to oversell it. The research shows that you can achieve about the same results with any split as long as you hit your volume target.[4]

Again, I don't recommend high-frequency, full-body training for anyone just starting. You can get great results with two or three full-body workouts a week. If you want to train more frequently, try an upper/lower split four days a week. Save the high-frequency option for when you're close to your genetic potential and need higher volume to get even closer.

If you're a good candidate for high-frequency, full-body training, here are a few ways to get the most out of it:

- Keep per-session volumes low. Generally, 3 to 5 sets per muscle per workout will be plenty.

- Keep RPEs in the 5 to 7 zone for the first one to two weeks of high-frequency training. Because you'll be training the same muscle groups on consecutive days, pushing too hard will just make you sore and interfere with your training the next day. Soreness impedes performance without contributing to muscle growth. (And you don't want to put that kind of stress on your joints before they're ready for it.) After a couple weeks of high-frequency training, a phenomenon known as the *repeated bout effect* will kick in, and you'll no longer get sore after training. You can then increase RPEs to the normal 7 to 10 zone.

- Organize your exercises strategically to include a mix of loads and rep ranges in each workout. Put another way, don't stack all your most challenging compound exercises on one day. For example, if you do barbell squats on Monday, you might want to do barbell bench presses and rows on Wednesday and save your deadlifts for Friday.

- You also want to strategically separate your heaviest exercises for each body part. So if your quad training includes squats, leg presses, and leg extensions, and you do squats on Monday, you could do leg presses on Wednesday and leg extensions on Friday. It would be less wise to do heavy squats on Monday and then heavy leg presses on Tuesday.

- As you can tell from the previous example, you don't *have* to hit each muscle group in every workout. Three exercises for quads are likely enough as long as the combined volume matches your target. The same goes for hamstrings and calves.

- Expect to do a lot of tinkering with your routine, especially in the first few weeks. Some combinations of exercises may be too much for your back, shoulders, elbows, or knees. You may find your hand and wrist muscles feel fried because you included too many grip-intensive exercises on consecutive days. Small tweaks to your workouts can yield big benefits in terms of performance and recovery.

You'll find a sample high-frequency, full-body routine in Chapter 15.

PUSH/PULL/LEGS (PPL) SPLITS

Push/pull/legs (PPL) splits have exploded in popularity in recent years, and for good reason! I think of the PPL split as a sort of upgraded body-part split. Instead of dedicating each training day to just one or two muscles, a PPL routine targets a limited combination of complementary muscles each day:

- **Push days:** You train chest, shoulders, and triceps on push days. Those muscles are primarily responsible for pushing something away from your body (like chest or shoulder presses) or pushing your body away from something (like push-ups and dips).

- **Pull days:** You train back, biceps, and rear delts on pull days. Those muscles are primarily responsible for pulling something toward your body (like rows and face pulls) or pulling your body toward something (like pull-ups and chin-ups). Some coaches include deadlifts on pull days because they activate the lats, traps, and lower back to different degrees. I think deadlifts usually fit better on leg days, given that lower-body muscles are the prime movers.

- **Leg days:** As you would guess, you train quads, hamstrings, glutes, calves, and any other lower-body muscles on leg day.

- **Abs:** Because abs don't fit neatly into any of these categories, I recommend doing them on whatever day has the shortest workout. Alternatively, you can spread your ab exercises across two or three days.

I also generally recommend running the workouts in this order: pull first, then push, then legs. That's simply because your back muscles will get hammered on pull day and then have to do a lot of stabilizing work on leg day, too.

Placing the push day between the pull day and the leg day gives your back muscles a full day of recovery before bracing for legs. Despite the reordering, I still call it a push/pull/legs split because that's the name the lifting community uses.

There are two ways to approach a push/pull/legs split. The most common option is to work out six days per week:

PPL split option 1	
Monday	Pull 1
Tuesday	Push 1
Wednesday	Legs 1
Thursday	Pull 2
Friday	Push 2
Saturday	Legs 2
Sunday	Rest

Six consecutive workouts with just one rest day isn't ideal for everyone. Even if your schedule allows you to spend that much time in the gym, your body may not be on board. The second option is to take a rest day after each three-workout cycle. It might look like this:

PPL split option 2	Week 1	Week 2	Week 3
Monday	Pull 1	Rest	Legs 2
Tuesday	Push 1	Pull 1	Rest
Wednesday	Legs 1	Push 1	
Thursday	Rest	Legs 1	
Friday	Push 2	Rest	
Saturday	Legs 2	Pull 2	
Sunday	Rest	Push 2	

	MONDAY	TUESDAY	WEDNESDAY	THURSDAY	FRIDAY	SATURDAY	SUNDAY
WEEK 1	1 PULL	2 PUSH	3 LEGS	4 (REST)	5 PULL	6 PUSH	7 LEGS
WEEK 2	8 (REST)	9 PULL	10 PUSH	11 LEGS	12 (REST)	13 PULL	14 PUSH
WEEK 3	15 LEGS	16 (REST)	17	18	19	20	21

As you can see, the drawback with option 2 is that your workout schedule changes every week. This may not be ideal for those who prefer set schedules. Some weeks, you'll be training on Monday, and other weeks, you'll be resting on Monday. This doesn't bother me, but my work schedule is quite flexible.

The third option is to set your training days in stone but be flexible with the workouts you do.

PPL split option 3	Week 1	Week 2
Monday	Pull 1	Legs 2
Tuesday	Push 1	Pull 1
Wednesday	Legs 1	Push 1
Thursday	Rest	Rest
Friday	Pull 2	Legs 1
Saturday	Push 2	Pull 2
Sunday	Rest	Rest

With this version, you work out and rest on the same days each week. Each Monday, you simply pick up where you left off.

The main advantage of all versions of the PPL split over the body-part split is that it allows you to train each muscle group twice weekly. (Or twice every eight days, in the case of options 2 and 3.)

You also have three or four days to recover before training the same muscles again, which means you don't need to manage fatigue and recovery as carefully as you do on a high-frequency full-body split.

The PPL split is similar to the upper/lower split in that you also have the opportunity to train with a slightly different emphasis earlier in the week versus later in the week. For example, on your first push day of the week, you could target your chest more; on your second, you could target your shoulders and triceps more. On your first pull day of the week, you could target the lats more; on the second, you could target the mid-traps more. On your first leg day, you could target your quads more; on the second leg day, you could target the hamstrings and glutes more. In practice, it could look something like this:

Leg day 1: Main emphasis quads; secondary emphasis hamstrings, glutes, and calves

Push day 1: Main emphasis chest; secondary emphasis shoulders, triceps, and abs

Pull day 1: Main emphasis lats; secondary emphasis mid-traps, biceps, and rear delts

Leg day 2: Main emphasis glutes and hamstrings; secondary emphasis quads and calves

Push day 2: Main emphasis shoulders; secondary emphasis chest and triceps

Pull day 2: Main emphasis mid-traps; secondary emphasis lats, biceps, and rear delts

However, there is a slight drawback with a PPL split: You're training upper-body muscles twice for every workout that trains lower-body muscles. This can make the PPL split slightly upper-body biased in practice. Of course, you shouldn't be concerned as long as your weekly volume is accounted for on the front end. Still, you may find that your leg days are longer than your push or pull days to get enough volume in and achieve a balanced routine.

Despite this, I can see why PPL splits are so popular. They give you the high volume and fun workouts of a body-part split with the frequency advantages of an upper/lower split.

HYBRID SPLITS

After reading about the splits I've discussed so far, you might have a logical question: If all the splits I've covered offer distinct advantages and disadvantages, why not build a Frankenstein's split by combining the best parts of each one? The answer is that you can. They're called hybrid splits.

HYBRID SPLIT 1

I can personally endorse this split, which Dr. Layne Norton popularized. It's the one I used to train for the 2012 Canadian Nationals in natural bodybuilding, where I won the lightweight class.

Dr. Norton's split combines the best of upper/lower and push/pull/legs splits:

Monday	Upper body
Tuesday	Lower body
Wednesday	Rest
Thursday	Push
Friday	Pull
Saturday	Legs
Sunday	Rest

In Dr. Norton's original routine, the upper/lower days early in the week target strength with relatively heavy weights and low to moderate reps. The push/pull/legs days are more hypertrophy focused with moderate weights and medium to high reps. You can find a sample routine for this split with the training programs in Chapter 15.

HYBRID SPLIT 2

This one, which I also like, combines a full-body routine with an upper/lower split for people who prefer to train three times a week:

Monday	Full body
Tuesday	Rest
Wednesday	Upper body
Thursday	Rest
Friday	Lower body
Saturday	Rest
Sunday	Rest

Because you hit all your muscle groups twice in your three workouts, it's a nice option for lifters who prefer to spend less time in the gym but still like the feel of a split routine. It also works great for older trainees who may need more time to recover between training sessions.

The drawback, of course, is that it's hard for intermediate to advanced lifters to pack all the volume they need into just three workouts. That problem is easy enough to resolve—just add another full-body workout in place of a rest day:

Monday	Full body
Tuesday	Rest
Wednesday	Upper body
Thursday	Lower body
Friday	Rest
Saturday	Full body
Sunday	Rest

DOUBLE-SPLIT ROUTINES

Professional athletes, people whose living depends on their ability to play a sport at the highest level, often train twice a day. The same is true of elite competitive bodybuilders. At that level, their training volume is so high, they sometimes need six ninety-minute workouts a week to reach their volume targets.

Some find that volume level more manageable with 12 weekly workouts—two daily, with a meal and perhaps a nap.

Here's what one day of upper-body training might look like on a double-split routine:

Monday morning (9:00 to 9:45 a.m.)
    Lat pulldown: 3 sets × 10 to 12 reps
    Flat dumbbell press: 3 sets × 8 to 10 reps
    Dumbbell lateral raise: 4 sets × 12 to 15 reps

Monday afternoon (3:00 to 3:45 p.m.)
    Chest-supported T-bar row: 3 sets × 12 to 15 reps
    EZ-bar biceps curl: 4 sets × 6 to 8 reps
    Overhead cable triceps extension: 3 sets × 10 to 12 reps
    Reverse pec deck: 2 sets × 15 to 20 reps

If you have all day to train (and recover from training), two forty-five-minute workouts might be a lot more appealing than a single ninety-minute session.

There's limited research on double-split routines.[5] This makes sense, given the small number of bodybuilders for whom they're both appealing and practical. The evidence from those studies doesn't make a strong argument for or against two-a-day workouts.

At the very least, I suspect double-split programs are equivalent to conventional splits as long as they're matched for volume. I know that's not exactly a ringing endorsement, but I do think they could be a game-changer for a few select people. If your schedule is flexible enough for you to try it, you can decide for yourself if it works better than a single daily workout.

MY FINAL WORD ON FREQUENCY (FOR NOW)

If you take away one message from this chapter, I hope it's that there's no "best" training split. They all work as long as you meet four conditions:

- You train with enough volume.

- You train with enough effort.

- You give your body enough time to recover.

- You do all of that consistently over time.

That doesn't mean every split I described is equally effective for everyone reading *The Muscle Ladder.* Different splits work better for different lifters at different stages of their training journey.

Even the heavily derided "bro" split works. A 2013 survey of competitive male bodybuilders found that more than two-thirds—69 percent—trained each muscle group just once per week.[6] The bro split lives!

Would these physique athletes have gotten better results doing upper/lower, PPL, or full-body splits?

It's hard to say. The best split for you, more often than not, is the one you enjoy the most or the one that allows you to keep training hard the longest. (As is often the case, all roads lead back to sustainability.)

As for training frequency, research tells us it's a relatively minor factor in the pursuit of hypertrophy.[7] Frequency is bookkeeping—how you organize your program. A well-organized program allows you to do the work you need to do with the time you have.

The next chapter turns its attention back to the individual exercise level. In fact, it addresses what may be the first question any lifter asks when approaching an exercise: "How heavy should I lift?"

CHAPTER 10

LOAD & REP RANGES

HOW HEAVY SHOULD I LIFT?

What is the best rep range for building muscle? Is it better to lift light weights for high reps? Or heavier weights for low reps? Or something in between?

Now that you've reached the seventh rung of the Muscle Ladder, you shouldn't be surprised when I say that the science on this topic is pretty straightforward. I've already explained that a wide range of rep zones are more or less equally effective for building muscle as long as you train hard enough and hit your volume targets.

That concept shouldn't be surprising if you understand what causes muscle to grow in the first place. Recall that high levels of tension must be reached for muscle to grow. Some people mistakenly interpret this to mean that heavier weights must be better because heavier weights generate higher levels of tension, but this isn't exactly right. It's true that heavier weights generate higher levels of tension faster than lighter weights. In other words, you reach higher levels of tension earlier in the set when lifting a heavy weight than you do when lifting a light weight. However, as long as you push the light weight sufficiently close to failure, the muscle recruits all available fibers and eventually reaches the same level of tension as what can be reached with the heavy weight.

Randomized controlled trials repeatedly bear this out: With an appropriate amount of volume, almost all the typical rep ranges can build muscle as long as you push yourself sufficiently close to failure.

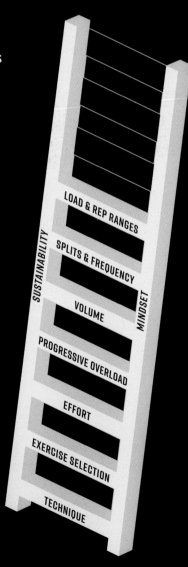

LOAD & REP RANGES

SPLITS & FREQUENCY

VOLUME

PROGRESSIVE OVERLOAD

EFFORT

EXERCISE SELECTION

TECHNIQUE

SUSTAINABILITY

MINDSET

REP RANGE RESEARCH

A 2016 study by Morton and colleagues compared a group doing 8 to 12 reps to a group doing 20 to 25 reps.[1] Participants took all 3 sets of each exercise to failure for twelve weeks. There was no difference in muscle hypertrophy between groups.

Another 2016 study compared a group doing approximately 8 reps to a group alternating rep ranges week to week by doing about 8 reps one week and 30 to 40 reps the next.[2] Once again, the participants took all sets to failure, and there was no difference in hypertrophy.

As a final example, a third 2016 study compared a group doing 8 to 12 reps to a group doing a broad mixture of rep ranges (one session in the 2 to 4 range, another in the 8 to 12 range, and a third session in the 20 to 30 range).[3] All sets were taken to failure, and, as you probably guessed, there was no difference in hypertrophy.

This is why lifters succeed with so many different types of routines. Given sufficient effort and volume, all routines can work.

Or I should say *almost* all of them work. Some weights really are too light to build muscle. For example, according to one 2018 study, 20 percent of your one-rep max (1RM) is too light.[4] What seems to happen with ridiculously light weights is that tension never quite gets high enough to force all your muscle fibers into action. Instead, your muscles cycle through the same fibers, no matter how many reps you do. (Think of it like line changes in a hockey game; the same players are never on the ice long enough to get completely fatigued.)

We don't know exactly where the cutoff is, but I think it's reasonable to say this: If you aren't on the brink of technical failure by your thirtieth rep, the weight is probably too light.

Some argue it works the same way at the other extreme: If you can't do at least 3 reps, that weight is too *heavy* to build muscle. I don't know if that's necessarily true on paper, but it often is in practice. There isn't enough evidence to say if really heavy sets of just 1 to 2 reps are actually worse for muscle growth when matched for volume, but they often do end up being less hypertrophic in practice because of recovery factors.

The available research suggests that any rep range from 3 to 30 can stimulate muscle growth to a similar degree, as long as effort and volume are matched. But think about how hard it would be to match effort and volume across that spectrum. Just because it's *possible* to build the same amount of muscle with low reps as with high reps doesn't mean it's a good idea to do a lot of work at either extreme.

High reps—15 to 30—make sense in some circumstances. Low reps—1 to 5—make sense in others. But in most circumstances, 6 to 15 reps is the most practical and productive range for hypertrophy.

HIGH-REP REALITIES

Let's start with the number one downside of high-rep training: It's exhausting. Think about doing a set of 6 squats to failure. I mean *true failure,* where you attempt a seventh rep but have to dump the weight because you're completely stuck at the bottom. Pretty hard, right?

Now, think about doing a set of 30 squats to true failure. You get the twenty-ninth rep but have to dump the bar on the thirtieth. Even if you've never done what I just described, you can most likely appreciate why the 30-rep set would feel much harder. I mean soul-crushingly hard. Not only that, the recovery demand is considerably greater.

What's the reward for putting yourself through that ordeal? The same as the reward for doing 6 reps to failure. It's just 1 set in your body's hypertrophic ledger, despite the enormous effort it took to perform the high-rep set and the outsized fatigue and muscle damage that follow.

Another issue with high double-digit repetitions: The higher your rep count, the harder it is to estimate RPE or reps in reserve. If you aim to finish your sets with just two RIR—RPE 8—how do you know when you've reached it? The higher your rep target, the more likely you stop shy of your RPE target because high-rep sets *feel* hard, even when you're not yet close enough to failure to maximize gains. If you consistently stop short, you aren't maximizing the muscle-building potential of your workouts.

Of course, this issue goes away if you take your high-rep sets all the way to failure, but then you're back to the first problem: High-rep sets are often unbearably fatiguing, with no additional benefit compared to lower-rep ranges.

That doesn't mean you should never train with high reps. Despite their limitations, they can offer distinct benefits when used strategically. For example, high-rep sets can lead to unbelievable pumps, which is a fun way to finish a workout. They also create higher levels of metabolic stress. That probably won't drive muscle growth on its own, but it may synergistically interact with other growth pathways.

High-rep sets can also be helpful when you're recovering from an injury. If heavy loads give you issues, strip the weight back and do higher-rep work instead. Assuming muscle building is the main goal, you can still get effective growth stimulus with pain-free lighter loads. As you recover, you can gradually increase the weight and decrease the reps again.

Finally, high reps simply work better on some exercises, especially those that isolate smaller muscles. Take your glute medius or your rear delts: Isolating them requires specific movement patterns. You can't easily do those movements with even moderate weights, much less heavy loads. If you try, your form quickly breaks down as you recruit bigger muscles to move the weight. But with high-rep hip abductions or reverse pec deck flies, you can generate a high level of tension in those smaller muscles.

So, while I don't think a hypertrophy program *requires* high-rep sets, I think it's wise to incorporate some work in the range of 15 to 30 reps, but they probably shouldn't comprise more than 10 to 20 percent of your total training volume.

LOW-REP REALITIES

When your goal is to build muscle, it's extremely challenging to hit your volume targets when you train with very low reps.

I'll call a set low-rep if it's in the 1- to 5-rep range. Like high-rep training, low-rep training comes with limitations.

The biggest issue with low-rep training from a muscle-building standpoint is that it makes training with sufficient total volume very challenging. Recall from Chapter 8 that you can use the concept of "hard sets" as a proxy for *rep volume* and *volume load* for hypertrophy purposes. However, this proxy starts to break down when reps are very low because if you're only doing, say, 1 rep as your set, it may technically count as a "hard set" (as long as it's close to a 1RM), but you only did one rep! The total amount of tension over time on a set of 1 rep is so drastically lower than a set of 10 reps that, if you're going to match volume between a 1-rep set and a 10-rep set, it makes more sense to use the original definitions of *rep volume* and *volume load.*

To match volume in this sense, you have to do way more low-rep sets to match the same volume as moderate-rep sets. Consider the volume load between 3 sets of a 1RM on the squat (option A) versus 3 sets of an 8RM on the squat (option B):

Squat option A: 3 sets × 1 rep × 315 lb = **945 lb of volume load**

Squat option B: 3 sets × 8 reps × 250 lb = **6,000 lb of volume load**

To match the volume of these two rep schemes, you'd have to do 19 sets of your 1RM on the squat. Even though volume load isn't a perfect predictor of hypertrophy, in this case, the discrepancy in volume load is too big to ignore.

A 2014 study from Dr. Brad Schoenfeld and colleagues bears this out.[5] This study compared moderate-rep training to very low-rep training. Half the participants did sets of 3 reps on a variety of exercises with heavy weight. The other half of the participants did sets of 10 reps on a variety of exercises with moderate weight.

To match volume load, the group doing 3 reps had to do 7 sets per exercise, whereas the group doing 10 reps only had to do 3 sets per exercise. In practice, this meant that the low-rep workouts took just over one hour to complete, whereas the moderate-rep workouts took an average of 17 minutes.

After eight weeks, the researchers found that the low-rep group gained significantly more strength on the bench press and a little more strength on the squat. No surprise there. Lifting heavy weights makes you better at lifting heavy weights. But both groups added about the same amount of muscle. So while you could interpret this study as showing that both low reps and moderate reps build the same amount of muscle (which they did), that interpretation needs to come with the caveat that the low-rep group had to do more than double the sets to match volume load, *and* their workouts took more than three times as long!

Here's another interesting difference: Two participants in the low-rep group left the study due to injury or fatigue compared to zero dropouts in the moderate-rep group. I don't want to make too much of that point; people leave studies for all kinds of reasons, and we have plenty of data affirming the safety of heavy lifting. I want to note that if you design a program where heavy, low-rep training dominates, the ability to recover may become strained.

Considering all that, I still think you can fit some low-rep training into a hypertrophy program without causing problems. That's especially true if you want to get stronger, which, in my experience, most lifters do. Gaining strength requires some heavy lifting.

It's also possible that low-rep training may potentiate future muscle-building. It seems reasonable to suppose that if you gain strength in the 1- to 6-rep zone, that strength will have some carry-over to more moderate-rep zones, allowing for more overload and, ultimately, continued progress. Granted, this is more of a personal hypothesis than a concept with strong empirical support. Even though some studies suggest that heavy strength training can potentiate muscle growth in future hypertrophy training phases, the findings are mixed.

So, I'll echo what I said in the previous section: When training for hypertrophy, low-rep sets in the 1 to 5 range should comprise about 10 to 20 percent of your total training volume.

THE PRACTICAL HYPERTROPHY REP RANGE

If high-rep sets (15 to 30 reps) make up 10 to 20 percent of your training volume, and low-rep sets (1 to 5 reps) make up 10 to 20 percent, that means moderate-rep sets (6 to 15 reps) should make up the remaining 60 to 80 percent.

If you're more interested in gaining strength, allocate more work to the low-rep zone. If you're less interested in gaining strength and more interested in hypertrophy and muscular endurance, allocate more work to the high-rep zone. See Figure 10.1 for a look at how these rep ranges could be distributed based on your focus.

As I said at the beginning of this chapter, all rep ranges (up to about 30 or 40) offer similar muscle-building potential. Six- to 15-rep sets should occupy most of your training because it's simply the most practical rep range.

Low-rep workouts take more time and may tax the joints more if overdone. High-rep workouts are psychologically challenging and physically exhausting if overdone. High-rep sets also make it harder to gauge RPE, meaning you run a greater risk of undershooting tension. Because of these practical programming concerns, doing more moderate-rep sets is better suited for handling the brunt of the volume. While it may be possible to maximize your muscular potential doing exclusively 6 to 15 reps, I would still recommend including at least some higher-rep work and some lower-rep work for novelty and variety.

Within the practical hypertrophy rep range of 6 to 15, your training can be further subdivided into a low-moderate range of 6 to 10 reps and a moderate-high range of 10 to 15 reps.

Figure 10.1

How to distribute volume across different rep ranges with the primary goal being hypertrophy

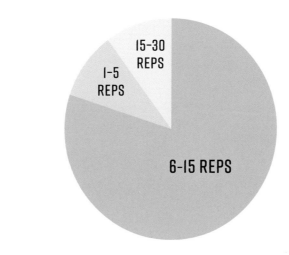

REP RANGES FOR PURE HYPERTROPHY

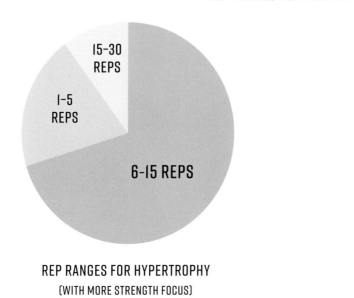

REP RANGES FOR HYPERTROPHY
(WITH MORE STRENGTH FOCUS)

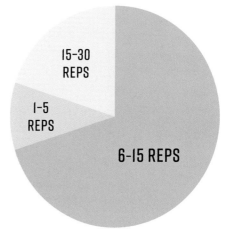

REP RANGES FOR HYPERTROPHY
(WITH MORE MUSCULAR ENDURANCE FOCUS)

Generally, the low end of the practical range—6 to 10 reps—works best with compound exercises that activate a lot of muscle mass. You can focus on improving your technique while also getting stronger on the exercises where you typically care about strength—squat, bench press, deadlift, and overhead press.

The high end of the practical range—10 to 15 reps—is better for exercises that target smaller muscle groups. That includes isolation exercises (like curls, pressdowns, and lateral raises) and some compound movements where you normally want to establish a mind-muscle connection (like face pulls and pulldowns).

A good workout typically includes a mix of both.

WHAT ABOUT STRENGTH?

Hypertrophy is known as a *nonspecific* adaptation. As the old saying goes, "There are many roads to Rome," and there are many ways to build muscle. High reps, low reps, moderate reps—they all can work, as long as you apply enough muscular tension over enough volume.

On the other hand, strength is a *specific* adaptation—one that requires a particular training style. To be more precise, strength is specific to the particular rep range you use. Training with sets of 10 builds your 10-rep max strength, but it probably won't do much for your 1-rep max on that exercise. You need to lift heavy stuff to get good at lifting heavy stuff.

I mean the "get good" part literally. Strength is both an adaptation and a skill, one that's specific to each exercise. To get strong, you need to practice the skill of being strong. Just like doing lay-up drills won't do much for developing your free throw in basketball, doing high-rep leg presses won't do much for increasing your max squat strength. Even though the same muscles are moving the weight, there's a huge gap in the skill required for a max-effort squat.

When training for maximum strength, I recommend allocating your rep ranges like this. (See Figure 10.2 for a visual breakdown.)

- **1 to 5 reps:** Fifty to 80 percent of total training volume. No surprise here; you have to train for the specific skill you want to improve.

- **6 to 15 reps:** Twenty to 40 percent of total training volume. A bigger muscle is usually a stronger muscle, so it makes sense to do some hypertrophy work.

- **15 to 30 reps:** Zero to 10 percent of total training volume. High-rep training doesn't translate well to maximum strength, so it isn't required.

Figure 10.2

How to distribute volume across different rep ranges with the primary goal being strength gain

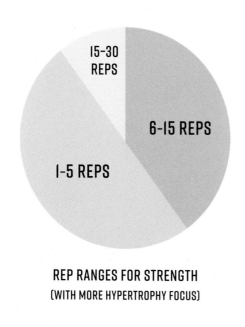

REP RANGES FOR STRENGTH
(WITH MORE HYPERTROPHY FOCUS)

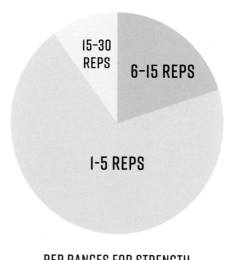

REP RANGES FOR STRENGTH
(WITH LESS HYPERTROPHY FOCUS)

DECIDING HOW HEAVY TO LIFT

As a beginner, deciding how heavy to lift is pretty simple. Start with a light weight and lift it through a complete range of motion until you're comfortable with the exercise. The amount of weight doesn't matter at this point. As I described in Chapter 7, your goal is to increase it over time.

How fast should you increase it?

You may come across detailed formulas based on how advanced you are and what exercise you're doing that tell you how much weight you should add each week. Sometimes, these formulas work, but because there are such big differences in strength between individuals (even of the same training status), I find general formulas too unreliable to recommend in practice.

Instead, I use a simple guess-and-check model. Start with a load you are 100 percent confident you can lift with good form. Once you feel you can confidently perform another 2 or 3 reps on the last set, try increasing the weight in your next workout. You're on the right track as long as you aren't sacrificing technique or range of motion to complete the target amount of sets and reps, and you're reaching a reasonable level of effort.

If you need to cheat to move the weight or reach blood-vessel-bursting levels of effort after the load increase, strip back to the weight you used before. Stick with that for a week or two as you continue to practice good form. After that, you can try the heavier weight again.

When doing relatively light exercises that are harder to overload with weight, remember that you can also try adding a rep to each set. This is where the double progression model I explained in Chapter 7 can be very useful.

I have two other ways to prescribe load for intermediate and advanced trainees: RPE and percentage of one-rep max.

RPE

As you probably recall from Chapter 6, RPE stands for rating of perceived exertion. It's a subjective way to estimate how close your set was to failure. RPE 10 means you couldn't have completed another rep. RPE 9 means you could've done one more, RPE 8 means you could've done two more, and so on.

In addition to telling you how hard you should push it, you can also use RPE to prescribe load. If you know your RPE and rep targets, figuring out how much weight to use is pretty straightforward. If you start too low and reach your rep target without getting close to your RPE target, increase the load for the next set. If you start too high, do the same thing in reverse.

You'll get better at matching your load to your RPE and rep targets over time, but no matter how much experience you have, you'll always have to do some trial and error. It works best if the "trial" part is a little too low. That way, your "error" becomes a warm-up set.

When you come in too hot on the first set and reach failure 2 or more reps short of your target, take some time to recover, reassess, and check your ego. After a solid rest period of at least three to five minutes, lower the weight and get back on track with your workout.

Here are a few ways to get closer the first time:

- Start by doing some warm-up sets to gauge your strength at that particular moment. Do 2 or 3 warm-up sets for compound exercises at the beginning of your workout and 1 warm-up set for smaller-muscle exercises later in the session.

  - If the warm-up sets feel light, you can be a little more assertive with the loads you select for your working sets.

  - If the warm-up sets feel heavy, ease into your first working set with a lighter load than usual. If you're stronger than you expected, no problem. Call it an extra warm-up set and return to your regularly scheduled training. If you hit your RPE and rep targets with the lighter weight, that's your first working set.

- After the first working set, ask yourself what the actual RPE was:

  - If it was within one point of the target RPE in either direction, you obviously selected the appropriate load. Use the same weight for the next set.

  - If the actual RPE was more than one point *higher* than the target RPE (it was too hard), decrease the load by 5 to 10 percent or whatever amount you think will get you in the correct RPE zone for the next set.

  - If the actual RPE was more than one point *lower* than the target RPE (it was too easy), increase the load by 5 to 10 percent or whatever amount you think will get you in the correct RPE zone for the next set.

Let's look at how I would select a weight at the beginning of a new program.

The program calls for 6 reps of barbell biceps curls at RPE 8. On a good day, I know I can usually get 6 to 8 reps with 100 pounds. So, I'll use that as my baseline, but the weight I use depends on what happens next.

I do my first warm-up set with 40 pounds for 6 reps. It feels easy, as I expect. My second warm-up set of 4 reps with 70 pounds also feels good.

For my first working set, I decide to go for 100 pounds. I get 6 reps, but it's a grinder. My target was RPE 8, which felt more like RPE 9 or 10. I was too ambitious, and that's okay.

After resting for about three minutes, I select 90 pounds for my second set. Once again, I get 6 reps, but it feels like RPE 7 to 8 this time. I probably could've gotten eight reps if there was $1,000 on the line. Maybe I could've hit 9 if I was willing to pop some blood vessels in an eyeball.

I rest another three minutes and do my third working set with the same 90 pounds. Because it's my last set, I push it to failure. This time, I blow past 6 reps and do 8, which gets me to RPE 9 to 10. The last rep took all my might, and I'm certain the ninth rep wouldn't have happened with good technique. That's perfect. I mark it in my notebook.

I also think ahead to my next workout. Because I read Chapter 7 of my book (I'm such a teacher's pet!), I went into this program with a progression plan in place. In this case, the plan is to increase reps from workout to workout while keeping RPE 8 as my target effort level, with the last set taken to failure.

RPEs, alas, are not a reliably precise metric. They can shift for any number of reasons—for example, where you are in your workout, how much cumulative fatigue you have from previous workouts, or how much fatigue or stress you have from work or home. Consequently, it's better to see an RPE target as a fuzzy zone rather than a clearly defined bull's-eye.

Although it's wise to have a progression scheme in mind to ensure progressive overload, you can't view load as a make-or-break factor in hypertrophy training. What matters is that you're stimulating the muscle with progressively more tension over a long time frame.

Try not to get too caught up in finding the perfect load for the perfect set. You're doing awesome as long as you're training hard and the general trend is upward.

PERCENTAGE OF ONE-REP MAX (%1RM)

The RPE-based approach works because it's autoregulated—that is, your loads can differ from your plan based on how strong you are on any particular day. The second method I use to prescribe load, %1RM, is more rigid. I tend to save this method for people who have powerlifting goals. If that's not you, feel free to skip ahead to the "Trusting the Logbook" section.

Although useful for strength coaching, determining load based on %1RM is less generalizable because you have to know your 1RM for the lift in question. Off the top of your head, how many lifts can you say that about? That's why I only use %1RM for primary exercises that lend themselves well to 1RM testing: squat, bench press, deadlift, and sometimes overhead press, but not EZ-bar biceps curl or reverse pec deck.

Once you know your 1RM for a lift and how many reps you want to do, Table 10.1 suggests the %1RM that a typical lifter would use for that many reps.

Table 10.1: Rep Targets at Varying %1RM Loads[6]

%1RM	Maximum Reps Possible*	Suggested Reps (at RPE 7 to 9)**
100%	1	N/A
95%	1 to 2	N/A
90%	2 to 4	1 to 2
85%	4 to 7	2 to 5
80%	6 to 10	4 to 8
75%	8 to 12	6 to 10
70%	10 to 15	8 to 12

* These are the reps possible at max effort (RPE 10) for an average lifter. Because of individual differences, you may be able to get more or fewer reps at any given %1RM.

** This column shows the rep count I would prescribe for each %1RM when I want a trainee to reach RPE 7 to 9.

A few notes about Table 10.1:

- You shouldn't be surprised to see that 100 percent of 1RM correlates to one possible repetition. If you can't get one, it's not your actual 1RM. And if you can do more than one, it's not your 1RM.

- Most people can get 2 to 4 reps with 90 percent of their 1RM. If your max squat is 315 pounds, 90%1RM is 283.5 pounds. However, without a complete set of microplates, you wouldn't use that exact load. You'd either go up to 285 (90.5 percent of 1RM) or down to 280 (89%1RM), neither of which should noticeably affect your rep count.

- For ease of loading and unloading, you might choose 275 pounds (87%1RM), with which you could probably get 4 to 6 reps on an all-out set.

- Most people can get 6 to 10 reps with 80%1RM. In this example, that would be 252 pounds. Again, the path of least resistance would be to round up to 255 (81% 1RM).

DETERMINING YOUR 1RM

You don't need to know your precise 1RM unless you're a competitive powerlifter. However, even if you're not into powerlifting, you might want to learn how to estimate how much you can lift for one all-out rep.

I know three ways to do it.

⚠ **CAUTION**

Always use a spotter when testing your max on the barbell bench press. When testing your barbell squat, use at least one spotter (get two if possible) and set the safety pins on the rack.

Option 1: The AMRAP Test

The first option for estimating your 1RM is to do an AMRAP (as many reps as possible) test. This is where you do one set for as many reps as possible with a reasonably heavy weight. If you have no idea what your current 1RM might be, you do the AMRAP test with a weight you think you can lift three to five times. Since the weight will be fairly close to your max, it's very important that you do a thorough warm-up before the AMRAP set by gradually building up in weight, as outlined in Table 10.2. Rest three to five minutes between each warm-up set.

Table 10.2: How to Warm Up to an AMRAP Test

Weight	Reps
Warm-up set 1: Empty bar	10
Warm-up set 2: 50% current estimated max	6
Warm-up set 3: 60% current estimated max	4
Warm-up set 4: 75% current estimated max	3
Warm-up set 5: 85% current estimated max	1
90% current estimated max	AMRAP

Plug the results of your AMRAP test into the free 1RM calculator on my website at jeffnippard. com/1repmaxcalculator. The calculated number is your working 1RM.

Option 2: The Recent Tough Set

The second way to estimate your 1RM is to use the results of a tough set. Find a set from a recent workout in which you got close to failure somewhere in the 3- to 6-rep range. Plug the weight you used and the reps you got in to the 1RM calculator at jeffnippard.com/1repmaxcalculator.

Option 3: The True One-Rep-Max Test

The final option is actually to test your 1RM. After a thorough warm-up, as shown in Table 10.3, do single repetitions with slightly more weight until you reach what you're pretty sure is your limit. *Maybe* you could get one more rep with a *tiny* bit more weight, but you're not confident enough to try it. Call that your 1 rep max.

Table 10.3: How to Warm Up for a True 1RM Test

Weight	Reps
Warm-up set 1: Empty bar	10
Warm-up set 2: 50% current estimated max	6
Warm-up set 3: 60% current estimated max	4
Warm-up set 4: 75% current estimated max	2
Warm-up set 5: 90% current estimated max	1
Warm-up set 6: 95 to 100% current estimated max	1
1RM test: 100 to 105% current estimated max*	1
*Continue the test until you don't feel confident attempting another lift with a heavier weight.	

That's close enough to establish your working 1RM for that lift.

This method is the most straightforward and accurate, and I wouldn't hesitate to recommend it for powerlifters and other experienced lifters who are used to hitting heavy singles. I would also recommend it to someone working with a credentialed strength coach.

If you aren't used to training this way, it's also the riskiest. That's why I made it the third option.

If you plan to use this option, I recommend considering it an RPE 9.5 max rather than a true 1RM, which would take you to RPE 10. Remember, you only need an estimate of your max to use the loading parameters in this chapter.

USING %1RM

Once you know your 1RM on the primary lifts, the next step is to use it to determine how much weight you should lift and for how many reps. This is where Table 10.1 comes in.

Let's say you want to do 3 sets of 4 to 8 reps on the squat at an RPE of 7 to 9. How heavy should you go?

The table shows that 4 to 8 reps at a 7 to 9 RPE corresponds to a load of around 80 percent of your 1RM. If your 1RM is 315 pounds, you'd load 80 percent, or 252 pounds (you can round down to 250).

Let's say your program asks for 1 set of 10 on the bench press, taken all the way to failure (RPE 10). How much weight should you load?

Using the same table, you can see that most people reach failure at 10 reps around 70 to 80 percent of their 1RM. If your 1RM is 315 pounds, load up 70 to 80 percent of that, or 220 to 250 pounds. Any weight in that range should have you getting close to failure around your tenth rep. If you get a few more or a few less reps, that's fine. Now you have more information about how you should adjust the load for the next workout.

TRUSTING THE LOGBOOK

I have a fourth option for deciding how much weight to use. Your training log will provide it.

If you've been tracking your workouts, you should have a clear record of how much weight you've used for various rep ranges on all your key exercises. You should also have some feedback from those previous workouts—not only how much you lifted but also how you felt while lifting.

So, if none of the previous options are practical or appealing to you, look at what you have lifted before to decide how much you should lift next.

Of course, once you've determined how much to lift, you can often use that same weight for multiple sets. And when you're doing multiple sets, you need to make sure to rest adequately between them, as I explain in the next chapter.

CHAPTER 11

REST PERIODS

HOW LONG SHOULD I REST BETWEEN SETS?

For years, traditional bodybuilding lore told us that short rest periods in between sets were the key to maximizing muscle growth. The idea was that forcing the muscles to work with limited recovery between sets would jack up metabolic stress, which was considered an important signal for hypertrophy.

How well does this "bro science" hold up against current science? That's what we'll explore on this eighth rung of the Muscle Ladder.

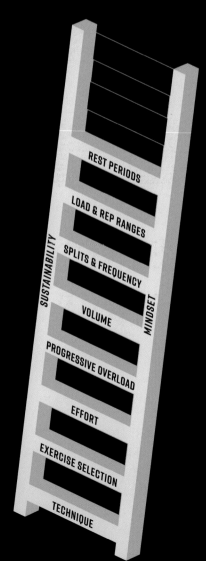

REST PERIOD RESEARCH

No need to tease this: Two areas of research debunk the idea that short rest periods are better for muscle growth. Not only does recent evidence downplay the role of metabolic stress in driving hypertrophy,[1] the metabolic stress you generate with limited recovery comes at the expense of mechanical tension. This is not good!

A 2007 study from Ratamess and colleagues found that both load and volume declined dramatically with rest periods of one minute or less.[2] A 2024 review looked at studies comparing short (less than one minute) and long (more than one minute) rest periods. While all nine studies only lasted between five to ten weeks (a relatively short duration for research designed to detect changes in hypertrophy), the results do still suggest a hypertrophic advantage with longer rest.[3]

The reason is straightforward enough: Longer rest periods allow more complete recovery between sets, which means you'll be able to generate higher tension deeper into your workout. That, in turn, means higher volume load and more muscle growth.

However, there are some downsides of longer downtime between sets:

With longer rest periods, you either do less work in the time you've allotted for your workout, or you need more time to do the same amount of work. Either option can make training take longer, which might be less enjoyable for some.

If you're easily distracted, longer rest periods can make you more susceptible to scrolling on your phone or getting drawn into a pointless conversation about whether sumo deadlifts are cheating. (They're not, by the way.) Those things challenge your focus and motivation, which can ultimately affect your results.

THE IMPORTANCE OF REST PERIODS

We have a name for continuous movement without rest: cardio (or, more formally, aerobic exercise).

Resistance exercise is primarily an anaerobic activity, which means your muscles don't need as much oxygen to perform. There's a limit to how long you can continue anaerobic work without stopping to recover.

Most of the benefits of a recovery period occur in the first minute. You catch your breath, your heart rate returns to whatever it was before you began the set, and you replenish your muscles' energy while clearing out some of the metabolic waste products you generated.

But everything I just described depends on what you did and how hard you pushed yourself to do it. A set of 10 squats at RPE 9 elevates your heart rate and challenges your breathing a lot more than a set of 10 pushdowns at RPE 7. You also burn through far more energy and create more metabolic waste.

Because of those conditions and nuances, think of my recommendations in this chapter less as firm rules and more as fuzzy lines. You always have to balance the potential benefits of additional rest with the downside of making your workouts longer or less engaging.

REST PERIOD RECOMMENDATIONS

Goldilocks was lucky: She only had three options, one of which was "just right." In the gym, it's easy enough to tell when rest periods are too short (you don't have enough gas in the tank for subsequent sets) or too long (you get bored and lose focus). But there's no obvious "just right" interval in between those extremes. Not only is it going to be different from exercise to exercise, it might be different for the same exercise from workout to workout.

These are my general guidelines for finding the sweet spot:

- **Isolation exercises:** Rest one to two minutes between sets.

- **Compound exercises (light):** Rest two to three minutes between sets.

- **Compound exercises (heavy):** Rest three to five minutes between sets.

When in doubt about how much recovery you need, consider these three factors:

- **The amount of muscle involved in the movement:** The more muscle mass involved, the more rest you need between sets

- **The technical demand of the exercise:** The more technically demanding the exercise, the more rest you need between sets

- **The amount of weight you're lifting:** The more weight you're lifting, the more rest you need between sets

Isolation movements (lateral raises, biceps curls, triceps pressdowns, and so on) involve fewer muscle groups, present little technical demand, and are typically performed with relatively light weights. Because of those factors, you won't need much time to recover between sets.

Lighter compound exercises (cable rows, lunges, lat pulldowns, and so on) go beyond isolation exercises on every factor. They involve more muscle and require more skill, and you'll typically perform them with heavier loads. But the weights aren't close to what you'd use for a deadlift or barbell squat. That's why the suggested rest periods—two to three minutes between sets—are in between those for isolation work and heavier compound lifts.

Heavy compound movements (barbell squat, bench press, deadlift, overhead press, and so on) are at the high end of every category. You'll deploy lots of muscle mass to move heavy weights in technically complex movements. Every rep requires your full attention and focus. It might take a minute at the end of a set just to catch your breath, and several more minutes of recovery before you're ready to go again.

That guideline doesn't apply to machine-based compound lifts (leg presses, hack squats, chest presses, etc.). Even though the loads may be even heavier than the ones you use with free weights, the exercises themselves require far less skill. Two to three minutes should be plenty of time to recover between sets.

Table 11.1 summarizes all the rest period recommendations.

Table 11.1: Recommended Rest Periods

Exercise Type	Rest Period
Isolation	1 to 2 minutes
Light compound	2 to 3 minutes
Machine-based compound	2 to 3 minutes
Heavy compound	3 to 5 minutes

REST PERIOD TRACKING

If you're a beginner, it might be useful to track rest periods. If nothing else, it helps you stay focused between sets. However, most lifters eventually learn to autoregulate recovery between sets. Your body tells you when you're ready.

Still, there are circumstances where an experienced lifter might choose to time their rest intervals. Someone who's naturally impatient might benefit from putting their recovery on the clock. That way, they force themselves to take more time between sets. Someone who's easily distracted could benefit from setting a timer between sets, which cuts down on wasted downtime and makes the session more efficient.

The goal in any circumstance is to make your workouts work better for you. It's good to have a rough idea of how long you've been resting, but except for the situations I just described, you rarely need to be ultra-strict about it. It's natural to feel better on some days than on others, and good lifters should be able to adjust their rest periods accordingly.

SUPERSETS

Here's a logical question: How do you manage rest periods when you do a superset—two exercises back to back, with no rest in between?

I'll start with a type of superset I don't recommend: pairing two exercises for the same body part, like bench presses with dumbbell flies or leg presses with leg extensions. A 2020 study found that force production suffered when participants paired exercises that used the same muscles.[4]

However, when participants paired exercises for separate, nonoverlapping muscles, they got the most from both movements. You can do that type of superset two different ways. Both of the following examples fall under the broader category of *separated supersets,* where you're supersetting exercises that train separate muscles:

- **Agonist-antagonist superset:** Pairing exercises for muscles performing the opposite movement patterns. Examples include supersetting shoulder presses and lat pulldowns (vertical push and vertical pull), bench presses and rows (horizontal push and horizontal pull), and leg extensions and leg curls (knee extension and knee flexion).

- **Alternate-peripheral superset:** Pairing completely unrelated exercises. The combinations can be as random as leg presses with lateral raises or lunges with biceps curls in a full-body workout.

The only real benefit of supersetting is that it cuts down on workout time. That's because one muscle is resting while the other is working, allowing you to whip through exercises more efficiently.

How long you should rest between supersets is fairly straightforward. Just arrange your supersets so that the guidelines from Table 11.1 still apply.

For example, if you superset two isolation exercises (like biceps curls and triceps extensions) ensure that both your biceps and triceps are getting one to two minutes of rest before working again. That series of supersets might look something like this:

> Superset 1A: Biceps curls, 10 reps
>
> Superset 1B: Triceps extensions, 10 reps
>
> Rest 30 seconds to 1 minute
>
> Superset 2A: Biceps curls, 10 reps
>
> Superset 2B: Triceps extensions, 10 reps
>
> Rest 30 seconds to 1 minute
>
> Superset 3A: Biceps curls, 10 reps
>
> Superset 3B: Triceps extensions, 10 reps
>
> Move on to the next exercise (or superset of exercises)

As you can see, because the biceps are resting while the triceps are working (and vice versa), you can reduce each rest interval between supersets to thirty seconds to one minute rather than the standard one to two minutes. This style of training probably doesn't offer any special advantage for hypertrophy, it just allows you to get through the workout a bit faster.

Similarly, if you're pairing two lighter compound exercises as a superset (such as bench presses and cable rows), you would just ensure that your pecs are getting two to three minutes of rest between sets of bench press. Same goes for your back.

I don't often recommend supersets on heavy compound exercises because you'll probably find that your strength performance is impeded unless you're in fantastic cardiovascular condition.

With that said, on any form of superset, you should certainly take more time if you need it. There's no point in doing supersets if fatigue causes you to perform less total work or lower-quality work.

MAKING SHORT REST PERIODS WORK

Even though the bulk of the science leans toward longer rest periods being better for muscle growth, there are two ways to use shorter rest periods in your workouts without killing your gains.

The first option is to do more volume. The best research on volume suggests that even though short rest periods seem to be worse for muscle growth at a fixed volume, you can compensate by doing more volume. How much more volume do you need to offset the potential gains lost by resting less? Probably more than you'd like to do. A deep dive literature review from James Kreiger suggests that you may need to do double the number of sets to get the same gains when doing short rest periods (generally less than sixty to ninety seconds between sets).[5] So, even though more volume with shorter rests is an effective option, it may not be a practical one if your goal is to make your workouts take less time.

A better, more practical option is to gradually reduce your rest periods over time. Rather than

starting on day 1 of week 1 with super short rest periods between sets, start with the guidelines given in Table 11.1 and gradually reduce them from there. (Again, the assumption is that your goal is to make your workouts more efficient.)

There is evidence showing that if you gradually reduce your rest periods over time, you can still maximize hypertrophy because your cardiovascular endurance improves, allowing you to recover faster between sets. In other words, you can start by resting, say, two minutes between sets in week 1 and then rest for fifteen seconds less in week 2 and fifteen seconds less again in week 3, until you eventually get down to just one minute rest in between sets.[6]

This approach should allow you to rest less in between sets and not necessarily compromise gains. However, if you find that you get to a point where your rest intervals have become so short that you're not able to sustain your strength performance from the previous week, that's a sign that you may be better off going back to taking a little more time between sets.

"THE BURN"

I have one final note about rest periods before you climb to the next rung on the Muscle Ladder.

The goal of resistance training, in the context of this book, is to look more muscular and/or perform better. Most of us, most of the time, are trying to build muscle and increase strength.

What we're not trying to do is flood the gym with our sweat, jack our heart rate to infinity, or "feel the burn." If your goal is to get leaner, let your diet do the heavy lifting. If it's to burn calories or improve your conditioning, do cardio.

When you're in the weight room, focus on getting bigger and stronger rather than on how many calories you can burn or how sore you can make yourself.

Your rest periods should be exactly as long as they need to be for you to get the most out of every set of every exercise in your program.

You've now reached a point on the ladder where all the training fundamentals have been covered. You have the knowledge you will rely on most throughout your lifting career. However, when you start to close in on your genetic ceiling for muscle growth, you'll want to climb up another rung to advanced training techniques.

CHAPTER 12

ADVANCED TECHNIQUES

HOW DO I KEEP DRIVING PROGRESS?

The true hallmark of an advanced lifter isn't how many years you've been training, or how much strength you've gained, or even the quality of your physique. It's your rate of progress. If you're still making progress from week to week, you're a functional beginner. Most of your gains are still ahead of you, and you have no idea what your ultimate potential might be.

If your progress has slowed, and it usually takes a month or three to see improvements in your strength, measurements, or photos, you're an intermediate. You're not exactly sure what your limits might be, but they're starting to come into focus.

If your genetic potential greets you every morning when you look in the mirror, and it takes a forensic analysis to detect any actual gains in your semiannual progress photos, you're ready for the advanced techniques you'll learn here, on the ninth and penultimate rung of the Muscle Ladder.

This rung is where the art of training often takes precedence over the science of training. Few studies are conducted on advanced lifters for the simple reason that few trainees at that level are available to researchers. Scientists make do with what they have, which is usually college students at the beginner or intermediate levels. Advanced lifters, in turn, have to make do with what they can learn from their own experiments. Their laboratories are their gyms and they are their own subjects.

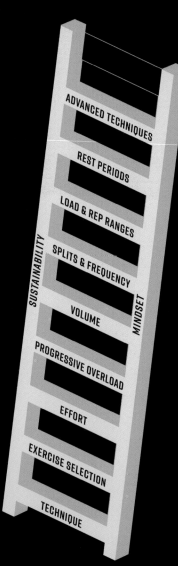

I've described strategies for advanced lifters throughout *The Muscle Ladder*—high-volume specialization phases and high-frequency training, for example.

This chapter will focus on advanced *intensity* techniques. These include partial reps, drop sets, myo-reps, forced reps, cheat reps, loaded stretches, and accentuated eccentric training. They all have one thing in common: They make training harder.

Most advanced lifters use intensity techniques to extend a set beyond the typical stopping point—that is, going "beyond failure." That isn't necessary for most trainees who can make progress in other ways. But as novel training stimuli, using intensity techniques can help experienced lifters get past the most stubborn plateaus.

PARTIAL REPS

Let's start with partial reps because I think they have the most scientific support of all the advanced hypertrophy techniques. There is a surprisingly large science base showing that training muscles in the more lengthened aspect of the range of motion is better for muscle growth than training muscles in the more shortened aspect of the range of motion.[1] Some evidence even suggests that emphasizing the stretched aspect of a lift could be better than using a full range of motion, at least for some muscles.[2]

As a quick refresher, partial reps are repetitions that don't use the entire range of motion (ROM). There are an infinite number of ways you can do a partial rep, but I'll confine this discussion to the most effective tactic: lengthened partials.

Lengthened partials (see Figure 12.1) are when you do partial reps while the muscle is stretched more. For example, you should be able to feel that your pecs are more stretched in the bottom half of a bench press. So a lengthened partial on a bench press would be when you go all the way down to your chest, but only about half way up to the top. Similarly, a lengthened partial on a squat would be when you go all the way down into the hole but only come about half way up. These can be contrasted with the less effective "shortened" partial, where you stay in the top half of the squat, only going about half way down. The key difference is that one type of partial is still a deep squat (you get the quads into a deep stretch) while the other type of partial is a shallow half-squat (where the quads don't get into a deep stretch).

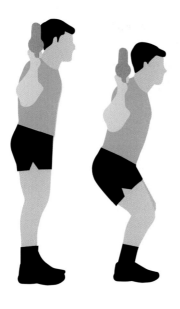
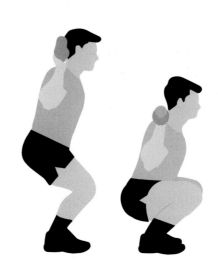

Figure 12.1

Shortened versus lengthened partials

Imagine you're doing dumbbell lateral raises. You reach the end of your final set feeling as if you have something left in the tank but not enough to complete another rep with a full ROM.

That's where partials reps come in. You can extend the set beyond your usual stopping point by continuing to raise the dumbbells out to the sides using only half or one-third of full ROM. This way, you might be able to get at least another four or five mini-reps. It's a fairly low-risk way to take the set beyond failure and exploit the remaining potential in your shoulders while they're in a more lengthened position.

If you've been paying attention, you know the difference between RPE 8 and RPE 10 is often small or undetectable in studies. So you can guess there's probably even less difference between RPE 10 and the RPE 10–plus you could reach with partial reps.

Still, I think they have their place, and I think they can be particularly effective on exercises with asymmetric strength profiles—where one part of the range of motion is much harder than another. The two muscles where this is most often the case are the hamstrings and the back.

For example, you've probably noticed that when you do lying leg curls, as you get to the final reps of your set, you can't quite get the foot pad all the way up to your glutes. However, you could probably keep going with another four or five partial reps if you wanted to. That's because the hamstrings are much stronger when they're more lengthened and much weaker when they're shortened, which means your hamstrings probably still have a lot more juice left in the tank, even once you've exhausted your ability to complete a full ROM. That's why I often extend my last set of leg curls with a few partial reps.

The same goes for most back exercises. On lat pulldowns, once you reach the point where you can't quite get the bar all the way down to your chest, you could still crank out another few partials.

So, on select exercises for the hamstrings and back, and for smaller muscles like the biceps and side delts, feel free to use some lengthened partials to extend the set. It might help you get a little more out of your training. Just be careful not to overdo it because beyond-failure training is very fatiguing.

I've also been experimenting with lengthened partials not as an end-of-set intensity technique to go beyond failure but on every rep of a set from start to finish. In this case, you do all your reps as normal, but instead of using a full ROM, you do lengthened partials on every rep. As I suggested in Chapter 4 on technique, I'm not sure the evidence on lengthened partials is strong enough to broadly recommend them on all reps of all exercises. However, based on my reading of the literature, they do seem to be equally effective at worst and marginally better at best. If you're stuck at a plateau for a stubborn body part, consider blasting it with some lengthened partials.

DROP SETS

Let's say you're doing leg extensions with 100 pounds. You barely squeeze out your tenth rep, suggesting you're about as close to RPE 10 as you can get. But instead of stopping, you drop the weight back and crank out another 4 or 5 reps with 70 pounds.

That's a drop set, and it's one of the most frequently used intensity techniques among bodybuilders. Despite its popularity, it doesn't have a particularly strong evidence base. A 2023 meta-analysis found no difference in hypertrophy when comparing drop sets to traditional sets.[3]

Surprising? Not really. As I discussed in Chapter 6, there isn't much difference between sets taken to failure (RPE 10) and those that stopped two reps short of failure (RPE 8). So why would going beyond failure offer a pronounced advantage over either of those stopping points?

The short answer is it probably doesn't—at least not for the subjects they reviewed in that study. But no one really makes that claim about any of these techniques. It's best to think of them as being useful in specific contexts, such as the following:

- Drop sets offer a way to increase high-tension rep volume without spending more time in the gym. You can tack on a few extra high-tension reps (high-tension because the muscle has already been to failure once), without the accompanying rest period that typically comes before doing more reps.

- Drop sets make training more challenging. For some of us, "more challenging" often means "more fun," and because fun is motivating, that makes the technique worth trying.

- Sometimes it's important to test your limits. Drop sets give you a chance to see what you're capable of. You may be disappointed, or you may be pleasantly surprised. There's only one way to find out.

- Drop sets may help advanced trainees bust through plateaus. Remember, most studies are carried out over a relatively short time frame and on relatively less-experienced trainees.

⚠ CAUTION

Because they're so fatiguing, drop sets work best in low-risk applications. I reserve them for isolation movements or machine-based exercises, and even then, I only ever do them on the final set for a body part.

Many people make the common mistake of dropping the weight back too much. Generally speaking, after reaching failure, I only drop the weight back by 20 to 30 percent, which allows me to do another 3 to 5 reps. If you do a drop set with a really big load reduction, you'll end up having to do many extra reps just to get close to failure again. I think it's smarter to do smaller drops and fewer total reps. That way, you get the extra stimulus from the extra reps without the added fatigue of what is essentially another high-rep set.

MYO-REPS

Don't feel bad if you've never heard of myo-reps. You're hardly alone. Their hype in science-based bodybuilding circles hasn't yet translated to widespread popularity in the gym.

The system was originally developed in 2006 by Børge Fagerli, a Norwegian engineer and bodybuilding coach. Here's how it works: After you take a set to failure, you rest for three to four seconds and then do 4 additional myo-reps. Rest for another three to four seconds, do 4 more myo-reps, and continue the cycle until you can no longer crank out those 4 myo-reps.

Fagerli's goal was to focus on "effective reps." The idea, put simply, is that the reps you do at the end of a set, when you're closer to failure, stimulate more hypertrophy than the initial reps, when you're nowhere near failure. Those initial reps are mostly a means to an end. They're not doing much to stimulate hypertrophy, but they get you to the ones that do.

Practically speaking, if you were doing a set of 15 biceps curls, the first 10 would serve as a gateway to the final 5, which are the truly effective reps. Conversely, if you were doing a set of 5 leg presses to failure, all 5 reps would be considered effective.

This framework isn't universally accepted, as you can imagine. For one thing, there's no evidence of a hard cutoff separating the ineffective reps on one side of the line from the effective reps on the other. Instead, as I've discussed, reps become increasingly conducive to muscle growth as you get closer to failure.

Everyone agrees that the reps closest to failure—the ones you do at RPE 8, 9, or 10—offer more hypertrophic stimulus than the ones you do at RPE 4, 5, or 6. Myo-reps give you a framework to perform more reps in that high-value zone.

Let's say you're doing a set of 10 biceps curls. Consider these two scenarios:

- **Scenario 1:** You reach failure on the tenth rep and end the set there. You've completed 5 effective reps, according to the theory.

- **Scenario 2:** You reach failure on the tenth rep, rest for three to four seconds, and do another 4 reps with the same weight. Then you rest for another three to four seconds and do another 4 reps. After another short rest, you get just 2 more reps before you hit the wall. Now you've completed 15 effective reps—5 in the original set, followed by 10 myo-reps.

Simple math tells us you get three times as many effective reps in Scenario 2 compared to Scenario 1. So, by the logic of those who promote myo-reps, they offer a clear hypertrophic advantage.

I want to emphasize that the advantage is entirely theoretical. As of now, there's no research comparing the muscle growth resulting from myo-reps versus standard reps. Nor is there any really convincing evidence that the last 5 reps in a set are the only effective ones.

So while I don't put myo-reps on a pedestal, I have used them in my training over the years. I also recommend them for intermediate to

advanced trainees with the goal of stimulating new growth in stubborn body parts.

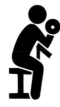

⚠ CAUTION

Similar to drop sets, myo-reps induce a deep level of fatigue and are best used in the same scenarios: the last set for a muscle group, as long as it's an isolation or machine-based movement.

FORCED REPS

Forced reps are yet another way to extend a normal set beyond the point where most lifters say "no mas."

In this case, you're doing a continuous set, usually with the help of a spotter who helps you force your muscles to crank out a few more reps. That sets them apart from drop sets, where you stop long enough to strip the weight back. The spotter performs that function by helping as much as you need to complete the reps.

Hypothetically, the advantage of forced reps is that you maintain constant tension on your muscles while extending a set beyond the typical termination point. Is that good? It's hard to say because there's no research comparing drop sets and forced reps.

One thing I can say from experience is that forced reps are more flexible and dynamic than drop sets. With forced reps, you can communicate with your spotter and tell them to take more or less weight into their hands depending on how much easier the weight becomes. As you fatigue beyond failure, the spotter can take incrementally more of the load. This is probably a good thing because it gives a more graded exposure to load reduction compared to the drop set, which is ultimately an arbitrary fixed load reduction.

Despite that slight potential advantage, I'm still hesitant to broadly recommend forced reps for several reasons:

- A lot depends on both verbal and nonverbal communication with your spotter. If the spotter fails to interpret your signals, you can find yourself trying to move more load than you expected. Even a good spotter can't know how much of the load they're controlling or

control the same amount from one workout to the next.

- Your ego can be your enemy with forced reps, especially on the bench press. A certain type of lifter will load the bar with more plates than they can handle on their own and leave it to the spotter to close the gap. A telltale sign your spotter is doing too much of the work is when their biceps pump is bigger than your chest pump.

- Overusing forced reps can make it hard to tell if you're actually getting stronger. Sure, you got 225 pounds for 10 reps on the bench press, but if your spotter had their hands on the bar for the final 5 reps, how much was "all you" and how much was "mostly them"?

With these drawbacks in mind, I recommend using forced reps sparingly. I occasionally do them if I'm training with someone, and we both feel motivated to push it on an exercise that lends itself to spotting—for example, chest presses, barbell curls, lat pulldowns, or leg presses.

They can make a workout a little more fun while also building chemistry between training partners, which almost certainly has a positive effect on your results.

However, they can also have the opposite effect, especially if they become a crutch for your ego by allowing you to imagine you're making progress. In reality, you may be setting yourself back by artificially extending sets instead of earning those reps the old-fashioned way.

Finally, as I've mentioned twice before, save this advanced technique for a muscle group's last set of the day.

CHEAT REPS

The more time you spend in the gym, the more pride you take in not just the muscle you've added or the strength you've built but also in your lifting skill.

That's why an experienced, conscientious lifter has a natural aversion to cheat reps and will often regard them as ego-driven reps. I agree that beginners and even most intermediate lifters should probably avoid cheat reps. In your first few years of training, it's really important that you learn and master proper technique. However, once you have that technique mastered, there are situations where I think cheat reps can make a difference in physique development.

One issue I see quite frequently is that people become so hyperfocused on maintaining "perfect" technique that they don't train as hard as they should be. They aren't able to maximize tension in the target muscle because they're so stiff and uptight. This causes them to stop their set at the first sign of extraneous movement.

Picture someone doing lat pulldowns with textbook form through their first 10 reps. Based on the consistent rep speed, it seems clear they could easily get at least one or two more. But because they felt themselves tempted to lean back a little on their tenth rep, they stop without attempting another.

Now picture a second person doing the same exercise with the same form through 10 reps. But instead of stopping there, they lean their torso back about 5 degrees further and crank out an eleventh rep. They lean forward and then pull back to hit their twelfth. Then they take a big breath and, with the help of a little extra momentum, crank out their thirteenth.

Who looked better? Many science-based lifters might say the first person, who finished their set without using any momentum or changing their form whatsoever. But who will build more muscle? If I had to bet, I'd put my money on the second lifter. Yes, their form changed on the last 3 reps, and they relied on a little momentum for the final 2, yet they were clearly in control through all 3 cheat reps.

But what if they hadn't stopped there? Things can get really ugly really fast. Like on the fourteenth rep, when they jerk their torso backward to generate momentum and still can't get the bar to their chest. Or the fifteenth, when they start with their torso perpendicular to the floor and finish close to parallel—and still barely pull the bar to where their chest would've been 3 reps ago.

Cheat reps can easily put you on a slippery slope. One moment loosening your form helps you increase the tension in your target muscles. but in the next, those muscles are relegated to a supporting role. So, how much cheating is okay, and how much is too much?

Well, like I said earlier, beginners and early intermediates shouldn't think about cheating at all. They need to lock in their form.

Advanced trainees can use some cheat reps on specific exercises. Back exercises like pulldowns and rows lend themselves well to mild cheating. A little momentum can go a long way on an exercise like dumbbell rows. You might get 5 more reps with a little torso rotation than you would with perfectly strict form. Over time, those extra reps can make a difference.

Here are some practical guidelines:

- When using cheat reps, always control the negative. The momentum is only meant to get the weight moving on the positive.

- Only use cheat reps if they allow you to get more reps with the target muscle doing the majority of the work. Stop the set when you feel the tension shifting to different muscles.

- Restrict cheating to *modest* alterations in form. For example, if you lean back 10 to 15 degrees on your first rep of lat pulldowns, you shouldn't lean back more than 15 to 20 degrees on your last rep. If you started a set of curls with a more or less perfectly upright posture, you shouldn't lean forward and back more than 5 to 10 degrees on your cheat reps.

- Save cheat reps for the last few reps of a set.

Based on those parameters, these are the most "cheat-friendly" exercises:

- Lat pulldowns

- Cable and dumbbell rows

- Barbell or dumbbell biceps curls

- Dumbbell lateral raises

That's a short list, as you can see. For the overwhelming majority of exercises, it's best to keep your form consistent from the first rep to the last.

STRETCHING

Stretching is an interesting type of exercise. Studies have shown that sedentary people who do a flexibility program will actually get stronger.[4] There's also some research suggesting that stretching a muscle in between sets may enhance muscle growth.[5] This shouldn't be incredibly surprising if you've been paying close attention because I've already talked about value in challenging the muscle in the stretched aspect of the range of motion.

The evidence on stretching a muscle when it isn't under load is still quite mixed, though. In a 2020 review, only two of the five studies that included resistance training showed a positive effect of stretching.[6] Both of those studies used

interset stretching—stretching between sets—rather than before or after the session.

This led the authors to speculate that stretching between sets could potentially be beneficial. Still, two studies is a far cry from a strong body of science, and a more recent 2021 study found no benefit of interset stretching on pec hypertrophy in trained subjects.[7] And another study from 2023 found no benefit of stretching the biceps in between sets.[8] The studies that do favor inter-set stretching have mainly found a positive effect for the quads and calves.[9] So while there is definitely reason to be skeptical of this approach, because there isn't any apparent downside (when incorporated properly) and there is a possible small upside (at least for some muscles), it could be worth trying out.

I don't do a lot of inter-set stretching these days, but when I do, it's usually for my lats, quads and calves. For example, I stretch my lats for twenty to thirty seconds in between sets of pulldowns. Every now and then, I'll do the same for my quads on leg extensions and my calves on calf raises. It probably doesn't make a big difference, but if I'm going to be resting in between sets anyway, I might as well get a bit of stretching in.

Also, in case you've heard of research showing that stretching reduces strength performance—don't worry—that only applies if you're holding the stretch for longer than sixty seconds.[10]

Bodybuilders also sometimes use loaded stretch training, where you hold a weight isometrically in a deep stretch. In practice, loaded stretch training doesn't lend itself well to many exercises. I use it most often for my pecs and occasionally for my triceps, hamstrings, and calves.

Here's how it works:

- After a hard set of chest presses, hold the weight in the stretched position—on or near your chest—for another ten to twenty seconds.

- On overhead triceps extensions, hold the stretched position at the bottom for ten to twenty seconds after completing a hard set.

- After your last rep of leg curls, just hold the stretched position with a slight bend in your knee for ten to twenty seconds.

- After your last rep of calf raises, hold the deep calf stretch under the same load for ten to twenty seconds.

Outside of these scenarios, it may be best to simply stretch the muscle the conventional way. For example, after a set of pull-ups, I wouldn't be able to hold the fully stretched position very long before my grip gave out. Even with straps, I wouldn't get the best stretch while hanging. A better strategy would be to stretch my lats between sets, holding each stretch for ten to twenty seconds.

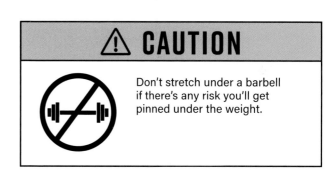

⚠ **CAUTION**

Don't stretch under a barbell if there's any risk you'll get pinned under the weight.

ACCENTUATED ECCENTRIC TRAINING

Every strength exercise, as you probably know, has two parts: the concentric phase, when you actually lift the weight, and the eccentric phase, when you lower it. Human physiology has evolved to make us much stronger on the latter than the former. That's why we can lower about 20 to 40 pounds more weight than we can lift.

Exercise scientists have studied eccentric contractions for decades. We know eccentric-only training creates far more muscle damage than conventional lifting. (That's why you get a lot more sore from running downhill than you do from running uphill.) We also have some mechanistic evidence that the eccentric phase may stimulate more muscle growth than the concentric.[11]

Accentuating the negative portion of a lift is relatively straightforward:

- You can have a training partner manually add resistance to the negative. For example, on a lying leg curl, you'd lift the weight the conventional way. Then, as you're lowering it, the other person would push down on the pad, giving you more work on the negative phase.

- You can lower a weight unilaterally on a bilateral exercise. On a leg extension, for example, you'd lift with both legs, lower it with just your left, lift it again, and then lower it with just your right.

- With the help of a training partner, you can load the bar or machine with a supramaximal load—a weight that's heavier than you could lift on that exercise. You'd lower the weight on your own, and then your partner would help you lift it back to the starting position.

The benefits of accentuated eccentric training are currently unclear. Only two of seven studies showed an advantage over traditional training for long-term strength gains.[12] For hypertrophy, studies show similar results for accentuated eccentrics and conventional lifts.[13]

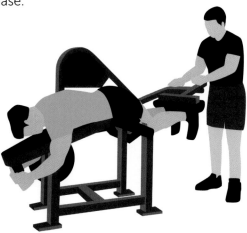

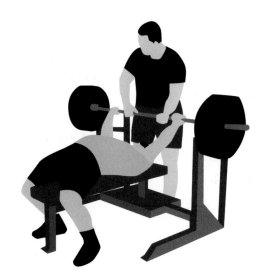

Tempo training offers a simpler alternative, and one you can do without a training partner. Just lift a weight at your normal speed and then take three to four seconds to lower it. However, as I discussed in Chapter 4, lifting tempo doesn't seem to have a meaningful effect on hypertrophy. That probably explains why its surge in popularity a few decades ago didn't last.

One final thought about eccentric training before I move on to the final rung of the Muscle Ladder:

No matter how slowly you lower a weight, it's extremely important to do it under control. That's true for lifters at every level, in almost every context. The only exception is when you're lifting extremely heavy weights with a primary focus on building strength. In those situations, slow eccentrics are a waste of energy and might even be dangerous if you're deadlifting with a near-max weight. But for everyone else, in every other context, your ability to lower weights under control will be a key factor in your long-term results.

It should be clear from this chapter that advanced intensity techniques are the cherry on top. And a small cherry at that. At this point, you have climbed up eight rungs that are important to handle first. Once those fundamentals are covered, the methods described in this chapter can be applied judiciously to break through plateaus as you nudge ever closer to your genetic ceiling.

You are ready to climb to the final rung of the Muscle Ladder: periodization. This is where you'll get to admire the view and focus on putting all of this knowledge into a cohesive program. So let's dive in—or climb up, I should say.

CHAPTER 13

PERIODIZATION

HOW DO I ORGANIZE TRAINING OVER TIME?

The first nine rungs of the Muscle Ladder focused on what you need to know to build muscle. Now, on the tenth and final rung, everything is fitting together in a coherent training program.

Periodization gives you a systematic way to organize training over time with the goal of maximizing your gains while minimizing the risk of injury or overtraining. In this chapter, I'll talk about how to plan your training across a full calendar year, when and how to use deloads to improve recovery, and how often you should switch training up to avoid plateaus and monotony.

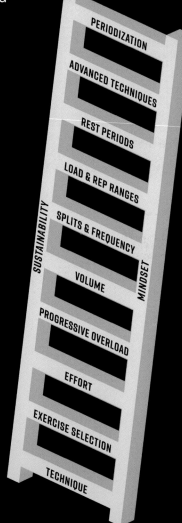

PERIODIZATION

ADVANCED TECHNIQUES

REST PERIODS

LOAD & REP RANGES

SPLITS & FREQUENCY

VOLUME

PROGRESSIVE OVERLOAD

EFFORT

EXERCISE SELECTION

TECHNIQUE

SUSTAINABILITY

MINDSET

Generally speaking, a periodized training plan will have three components: the macrocycle, the mesocycles, and some microcycles (see Figure 13.1).

The *macrocycle* is the whole enchilada. If your goal is to get shredded for summer, your macrocycle might begin with a higher-volume training phase in January and conclude with a lower-volume phase from May to June when caloric intake is also lower. For a competitive bodybuilder or powerlifter, the macrocycle might begin with your recovery from one major contest and end with achieving peak form for the next one. A team-sport athlete's macrocycle would cover twelve months—preseason, regular season, postseason, and offseason. An Olympic-level athlete might have a four-year macrocycle, one that begins with their first training session after the most recent Games and concludes forty-eight months later with their final prep for the next one.

Within that macrocycle are at least two *mesocycles.* Each mesocycle focuses on a key goal and lasts one to three months. If you're doing Arnold's eight-week arm-blaster program (that may or may not be a real thing), that's your mesocycle.

Within each mesocycle are several *microcycles.* A microcycle typically lasts a week and refers to how individual workouts are laid out throughout the week. For example, if you're running an upper/lower split with four workouts per week, your microcycle spans one week's worth of upper/lower workouts. In the asynchronous push/pull/legs split I discussed in Chapter 9, your microcycle repeats every eight days instead of seven.

For the rest of this chapter, I'll talk about each of the components in detail.

Figure 13.1

Breakdown of macrocycle, mesocycle, and microcycle

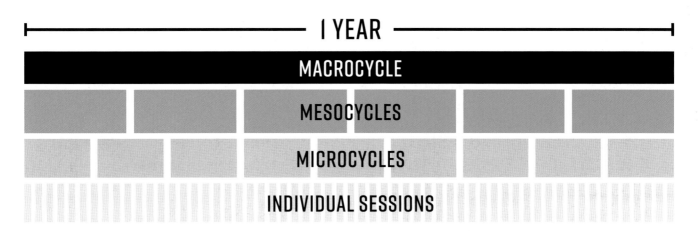

THE MACROCYCLE

Not every lifter wants or needs to preplan their entire training schedule across a full macrocycle. Indeed, you can apply everything you've learned in *The Muscle Ladder* without organizing your training into cycles and still make incredible progress. I think macrocycle-level planning is most relevant for those who compete in bodybuilding or powerlifting and lifters who like to have more structure in their training. There are also basic programming principles that any dedicated trainee can borrow and apply; you don't have to be preparing for a competition to use macrocycle planning.

BODYBUILDING

If you're a competitive bodybuilder, you'll likely prioritize higher-volume training in the offseason, when muscle *growth* is your top priority. You'll want to be in a caloric surplus, both to have the energy to train and for the raw materials to build bigger muscles.

Later in the macrocycle, as the competition season approaches, achieving low body fat is your top priority. Your diet goes from a caloric surplus to a deficit, and your workouts may need to shift from higher to lower volume. In the later stages of contest prep, as your body fat approaches dangerously low levels, it can become nearly impossible to manage recovery and prevent injury with the same level of volume you used in the offseason.

Table 13.1 is an example of a macrocycle for a competitive bodybuilder. The full calendar year is split into four quarters (three months each) to prepare for a bodybuilding competition on October 1.

Table 13.1: Macrocycle for October 1 Bodybuilding Competition Prep

	Q1: January to March (offseason)	Q2: April to June (transition)	Q3: July to September (precontest)	Competition	Q4: October to December (post-contest)
Goals	Build muscle, gain strength, bring up weak body parts	Shift from offseason to contest prep	Maintain as much muscle as possible while getting shredded	Hit the stage with single-digit body fat	Recover mentally and physically and prepare for offseason
Training notes	Heavier strength training can be included. Recovery ability is high, so failure training can be more frequent. If high volumes are tolerated, they can be pushed higher. Option to dabble in powerlifting. Wide variety of rep ranges can be used (1 to 5, 6 to 12, 12 to 20+). Split should prioritize weak points; it's time to improve!	Transition into more "contest-prep-friendly" training. Prioritize moderate rep ranges (use 1- to 5-rep and 12- to 20+-rep sets more sparingly). Failure training can still continue if recovery is good. Volume can remain the same as long as it is well tolerated and being recovered from.	Lower-volume workouts. Moderate-high effort. Avoid excessive failure training to preserve recovery. Avoid exercises that may increase the risk of injury. Choose exercises that are less fatiguing. Include more machine work. Consider eliminating low reps (1 to 5 reps). Consider a full-body split to avoid gruesome leg days.	Bodybuilding competition on October 1.	Prioritize fun training with plenty of flexibility to recover from the mental demands of contest prep. Gradually increase volume post-competition as ability to recover improves. Consider push/pull/legs split to promote better pumps, fueled by overfeeding.

POWERLIFTING

If you're a competitive powerlifter, your offseason is a good time to emphasize exercise variation and higher-rep training with the goal of promoting hypertrophy and improving weak points in your lifts. As you get closer to the meet, you'll become much more specific with your training, prioritizing the squat, bench press, and deadlift with heavier loads as you reduce the volume on accessory lifts.

Table 13.2 presents a sample macrocycle for a competitive powerlifter.

Table 13.2: Macrocycle for October 1 Powerlifting Meet Prep

	Q1: January to March (offseason)	Q2: April to June (transition)	Q3: July to September (meet prep)	Meet	Q4: October to December (post-meet)
Goals	Build work capacity, build muscle, and improve weak points	Shift into more powerlifting-specific training.	Peak for maximum strength on meet day.		Recover from the meet and transition into a new macrocycle.
Training notes	Higher-volume training can be included. Use plenty of exercise variation. Focus on building weak points (e.g., if your triceps are limiting your bench, do plenty of triceps isolation work). Combine heavier and lighter weights. All rep ranges can be used.	Training loads are gradually increased. Volume may begin to gradually decrease. Less exercise variation. Gradually increase emphasis on the squat, bench press, and deadlift. Gradually reduce high-rep work.	Training loads should be gradually increased. Minimal exercise variation: focus on the squat, bench, and deadlift. Regular heavy strength work on the squat, bench, and deadlift. Volume may slightly taper at this stage. Most sets should be in the 1- to 5-rep range. Prepare for the meet environment by facing away from a mirror while lifting and practicing referee commands.	Powerlifting meet on October 1.	Decrease training loads to promote recovery. Prioritize fun training with plenty of flexibility to recover from the mental demands of meet prep. More exercise variation is allowed. All rep ranges can be used. Don't overdo heavy sets and avoid max effort powerlifts.

POWERBUILDING

As the name suggests, *powerbuilding* combines bodybuilding and powerlifting goals—bigger muscles and bigger numbers on the squat, bench, and deadlift.

Table 13.3 outlines how you might accomplish both goals within a powerbuilding macrocycle.

Table 13.3: Macrocycle for Powerbuilding

	Q1: January to March (hypertrophy and strength)	Q2: April to June (more hypertrophy)	Q3: July to September (more strength)	Q4: October to December (more hypertrophy)
Goals	True powerbuilding: build strength and size evenly.	Focus more on hypertrophy while putting strength work at maintenance levels.	Focus more on strength while putting hypertrophy work at maintenance levels.	Focus more on hypertrophy while putting strength work at maintenance levels
Training notes	Training should consist of a roughly even mix of low reps (1 to 5) and moderate to high reps (6 to 12+). The squat, bench press, and deadlift are prioritized above other exercises, but there is still considerable exercise variation.	Training should consist primarily of moderate and high reps to promote hypertrophy. Low-rep strength work is still included but is more limited. The squat, bench press, and deadlift are still included, but there will be an increase in variations of those lifts—hack squats, RDLs, etc.	Training should focus much more on heavier, lower-rep training to promote strength gains. Moderate- and high-rep work is still included but is more limited. The squat, bench press, and deadlift are highly prioritized and likely will be trained multiple times per week.	This can be a repeat of the Q2 block of training. At this point, you may want to focus more on developing specific weak points before returning to another "true powerbuilding" phase. For example, if biceps are a weak point from a bodybuilding standpoint, you can train biceps at a higher frequency. If the bench press is a weak point, you can increase bench frequency as well.

COMBINING HYPERTROPHY AND ENDURANCE

It's easy enough to improve your endurance by combining some cardio with your typical training routine. Done strategically, the cardio shouldn't interfere with your muscular development and may even help you recover between strength workouts. But when your goal is to develop endurance at a high level while simultaneously building muscle mass, you really need a long-term plan.

Table 13.4 offers an example of a combined endurance and hypertrophy macrocycle.

Table 13.4: Macrocycle for Hypertrophy and Endurance

	Q1: January to March (more hypertrophy)	Q2: April to June (hypertrophy and endurance)	Q3: July to September (more endurance)	Q4: October to December (hypertrophy and endurance)
Goals	Focus on hypertrophy, while endurance work is at maintenance levels.	Develop muscle size and endurance concurrently.	Focus on endurance, while hypertrophy work is at maintenance levels.	Develop muscle size and endurance concurrently.
Training notes	Lift weights three to five times per week. Low-, moderate-, and high-rep ranges can be used. Cardio should be performed two to four times per week after training sessions and/or on rest days between weight workouts. If possible, try to include lower-impact cardio modes, like swimming and cycling, to minimize interference with resistance training.	Lift weights two to three times per week. Prioritize moderate- and high-rep weight training, which will improve muscular endurance more than low-rep training. Cardio should be performed three to four times per week after training sessions and/or on rest days between weight workouts. If possible, try to include lower-impact cardio modes, like swimming and cycling, to minimize interference with resistance training.	Do cardio four to six times per week. When possible, do cardio after lifting or on separate days. Reduce weight training to maintenance levels (one to three full-body workouts per week). Prioritize higher-rep weight training. With reduced lifting frequency, it'll be easier to recover from higher impact cardio, such as running.	This phase of training can be a return to Q2. Prioritize moderate- and high-rep weight training. Lift with weights two to three times per week. Cardio should be performed three to four times per week after training sessions and/or on rest days between weight workouts. If possible, try to include lower-impact cardio modes, like swimming and cycling, to minimize interference with resistance training.

THE PLATEAUED ADVANCED TRAINEE (SPECIALIZATION PHASES)

If you're an advanced lifter who's encountered a plateau in your muscular development, just about anything you try to make progress will come with significant trade-offs. For example, let's say you go from 20 to 30 sets per week for your quads. It could certainly stimulate new growth, but there's a high risk of overtraining if you don't lower volume somewhere else.

This is where periodization offers a unique benefit. With strategically planned specialization phases, you can blast key body parts with higher volume while reducing volume for other muscles.

It works because it takes more volume to build new muscle than to maintain what you already have. That means you get the benefit of gains in one muscle group without the penalty of impairing your gains elsewhere. You can program specialization phases for different body parts within a macrocycle, giving you the ability to turn up and dial back volume to maximize gains with minimal risk of injury, overtraining, or stagnation.

Table 13.5 shows one example of how an advanced trainee could periodize a year of specialization phases with the goal of breaking plateaus and driving progress.

Table 13.5: Macrocycle for Breaking Through a Plateau

	Q1: January to March (chest specialization)	Q2: April to June (back specialization)	Q3: July to September (quad specialization)	Q4: October to December (arm specialization)
Goals	Increase chest size while maintaining or slow-gaining other muscles.	Increase back size while maintaining or slow-gaining other muscles.	Increase quad size while maintaining or slow-gaining other muscles.	Increase arm size while maintaining or slow-gaining other muscles.
Training notes	Increase chest volume by 20 to 50 percent. Perform 20 to 30 sets for your chest per week while reducing volume for lower-priority body parts. Potential exercise overlap: Consider reducing isolation work for triceps and shoulders.	Increase back volume by 20 to 40 percent. Perform 25 to 35 sets for your back per week while reducing volume for lower-priority body parts. Potential exercise overlap: Consider reducing isolation work for biceps and rear delts.	Increase quad volume by 20 to 50 percent. Perform 20 to 30 sets for your quads per week while reducing volume for lower-priority body parts. Potential exercise overlap: Consider reducing isolation work for glutes.	Increase biceps and triceps volume by 20 to 50 percent. Perform 20 to 30 sets for your biceps and 20 to 30 sets for your triceps per week while reducing volume for lower-priority body parts. Potential exercise overlap: Consider reducing isolation work for forearms and front delts.

NONCOMPETITIVE LIFTER

As a noncompetitive lifter, the idea of periodized training may not be very compelling. That's especially true if you're still making steady progress.

But what if you're training for multiple goals—some combination of strength, hypertrophy, athletic performance, and/or endurance? Or you want to reach peak condition for some specific event—a wedding, reunion, or beach vacation? Or you know your training will need adjustments because of foreseeable changes to your life or work—the arrival of a new baby, or extensive job-related travel? Or you're a student, and you know you'll have a lot more freedom to lift during summer break than you do while managing a full course load?

In each case, macrocycle-level planning can help you adjust your training as required for your goals or nontraining priorities:

- If you're training for multiple goals, a periodized plan can help you focus on each of them sequentially rather than spreading your efforts around and not making satisfactory progress toward any of them.

- If your goal is to hit peak "which way to the beach?" shape, a six-month version of a competitive bodybuilder's macrocycle can help you first build up and then lean out in time for the event.

- If you know your training will soon be disrupted, you can set up a macrocycle that allows you to crank up the volume while your schedule allows it and then downshift to lower frequency and volume when duty requires.

- Conversely, if you're a student, your macrocycle can begin when classes end, when you'll have the freedom to train with higher volume and frequency without compromising recovery. Then you can downshift to maintenance workouts at the start of the next semester.

Those are just a few ways you can plan your training around the seasons of your life.

THE MESOCYCLE

Every situation I described in the previous section includes some suggested mesocycles—the phases of training that typically last one to three months and build toward the overall goal of the macrocycle. In this section, I'll focus specifically on bodybuilding.

Mesocycles for bodybuilding are generally straightforward: You build up, and then you deload (see Figure 13.2). That's it. Build up volume, intensity, or both across four to eight weeks of training, deload for a week, and then begin the next mesocycle.

Figure 13.2

Mesocycle: build and then deload

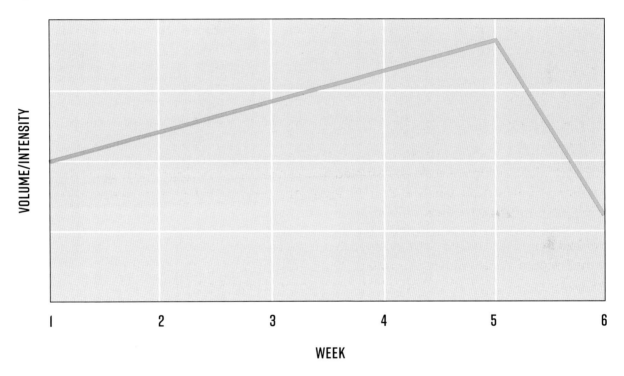

In the next sections, I give you some sample mesocycles.

BASIC PROGRESSIONS

The buildup phase of a bodybuilding mesocycle applies the principles of progressive overload. You're progressively increasing one or more of the variables I discussed in Chapter 7—weight, volume, and so on.

Table 13.6 shows a six-week mesocycle—a five-week buildup followed by a one-week deload—for someone trying to increase their pec size and bench press strength. This mesocycle and the next one are based on linear progressive overload.

Table 13.6: Mesocycle Example 1a: Linear Progression on the Bench Press

Buildup					Deload
Week 1	Week 2	Week 3	Week 4	Week 5	Week 6
180 lb × 6 reps	185 lb × 6 reps	190 lb × 6 reps	195 lb × 6 reps	200 lb × 6 reps	170 lb × 6 reps

As you can see, you're simply adding five pounds to the bar every week but keeping the same rep count until you deload in Week 6.

The next six-week mesocycle, shown in Table 13.7, continues the same progression scheme.

Table 13.7: Mesocycle Example 1b: Linear Progression on the Bench Press

Buildup					Deload
Week 7	Week 8	Week 9	Week 10	Week 11	Week 12
205 lb × 4 reps	210 lb × 4 reps	215 lb × 4 reps	220 lb × 4 reps	225 lb × 4 reps	200 lb × 4 reps

After Week 12, you switch to a double-progression model, as shown in Table 13.8.

Table 13.8: Mesocycle Example 1c: Double Progression on the Bench Press

Buildup						Deload
Week 13	Week 14	Week 15	Week 16	Week 17	Week 18	Week 19
225 lb × 4 reps	225 lb × 5 reps	225 lb × 6 reps	230 lb × 4 reps	230 lb × 5 reps	230 lb × 6 reps	210 lb × 4 reps

This time, you're progressing both reps and load—going from 4 reps in Week 13 to 6 reps in Week 15, then adding weight in Week 16 while dropping back to 4 reps.

You can also base your mesocycle on gradually increasing RPE, as shown in Table 13.9.

Table 13.9: Mesocycle Example 2: Increasing RPE (Any Compound Exercise)

Buildup				Deload
Week 1	Week 2	Week 3	Week 4	Week 5
3 sets × 6 to 8 reps RPE of 7 to 8	3 sets × 6 to 8 reps RPE of 8 to 9	3 sets × 6 to 8 reps RPE of 9 to 10	3 sets × 6 to 8 reps RPE of 10 (plus optional drop set after the final set)	2 sets × 6 to 8 reps RPE of 6 to 7

The idea is to work progressively harder until you take each working set to true failure in Week 4. And if that's not difficult enough, you have the option to add a drop set after your third set. You'll recover from that effort with a full deload in Week 5, when you drop down to RPE 6 to 7.

How you increase your RPE each week is up to you. You can add weight while keeping reps the same, increase reps while using the same weight, or do some combination. Since this is an autoregulated approach, you may end up hitting your RPE target with fewer reps than you anticipated. It doesn't matter. As long as you reach a progressively higher RPE each week, you've accomplished your objective.

Here's yet another way to structure a mesocycle: adding sets, as shown in Table 13.10.

Table 13.10: Mesocycle Example 3: Adding Sets (Any Exercise)

Buildup				Deload
Week 1	Week 2	Week 3	Week 4	Week 5
2 sets × 8 to 10 reps	3 sets × 8 to 10 reps	4 sets × 8 to 10 reps	5 sets × 8 to 10 reps	2 sets × 8 to 10 reps

Remember that because adding sets increases volume very quickly, you should consider adding them a more advanced periodization strategy—one that should be reserved for low-load exercises and movements where other forms of progression are more difficult to achieve week to week. For example, I sometimes add sets when a trainee has fully plateaued their lateral raise progression.

ADVANCED PROGRESSIONS

For those interested in digging yet another layer deeper, let's consider some more advanced mesocycle examples using linear periodization, reverse linear periodization, and weekly undulating periodization.

LINEAR PERIODIZATION

Linear periodization is when the intensity (load) goes up while the volume goes down. As you can see in Table 13.11, as the weight increases, the reps decrease from week to week. Linear *periodization* should not be confused with linear *progression*. Linear periodization is when the load goes up while the reps go down. Linear progression is when either the load, the reps, or both go up by using progressive overload.

Let's consider what linear periodization might look like for someone trying to increase their squat max across a seven-week mesocycle.

Table 13.11: Advanced Linear Periodization: Strength Focus

Buildup						Deload
Week 1	Week 2	Week 3	Week 4	Week 5	Week 6	Week 7
295 lb × 8 reps	315 lb × 6 reps	325 lb × 4 reps	345 lb × 3 reps	365 lb × 2 reps	385 to 395 lb × 1 rep	315 lb × 4 reps

Now take a look at Table 13.12, which shows how someone might use the barbell biceps curl to increase their arm size and strength using linear periodization.

Table 13.12: Advanced Linear Periodization: Strength Focus

Buildup					Deload
Week 1	Week 2	Week 3	Week 4	Week 5	Week 6
3 sets × 14 reps RPE of 9	3 sets × 12 reps RPE of 9	3 sets × 10 reps RPE of 9	3 sets × 8 reps RPE of 9	3 sets × 6 reps RPE of 9	2 sets × 10 reps RPE of 6 to 7

In this example, you're doing fewer reps each week at the same RPE, which means you'll work with progressively heavier weights.

The next two examples show reverse linear periodization, which is exactly what the name implies.

REVERSE LINEAR PERIODIZATION

In linear periodization, the weight goes up while the volume goes down. In reverse linear periodization, the weight goes down while the volume goes up. Table 13.13 outlines an example of what this might look like for someone trying to increase their work capacity on the squat across a six-week mesocycle.

Table 13.13: Reverse Linear Periodization: Strength and Work-Capacity Focus on the Squat

Buildup					Deload
Week 1	Week 2	Week 3	Week 4	Week 5	Week 6
3 sets × 2 reps RPE of 8	3 sets × 4 reps RPE of 8	3 sets × 6 reps RPE of 8	3 sets × 8 reps RPE of 8	3 sets × 10 reps RPE of 8	2 sets × 6 reps RPE of 6 to 7

For a bodybuilder, this type of periodization can be useful for increasing your ability to train with higher volume. As the reps go from 2 in Week 1 to 10 in Week 5, you will be presented with a massive overloading stimulus for quad hypertrophy. For a powerlifter, reverse linear periodization is an effective way to build muscle in the offseason while maintaining specificity on the squat, bench, and deadlift.

Table 13.14 shows how you might use reverse linear periodization with the close-grip bench press to increase your volume tolerance and triceps size.

Table 13.14: Reverse Linear Periodization: Hypertrophy Focus Using the Close-Grip Bench Press

Buildup					Deload
Week 1	Week 2	Week 3	Week 4	Week 5	Week 6
3 sets × 4 to 6 reps RPE of 9	3 sets × 6 to 8 reps RPE of 9	3 sets × 8 to 10 reps RPE of 9	3 sets × 10 to 12 reps RPE of 9	3 sets × 12 to 14 reps RPE of 9	2 sets × 8 to 10 reps RPE of 7 to 8

In Table 13.14, you can see that the rep count again increases from week to week and the weight you're using decreases to maintain the same RPE of 8. By the end of the build-up phase, this trainee will have built up a significantly higher volume tolerance for their close-grip bench press and will have built up their triceps size as well.

WEEKLY UNDULATING PERIODIZATION

The final advanced progression is weekly undulating periodization, or WUP, which is one of the more entertaining acronyms in exercise science. (DOMS—delayed-onset muscle soreness—is also high on the list.)

Undulating means "moving up and down in waves." Thus, WUP means your sets, reps, and/or loads go up and down in a rhythmic fashion from week to week.

It's distinct from daily undulating periodization, or DUP (another world-class acronym). DUP, which I'll return to later in this chapter, has you doing different combinations of sets and reps in every workout in any given week. With WUP, you're doing the same set-rep combos throughout the week rather than doing something different each day.

WUP is a bit more chaotic than the other models we've covered, which makes it ideal for a lifter who's stagnated with other progression models or who's easily bored and thrives on novelty. I sometimes use it in programs for powerlifters who I think would benefit from something less predictable.

The example shown in Table 13.15 is for a hypothetical powerlifter who's stuck on a max bench press of 315 pounds.

Table 13.15: Weekly Undulating Periodization: Strength Focus on the Bench Press

Buildup				Deload
Week 1	Week 2	Week 3	Week 4	Week 5
3 sets × 8 reps × 235 lb (~75% 1RM)	3 sets × 4 reps × 265 lb (~85% 1RM)	3 sets × 6 reps × 250 lb (~80% 1RM)	3 sets × 2 reps × 280 lb (~90% 1RM)	2 sets × 5 reps × 235 lb (~75% 1RM)

As you can see in Table 13.15, the load goes up in Week 2, down in Week 3, up again in Week 4, and then down again for a deload in Week 5. This is the wave-like pattern I referred to earlier. Again, this type of periodization may be unnecessary for most lifters, but the variety can be useful for busting through strength plateaus.

Now look at Table 13.16 to see what WUP might look for hypertrophy.

Table 13.16: Weekly Undulating Periodization: Hypertrophy Focus on the Bench Press

Buildup				Deload
Week 1	Week 2	Week 3	Week 4	Week 5
3 sets × 10 to 12 reps RPE of 9	3 sets × 6 to 8 reps RPE of 9	3 sets × 8 to 10 reps RPE of 9	3 sets × 4 to 6 reps RPE of 9	2 sets × 6 to 8 reps RPE of 7 to 8

Once again, the rep range goes down, then up, then back down before the deload. If this type of periodization were suitable for an advanced trainee, you would then extend the WUP model out across another five weeks as shown in Table 13.17 to complete a ten-week training program.

Table 13.17: Weekly Undulating Periodization: Hypertrophy Focus

Buildup				Deload
Week 6	Week 7	Week 8	Week 9	Week 10
3 sets × 10 to 12 reps RPE of 9 (aim to add weight or reps from Week 1)	3 sets × 6 to 8 reps RPE of 9 (aim to add weight or reps from Week 2)	3 sets × 8 to 10 reps RPE of 9 (aim to add weight or reps from Week 3)	3 sets × 4 to 6 reps RPE of 9 (aim to add weight or reps from Week 4)	2 sets × 6 to 8 reps RPE of 7 to 8

As you can see, it's the same mesocycle as the first five weeks but with added weight or reps. You can visualize this sequence as the waves getting progressively bigger from mesocycle to mesocycle. Extended across several months of training, it would look something like Figure 13.3.

Figure 13.3

Undulating mesocycle

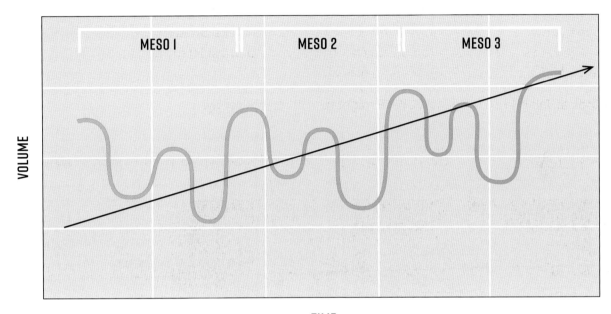

PUTTING IT ALL TOGETHER

The detailed mesocycles shown in Tables 13.11 through 13.17 may be unnecessary for most lifters simply seeking muscle growth, but they can be useful for advanced lifters who've stalled on simpler progression schemes. They also might be worth trying for intermediates who thrive on novelty and variety.

I decided to cover them here for the sake of completeness and because of their popularity among exercise scientists. Including them also helps me make an important point: You can find virtually unlimited ways to structure a program. You're only limited by your curiosity and imagination. Just keep in mind that, for all their complexity, the goal is basic and fundamental: progressive overload. If you like nerding out on these different models, that's awesome. Me too! If not, don't let it bog you down. Periodization is on an upper rung and toward the back of the book for a reason.

If your current routine allows you to make progress, you're doing great. If your progress is slowing down, or you've hit a dead end, it could be time to consider some of these periodization options.

DELOADS

A deload is a period of training where the load, volume, or both are decreased for a short period, usually a single week. The purpose of a deload is to reduce fatigue, promote recovery, and allow a brief mental break so that the more challenging training phases can be maximized more effectively.

In most sports, athletes and coaches realize that you need to have periods of rest and lighter training to optimize performance over the long haul. For many lifters, it's "go hard or go home" fifty-two weeks a year—which, alas, is a surefire formula for burnout, injury, or long and frustrating plateaus.

It's much smarter to organize your training in a way that combines buildup periods of progressively harder training with deload weeks in which you give your body a break with lighter, easier workouts. Slowing down for a week or two doesn't just give your muscles and joints time to recover; it also gives your mind a chance to reset.

That sets you up to train harder and more effectively in the next block of training.

Generally speaking, I schedule a deload once every four to twelve weeks. More advanced trainees pushing their limits with harder sets and heavier loads generally need deloads more often. Less advanced trainees who don't need to push as hard or heavy to make progress usually don't need to deload as frequently. Obviously, if you're not actually training hard yet, you don't

need a deload at all. Focus on training harder first.

For those who prefer to plan, you can schedule your deload weeks at regular intervals. I typically plan a deload every eight weeks or so, depending on the exact goal of the program. The other option is to do less planning and be more flexible, taking a deload whenever your body tells you it's time for one. If you notice weights feeling brutally heavy, your sleep is lacking, and your motivation to train is waning, you're probably due for one.

THE FULL TRAINING BREAK

There was a time, not so long ago, when bodybuilders would stop training for a full week or two after a major competition. Even though that practice is less popular these days, it still makes some sense. Research shows most people won't lose significant size or strength until at least two or three weeks of complete detraining.[1]

In my experience, the biggest risk of a complete break is what it does to your momentum. I've found the weights tend to feel heavier when I return, and I struggle to get back into my routine.

But with a deload, which I'll discuss in a moment, I can maintain my routine while still giving my body and brain a chance to regroup. It's not unusual for me to feel even stronger when I restart hard training after the deload week. That's why I don't often recommend a complete break from training unless you need to. The deload accomplishes the same goals with less disruption.

That said, there's nothing wrong with stepping away from your workouts when circumstances call for it. Let's say you're on vacation. Maybe you can find a local gym and continue your workouts. However, if you don't, taking a week off definitely won't kill your gains, and there's nothing wrong with taking a full mental break every once in a while.

The best vacations are the ones where you leave your routines behind. See new things, try different foods, and enjoy new and different ways to be active. If you want a break, know that the gym will be there when you get back.

THE CALCULATED DELOAD

A deload works best with moderate decreases in volume and intensity, based on the following guidelines:

- Drop volume by 30 to 50 percent. In practice, this typically means cutting one or two sets per exercise.

- Reduce effort by around 10 to 30 percent or about one to three points of RPE. How much you drop back depends on the exercise. If you've been training at RPE 9 with a primary exercise, for example, you'd want to use RPE 6 or 7 for your deload week. However, if you've been at RPE 7 with an accessory exercise, you probably don't want to pull back that far. You'll still get the benefits of a deload at RPE 6 because you're also reducing volume.

- If your intensity is based on a percentage of your one-rep max, reduce your %1RM by 5 to 10 percent for your deload. In your final loading week, let's say you're doing 6 reps with 80 percent of your 1RM in the bench press. You might deload with 6 reps at 70 to 75 percent of your 1RM. You also might want to cut 1 or 2 reps from each set in addition to cutting 1 or 2 sets and reducing the %1RM.

THE INSTINCTIVE DELOAD

The good thing about a calculated deload is that it gives you a systematic way to scale back your volume and intensity. If this is the first time you've included deloads in your training, I recommend figuring it all out in advance.

But predetermined set, rep, and load targets may not reflect how you feel when you get to the deload week or what your body needs.

The alternative is to let your instincts and experience guide your decisions. You'll still go into it with the goal of having a "light week" but with a more flexible idea of what that will entail. It's a given that you'll do 1 or 2 fewer sets per exercise and stop each set a little further from failure, but you'll give yourself the option to make other adjustments. For example, you might swap out an exercise that felt like a grind during the last week or two of your mesocycle. Another way you can be flexible is to use dumbbells instead of a barbell on bench presses or curls or cables or machines instead of free weights. Because you're trying to be instinctive, you don't want to overthink it.

With either type of deload, calculated or instinctive, it's important to remember what you're *not* doing. You're *not* using your deload week as an excuse to sandbag your workouts or blow off your workouts entirely. You're still training with attention and focus.

Some coaches I know refer to deloads as "technique weeks," reframing them as a temporary shift in focus, rather than a step backward. Whatever you call that week, you'll still use lighter loads and reduced volume. You're also still minimizing fatigue and maximizing recovery, but you'll also take advantage of the lighter loads and reduced fatigue to refine your technique or improve your mind-muscle connection.

THE MICROCYCLE

The third and final element of periodization is the microcycle, usually a single week's worth of training. How you set up your microcycles is similar to choosing a training split. I won't rehash the details of each split here, or their specific advantages and disadvantages. (Feel free to review Chapter 9 if you need a refresher.) Any of them can work in a microcycle.

What I'll do instead is focus on two general principles you'll apply in your microcycles: prioritization and variation.

PRIORITIZATION

You prioritize key exercises by placing them either earlier in the week or earlier in a training session. You also prioritize the muscles that require the most effort to build or the ones you consider weak points. The goal is to work on them when you have the most energy and focus and the least residual fatigue.

For most people, leg workouts hit the trifecta:

- Exercises like squats and deadlifts are the most technically challenging and physically exhausting.

- Leg muscles are often the hardest to build.

- If you ignored your legs for your first year or two in the gym, your quads, hamstrings, and/or glutes probably lag behind your arms, chest, and shoulders.

Table 13.18 shows how you could prioritize legs with a push/pull/legs split with your most challenging workout on Monday, following a rest day.

Table 13.18: Sample Schedule for Push/Pull/Legs Split with Leg Prioritization

Day of the Week	Focus
Monday	Legs (hardest, highest-volume workout)
Tuesday	Push
Wednesday	Pull
Thursday	Legs (lighter workout)
Friday	Push
Saturday	Pull
Sunday	Rest

Granted, this structure won't be ideal for everyone. For example, if you're a bartender who works late shifts all weekend, Monday could be the *worst* day of the week for a leg workout. It might make more sense to schedule that workout for Tuesday after you've had a chance to catch up on your sleep.

Whatever your circumstances at work or home, it's smart to set up your workout schedule so you minimize overlapping types of stress.

Table 13.19 has another example for someone who prefers an upper/lower split and whose chest is a glaring weak point.

Table 13.19: Sample Schedule for Upper/Lower Split with Chest Prioritization

Day of the Week	Focus
Monday	Upper (hit chest first)
Tuesday	Rest
Wednesday	Lower (hardest leg day)
Thursday	Rest
Friday	Upper (hit chest first)
Saturday	Lower
Sunday	Rest

As you can see, both upper-body workouts follow rest days (as does your hardest leg session of the week). You'll further prioritize chest by hitting it first on those two days.

VARIATION

According to a wonderful 2012 review paper by John Kiely, "training variation is a critical component of long-term planning, but if adaptive energy is too widely distributed, gains may be excessively diluted."[2]

It's among my favorite quotes about training in general, and it's by far my favorite about periodization. It confirms that variety is good as it warns against too much of it. You can turn it around to say that repetition is good because it gives you a way to make and measure progress, but too much repetition leads to boredom and stagnation.

You have two primary ways to create variety within a microcycle: DUP and exercise variation.

DUP

DUP, as you may recall from earlier in this chapter, stands for daily undulating periodization. It's probably the most popular periodization model among coaches and lifters. Even if you haven't heard of DUP, you may have some sense of how it works.

Undulating refers to a wavelike motion. The "daily" part means your sets, reps, and/or loads are somewhat different in each workout.

Let's use the example of someone who's training their biceps three times per week:

Monday	Wednesday	Friday
3 sets × 10 reps × 60 lb	3 sets × 6 reps × 80 lb	3 sets × 15 reps × 40 lb

As you can see, with a DUP setup, the reps undulate within the week. The week starts with moderate reps, drops to low reps mid-week, and then increases to high reps at the end of the week. When you repeat the workouts the following week, you'd follow the same pattern but still want to ensure that you're applying progressive overload by adding a rep or some weight.

The basic principle of DUP also can be applied to body parts being trained only twice a week. Here's how it might look for someone who squats twice a week. In this case, the first workout focuses on strength development, and the second is designed for hypertrophy:

Monday	Tuesday	Wednesday	Thursday	Friday
3 sets × 3 to 5 reps RPE of 7 to 8			3 sets × 6 to 8 reps RPE of 7 to 8	

As you can see, there are two different rep ranges being used within the same week for the squat. Earlier in the week is a heavy leg day, and later in the week is a lighter leg day. Even this simple structure counts as DUP because when it's expanded over time, the reps go up and down and up and down in waves as you move toward a gradual increase. For progression using this example, you may want to increase your loads from week to week in the Monday workout, whereas you focus more on adding reps in the Thursday workout.

Here's an example of how a powerlifter might use DUP for the bench press:

Monday	Tuesday	Wednesday	Thursday	Friday
Bench press (hypertrophy focus) 3 sets × 8 to 10 reps RPE of 8 to 9		Bench press (strength focus) 3 sets × 3 to 5 reps RPE of 7 to 8		Bench press (power focus)* 3 sets × 2 to 4 reps RPE of 5 to 6
* Focus on moving the bar with maximum concentric speed (explosive power)				

The Monday workout uses moderate reps to build the chest, shoulders, and triceps. The Wednesday workout uses lower reps to emphasize pure strength development. On Friday, you train for power by moving relatively light weights as explosively as possible.

The mechanism by which DUP works isn't perfectly clear. Is there a physiological mechanism that rewards you for training for two or three distinct but complementary adaptations within each microcycle? Or does the value come from simply not doing the same thing in every workout? Personally, I lean toward the second idea. I suspect the main benefit of DUP is psychological—you simply enjoy training more when it includes some variety.

EXERCISE VARIATION

Most strength coaches consider DUP as a method for varying sets, reps, or load within a week on a given exercise. However, you can also create variety throughout a training week by varying the exercises themselves. Recall the 2014 Fonseca study from Chapter 5, where participants who did a combination of squats, leg presses, and lunges gained more muscle across all heads of the quadriceps compared to those who did squats exclusively. With that in mind, here are a few ways to vary exercises within a microcycle:

- If you do back squats in your first lower-body workout, do front squats or hack squats in the second one.

- If you do barbell bench presses in your first upper-body workout, do close-grip or incline dumbbell presses in the next one.

- If you do traditional deadlifts from the floor one day, do Romanian deadlifts or pull from blocks on another.

- If you do EZ-bar curls early in the week, try preacher or incline dumbbell curls later in the week.

And with that, we have arrived at the top of the Muscle Ladder. After climbing all ten rungs, you now have all the tools you need to get jacked using science.

Before you climb back down, read on for three more important and often neglected elements of a successful training program: nutrition, supplements, and cardio.

A VERY BRIEF PRIMER ON CALORIES-IN, CALORIES-OUT (CICO)

CICO—calories-in, calories-out—is the consensus model of energy balance among nutrition scientists.

Calories, as you probably know, are units of energy. If you consume more calories than you burn, you're in a *caloric surplus.* Do that over time and you'll gain weight. If you burn more calories than you consume, you're in a *caloric deficit,* which leads to weight loss over time. If you're in *energy balance,* your weight should remain stable.

There's only one way to consume energy: eat something that contains calories. However, you have four ways to burn energy. Together, these four categories determine how many calories you burn each day—your total daily energy expenditure (TDEE):

- **Resting energy expenditure (REE):** Sometimes referred to as your basal metabolic rate (BMR), it accounts for as much as 70 percent of your total daily energy expenditure (TDEE). Even though you're motionless, your body is still busy keeping you alive. Your brain and liver each account for about 20 percent of your resting energy expenditure, while your heart, lungs, and kidneys also punch above their weight in terms of energy use.

- **Exercise activity thermogenesis (EAT):** Exercise burns fewer calories than most people expect—only around 5 to 10 percent of TDEE for someone who lifts weights a few days a week. (It would be much higher for an endurance athlete training or competing for several hours a day.) That's because your basic functions still account for most of your energy expenditure, even when you're working out.

- **Non-exercise activity thermogenesis (NEAT):** Most of your daily activities—anything from washing dishes to walking to the bathroom—don't qualify as exercise. NEAT includes any daily activity other than formal exercise—stuff like bringing in groceries, playing guitar, and tapping your feet at your desk. NEAT burns more calories than many people expect but can vary drastically between individuals. It typically falls somewhere around 15 percent of the daily total burn, but can be a lot higher for someone who's extremely fidgety—constantly tapping their feet or squirming around. Or it could be lower for someone who burns a lot of energy in training and then moves less while recovering.

- **Thermic effect of food (TEF):** It takes energy to process energy. About 10 percent of your TDEE comes from digesting the food you eat. Protein has the highest thermic effect, whereas fats have the lowest. Carbs burn a little more than fat but much less than protein. No known foods have a TEF high enough to cost more energy than they contain. Thus, there's no such thing as a food with "negative calories." Even if they did, TEF is not a major contributor, typically checking in at around 5 percent of the total daily burn.

Figure 14.1 shows a breakdown of the components of TDEE.

Figure 14.1

The four components of total daily energy expenditure (TDEE)

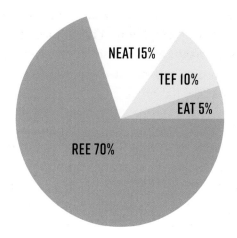

NEAT 15%
TEF 10%
EAT 5%
REE 70%

What's confusing about metabolism is that all the components of TDEE are in constant flux, depending on what's going on with the other components. That's why it's so hard to lose weight from exercise alone. Your body may adjust to your increased EAT by increasing your appetite, downregulating other parts of your metabolism, or some combination of adjustments.

That's a major source of confusion, not to mention frustration, for someone trying to lose weight. And it's a big part of the reason why diet is so important for fat loss. The following sections describe a few more ways your body weight doesn't always do what you expect.

WATER FLUCTUATIONS

Your body is about 65 percent water. But it's distributed in crazy ways. Water makes up about three-quarters of your muscle mass but as little as 10 percent of your fat. This means even small, normal daily fluctuations in water weight can have a noticeable impact on how your body looks, feels, and weighs.

Your body can retain water for any number of reasons—eating more salty food than usual, consuming more carbs, drinking more fluids. It could be related to your menstrual cycle or stress level. You can also drop water weight for similarly transitory reasons.

Small daily variations don't matter. As I explained in Chapter 3, your focus should be on the long-term trend line. If it's moving up, you're in a caloric surplus (which is a good thing when you're trying to add muscle). If it's moving down, you're in a caloric deficit. Figure 14.2 shows an example of the daily fluctuations in weight that can occur due to water fluctuations.

Figure 14.2

Weight loss with fluctuations due to water weight

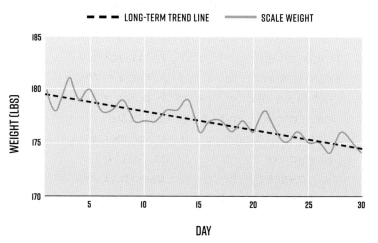

WEIGHT LOSS WITH FLUCTUATIONS DUE TO WATER WEIGHT

- - - LONG-TERM TREND LINE ——— SCALE WEIGHT

WEIGHT (LBS)

DAY

METABOLIC ADAPTATION

Another reason it's hard to manipulate your weight is *your weight doesn't want to be manipulated.*

When you eat less, your metabolism slows down. It adapts to lower energy consumption with lower energy expenditure. When you do lose weight, your body becomes more metabolically efficient, conserving more calories both at rest and during exercise. Your REE and EAT go down because your body is smaller. Your TEF goes down because you're eating less. And your NEAT might also decline if cumulative fatigue from your workouts and caloric deficit means you fidget less or move around less.

Collectively, these changes result in fewer calories burned than you were burning at the start of your diet. In other words, your maintenance calories decrease throughout the course of your diet due to metabolic adaptation.

Some people interpret these changes to mean that CICO isn't working because they aren't losing weight at the rate that they expected. The reality is that the calories-out side of the equation has changed. So to keep up with your target rate of weight loss and account for metabolic adaptation, you may need to either decrease your caloric intake further or accept a slightly slower pace of weight loss than you initially anticipated.

Metabolic adaptation also occurs in response to a caloric surplus for the same reasons. When you eat more calories, your body burns more calories. Your REE and EAT go up because your body is getting bigger. Your TEF increases because you're eating more food. And NEAT might increase for the simple reason that you have more energy to burn with extraneous movement.

NOT ALL CALORIES ARE CREATED EQUAL

You might also hear people say a calorie is not really a calorie because calories from different food sources have different metabolic effects. That idea makes as much sense as saying a mile isn't really a mile because it's harder to walk uphill than on flat ground.

A calorie is simply a unit of energy, just as a mile is a unit of distance. Still, there's a hint of truth, as obviously not all foods have the same impact on the body. Foods with lots of fiber or water make you feel full faster than highly processed foods. Foods with a lot of protein are typically more satiating, which means you'll be less hungry between meals. Foods rich in vitamins and minerals offer important health benefits you can't get from foods with fewer nutrients.

So two things can be true at once: Different food sources can have different effects on your health, appetite, mood, and performance, and energy balance determines long-term weight changes.

SETTING UP YOUR CALORIES

How many calories you should eat per day depends on your primary goal: lose fat, build muscle, or do both. The latter goal, body recomposition, is theoretically possible for anyone, but it's most realistic when you're

- New (or relatively new) to weight training

- Returning to the gym after an extended layoff

- Using a well-designed training program for the first time

- Carrying a lot of body fat

- Using anabolic steroids

Progress made by people in these categories are similar to newbie gains. (Steroids typically have the most dramatic effects when someone uses them for the first time.) But if you're not in one of these categories, it makes more sense for you to focus on one goal at a time.

MAINTENANCE CALORIES

It's easy enough to create a caloric surplus or deficit. Just eat more or less. But at some point, you'll probably want a more precise approach. To do that, you need to start with an estimate of your *maintenance* calories—the amount of food you need to stay at your current body weight.

I typically recommend one of three ways to calculate maintenance calories:

- A super quick and dirty method

- A *somewhat* quick and dirty method

- A not-quick, not-dirty, frankly laborious method

The two quick and dirty methods, as you guessed, are less accurate than the calculations behind Door Number Three, but they're good enough to get the job done for most people.

QUICK AND DIRTY METHOD: A VERY ROUGH FORMULA

You want easy? It doesn't get easier than this: multiply your body weight by a number between 14 and 18:

- If you're younger than 40 and generally active outside the gym, multiply your body weight by 17 or 18. So if you weigh 180 pounds, your maintenance calories would be somewhere between 3,060 and 3,240 a day.

- If you're older than 40 and generally inactive at home and at work, multiply your body weight by 14 or 15. So if you weigh 200 pounds, you'd maintain your current weight with between 2,800 and 3,000 calories a day.

- If you aren't sure how to define your activity level, multiply your body weight by 16 and see what happens.

SOMEWHAT QUICK AND DIRTY METHOD: THE MIFFLIN-ST. JEOR EQUATION

The Mifflin-St. Jeor equation, developed in 1990, is still considered by many to be the most accurate way to estimate daily energy expenditure.

To begin, you need to know your weight in kilograms (divide your weight in pounds by 2.2) and your height in centimeters (multiply your height in inches by 2.54). Then follow these steps:

1. Calculate your basal metabolic rate (BMR), which is the number of calories you burn at rest:

   BMR (male): [10 × weight (kg)] + [6.25 × height (cm)] − [5 × age (years)] + 5 = calories per day.

   BMR (female): [10 × weight (kg)] + [6.25 × height (cm)] − [5 × age (years)] − 161 = calories per day.

2. Multiply your BMR by the physical activity multiplier from Table 14.1 that best applies to you.

Table 14.1: Activity Multipliers Based on Activity Level

Activity Level	Example	Activity Multiplier
Sedentary	Work a desk job, very little activity outside of lifting weights	1.2 to 1.5
Lightly active	Work a desk job, take pet for a walk most days in addition to lifting weights	1.5 to 1.8
Moderately active	Work as a full-time restaurant server, occasionally play tennis in addition to lifting weights	1.8 to 2.0
Highly active	Work in construction or another physically demanding field or train and compete in a sport like soccer or basketball in addition to lifting weights	2.0 to 2.2

As an example, let's consider a 5'7", 150-pound male named Max.

Using the Mifflin-St. Jeor equation, we calculate his BMR to be 1,639 calories per day.

He works a desk job and walks his dog most days. He also lifts weights three to five days a week. According to Table 14.1, he falls into the lightly active category, which means his activity multiplier is 1.5 to 1.8. Let's pick 1.6.

Maintenance calories = BMR × activity multiplier = 1,639 × 1.6 = 2,622.

So if Max eats in the neighborhood of 2,622 calories per day, he should maintain his current weight.

LABORIOUS METHOD: GUESS AND CHECK

Because the guess-and-check method allows you to collect data directly from your body, it's more accurate than the other two, which is good. It has a downside, though: It takes at least two weeks to complete.

But here's why you might consider it anyway:

The two easy (or easy-ish) calculations are accurate for most people, so by definition, they're also inaccurate for some people. If you're one of the people for whom the quick methods are inaccurate, the estimates could be off by hundreds of calories in either direction.

Here's how the guess and check method works:

- Week 1: Track your body weight and caloric intake every day. Calculate your average daily calories and average body weight for that week.

- Week 2: Do the exact same things for the next seven days and calculate your averages.

  Note: Make sure the two weeks you track are relatively typical for you. The experiment won't work if one of the weeks includes travel, holiday or birthday parties, interrupted sleep, or an unusual amount of stress at work or home.

- Determine the average weight you gained or lost from Week 1 to Week 2.

- For example, if your average weight for Week 1 was 190.4 pounds and your average weight for Week 2 was 191.4 pounds, then you gained 1 pound on average.

- Determine your maintenance calories based on the weight change. Assume that you need about a 500-calorie deficit per day to lose 1 pound of weight per week and a 500-calorie surplus per day to gain 1 pound of weight per week.[1] (Note these numbers aren't perfectly accurate, but they work great for estimating maintenance calories and roughly predicting weight gain and weight loss.)

  - If you maintained your average weight from Week 1 to Week 2, then whatever your average caloric intake was can be set as your maintenance calories.

- If you lost between 0.5 and 1 pound, then your maintenance calories will be roughly 250 to 500 calories more than your average calories. If you lost 1 to 2 pounds, then your maintenance calories will be 500 to 1,000 calories more than your average calories.

- If you gained 0.5 to 1 pound, then your maintenance calories will be roughly 250 to 500 calories less than your average calories. If you gained 1 to 2 pounds, then your maintenance calories will be 500 to 1,000 calories less than your average calories.

Here are few examples:

If you ate 3,000 calories per day on average and lost 1 pound from Week 1 to Week 2, then your maintenance would be 3,500 calories (3,000 + 500 = 3,500).

If you ate 2,000 calories per day on average and lost 0.4 pound from Week 1 to Week 2, then your maintenance would be 2,200 calories (2,000 + 0.4 × 500 = 2,000 + 200 calories = 2,200).

If you ate 3,000 calories per day on average and gained 1.2 pounds from Week 1 to Week 2, then your maintenance would be 2,400 calories (3,000 − 1.2 × 500 calories = 3,000 −600 = 2,400).

If you ate 2,600 calories per day on average and gained 0.4 pound from Week 1 to Week 2, then your maintenance would be 2,400 calories (2,600 − 0.4 × 500 = 2,600 − 200 = 2,400).

BULKING, CUTTING & RECOMP CALORIES

Once you have an estimate of your maintenance level (remember, these methods only give you an educated guess), you can add or cut calories, depending on your primary goal.

To lose a pound a week, you would need a caloric deficit of roughly 500 calories a day. To gain a pound a week, you'd need the opposite: a 500-calorie-a-day surplus.

But remember what I mentioned earlier: Any change in your energy intake will provoke changes to your energy expenditure.

If you're disciplined enough to maintain that new diet long enough, what was once a caloric deficit or surplus will eventually become your maintenance level. Your body will see it as your new normal, and your metabolism will adjust to accommodate it. To keep your weight moving in the direction you want it to, you'll need to periodically adjust your calories to keep up with your moving maintenance. You can do this yourself by paying attention to your average trends in weight and caloric intake or you can hire a coach who understands metabolic adaptation. Or you can use an app like MacroFactor, which uses algorithms to detect changes to your metabolism and update your calories over time. (Disclaimer: I'm a part owner of the app.)

Use Table 14.2 as a guide for setting up your calories, based on your maintenance calories and your main goal: building muscle (bulking), losing fat (cutting), or building muscle and losing fat at the same time (body recomposition or recomp).

Table 14.2: Setting Up Caloric Intake Based on Goal

Main Goal	Caloric Target	Example	Notes
Bulking	Lean/slow bulk: Set calories at 5 to 10 percent above maintenance calories.	If your maintenance level is 3,000 calories, you would lean bulk on 3,150 to 3,300 calories per day.	Aim to add around 0.5 to 1 percent to your body weight per month, which is typically about 0.5 to 2 pounds.
	Standard bulk: Set calories at 10 to 20 percent above maintenance calories.	If your maintenance level is 3,000 calories, you would standard bulk on 3,300 to 3,600 calories per day.	Aim to add around 1 to 1.5 percent to your body weight per month, which is typically about 1 to 3 pounds.
Cutting	Set calories at 10 to 20 percent below maintenance.	If your maintenance level is 3,000 calories, you would cut on 2,700 to 2,400 calories per day.	Aim to lose around 1 to 3 percent of your body weight per month, which is typically about 2 to 7 pounds. That comes out to about 0.5 to 2 pounds of weight loss per week, on average.
Body recomposition	Set calories at approximately maintenance intake.	If your maintenance level is 3,000 calories and you hope to stay at or near your current weight while losing fat and gaining muscle, you would recomp on about 3,000 calories per day.	If you're more focused on building muscle, aim for a small caloric surplus—about 5 percent more than your maintenance level. If fat loss is a higher priority, aim for a small caloric deficit of 5 to 10 percent.

USING REFEEDS

Refeeds on a diet are analogous to deloads on a training program. You eat more food for a limited time (usually just one or two days a week) with the goal of improving your long-term results.

Higher-calorie days offer a psychological break from the diet similar to the physical benefits of deloads when you give your muscles and joints a chance to recover from the strain of heavy training. If you're doing an extreme cut, a refeed also has the physical benefit of replenishing glycogen, giving you more energy to train.

You don't need a refeed during a bulk or recomp phase, for the obvious reason that you're neither straining your willpower nor draining your glycogen. Even when you're cutting, refeeds are optional.

In my experience, some people do better with refeeds. Getting to eat more food and different types of food is like releasing a pressure valve. Other people do better with the consistency of continuous dieting. And yet another group does better with continuous dieting in the early stages of a diet and switching to using refeeds in the later stages as their body-fat percentage reaches the low single digits.

Table 14.3 shows three ways to approach a cutting diet. In this example, the goal is to average 2,000 calories a day—a 20 percent deficit from a maintenance level of 2,500 calories a day. The first column shows a continuous target of 2,000 calories a day. The others show how much you'd eat each day with either one or two refeeds a week.

Table 14.3: Refeed Schedules Based on a 20 Percent Average Caloric Deficit

	Continuous Diet (No Refeeds)	One Refeed Day	Two Refeed Days
Monday	2,000 calories	1,875 calories	1,800 calories
Tuesday	2,000 calories	1,875 calories	1,800 calories
Wednesday	2,000 calories	1,875 calories	1,800 calories
Thursday	2,000 calories	1,875 calories	1,800 calories
Friday	2,000 calories	1,875 calories	1,800 calories
Saturday	2,000 calories	1,875 calories	2,500 calories
Sunday	2,000 calories	2,750 calories	2,500 calories
Average Deficit	−20%	−20%	−20%

SETTING UP YOUR PROTEIN

How much protein you should eat per day depends on your primary goal. In general, you want more protein when you're in a caloric deficit, and less when you're bulking or recomping, as shown in Table 14.4.

For most people, an intake in the middle of the ranges outlined will be plenty to maximize muscle growth or muscle retention. If you're exceptionally lean, you may want to use the upper end because muscle makes up a higher percentage of your body mass, and you need more protein per unit of body weight. If you're at a high body fat percentage, use your goal weight instead of your current weight when determining your protein intake.

Table 14.4: Setting Up Protein Intake Based on Goal

Main Goal	Protein Target	Example
Bulking	0.7 to 1 gram of protein per pound of body weight (1.6 to 2.2 grams per kilogram)	If you weigh 190 pounds, you should eat between 133 and 190 grams of protein per day.
Cutting	0.8 to 1.2 grams of protein per pound of body weight (1.8 to 2.7 grams per kilogram)	If you weigh 190 pounds, you should eat between 152 and 228 grams of protein per day.
Body Recomposition	0.7 to 1 gram of protein per pound of body weight (1.6 to 2.2 grams per kilogram)	If you weigh 190 pounds, you should eat between 133 and 190 grams of protein per day.

As you can see, this table offers pretty broad ranges for protein intake. Anything within the range is considered optimal. Most people can simply aim toward the bottom to middle of the range and not need to worry. Those who are leaner or more advanced or simply prefer to eat more protein can aim for the higher end of the range.

SETTING UP YOUR FATS

Fats play many roles in your overall health. Here are just two examples: They're essential for your hormones to function properly and also an important source of energy. Most lifters, no matter their primary goal, do well with between 20 and 35 percent of their total calories from fat.

Let's say you're in a cutting phase and eating 2,200 calories per day. You'd want between 440 and 770 of those calories from fat, or about 49 to 86 grams of fat per day. (One gram of fat contains about nine calories, whereas protein and carbohydrate have about four calories per gram.)

So if your fat target is 30 percent of total calories, here's how you'd calculate it:

$$2{,}200 \times 0.3 = 660 \text{ calories}$$

$$660 \text{ calories} \div 9 \text{ calories per gram} = 73 \text{ grams of fat per day}$$

SETTING UP YOUR CARBS

Unlike protein and fat, your body doesn't *need* carbohydrates, but it's challenging for most people to function optimally without them. Not only are carbs your primary fuel source during training sessions, carbohydrate-rich foods provide many of the most important vitamins and minerals. On top of all that, carbs make your meals more satiating and enjoyable.

You determine the proportion of carbs in your diet by calculating how many calories remain after accounting for protein and fat. Table 14.5 shows how it works.

Table 14.5: Examples of Carb Intake Based on Calorie, Protein, and Fat Targets

	Weight	Main Goal	Calories	Protein	Fat	Carbs
Example 1	190 lb	Recomp	3,000	160 g (640 calories; 21 percent of total)	90 g (810 calories; 27 percent of total)	390 g (1,560 calories; 52 percent of total)
Example 2	210 lb	Lose fat	2,600	170 g (680 calories; 26 percent of total)	75 g (675 calories; 26 percent of total)	310 g (1,240 calories; 48 percent of total)
Example 3	130 lb	Bulk	2,500	120 g (480 calories; 19 percent of total)	70 g (630 calories; 25 percent of total)	275 g (1,390 calories; 56 percent of total)

I rounded up some of the numbers to keep it simple, which means the sum of calories from protein, fat, and carbs differs slightly from the target calories. Also note that the macros in these examples aren't necessarily what I'd recommend for every trainee with these goals.

FIBER

Fiber is a complex carbohydrate that can't be fully digested by humans, which means it doesn't provide as much energy as other types of carbs. But it does slow down digestion, which helps you feel full longer between meals. That's hugely valuable during a fat-loss phase, when your diet sometimes pushes your self-control to the limit.

Fiber is linked to long-term health benefits, including a lower risk of heart disease, type 2 diabetes, and colorectal cancer.[2] In addition, fiber has a higher thermic effect than other carbs.

Still, despite its many benefits, more fiber is not necessarily better. Excessive fiber intake can lead to bloating, nutrient absorption issues, and irregular bowel movements.

How much fiber should you get? It depends on how many carbs you typically eat, as you can see in Table 14.6.

Table 14.6: Recommended Fiber Intake Based on Carb Intake

Total Daily Carb Intake	Recommended Daily Fiber Intake
Less than 100 g carbs	About 20 g fiber
100 to 200 g carbs	20 to 30 g fiber
200 to 300 g carbs	30 to 40 g fiber
300 to 400 g carbs	40 to 50 g fiber
400 to 500 g carbs	50 to 60 g fiber
500 g carbs or more	60 to 70 g fiber

BEING FLEXIBLE

So far in this chapter, I've discussed calories and macros as a series of math equations, but I don't want to leave you with the idea that you have to quantify every gram of every nutrient in every meal to reach your goals. In fact, it's usually better if you don't.

As you may recall, in Chapter 3, I said you're more likely to achieve long-term success with a flexible approach. This is as true for nutrition as it is for your training.

Your daily calories are going to fluctuate day to day. Even if you track all your calories meticulously, there's a certain margin of error associated with food labels. Same goes for your energy expenditure; even if you have the most predictable of lifestyles, you won't move the exact same amount each day. You may as well give yourself some wiggle room to accommodate that reality. If you consistently get within 50 to 100 calories of your target in either direction, you're doing great.

What matters is your energy balance over time. If your average intake results in a long-term caloric surplus, you'll gain weight. If your average intake results in a long-term caloric deficit, you'll lose weight. Focus on the trendline, not the individual data points.

For protein, I like to be within 10 to 20 grams of my target. For carbs and fats, I'm generally much more flexible. Honestly, I don't pay close attention to my exact carb and fat numbers on a daily basis. As long as I'm making reasonable food choices and not purposefully skipping on fat sources, the carbs and fat in my diet mostly take care of themselves.

The approach I just described—tracking calories and protein, but not the other two macros—is practical for most of us. It's also effective because calories and protein do more to determine body composition than carbs or fat.

The key, I've found, is to be relatively consistent with your fat. If you regularly stray above or below the recommended range of 20 to 35 percent of total calories, your carbs will also be all over the place. That's going to make it much harder to manage your appetite and energy levels and may even affect your training.

All that said, if you prefer to track all three macros, I suggest staying within 10 grams of your daily fat target and 20 to 30 grams of your target carbs (while keeping within your target calorie range, of course).

USING NONTRACKING APPROACHES TO DIET

It's possible to reach your goals without ever tracking anything. In a moment, I'll explain a few ways to get around doing it.

First, though, I want to make the case that every lifter should give tracking what they eat a shot, at least for a while. You may find you like it. I know I do. I still track my food most days of the week using my nutrition app, MacroFactor. It only takes me about five to ten minutes a day. The longer you do it, the easier it becomes.

Many of the benefits come from the process rather than the results. Tracking what you eat and how much of it raises your nutritional IQ. But you don't just learn what your food is made of, as important as that is. You also gain valuable insights into your eating behaviors. How do different foods, or combinations of foods, affect you? What impact do they have on your hunger levels or the quality of your workouts?

If you've never tracked your food before, I encourage you to try it to see what happens. If you have tried it and found it too tedious or annoying to continue, I have some nontracking options to suggest. Here are a few strategies for a fat-loss diet:

- Use your average weekly body weight as your primary metric. If progress is too slow, or if you're not making any progress at all, identify the highest-calorie foods you eat on a regular basis and look for reasonable alternatives. By "reasonable," I mean lower-calorie foods you like that satisfy your appetite in a similar way. It's hard to go wrong with lean protein, fruits, and vegetables.

- Eat three to five balanced discrete meals rather than picking throughout the day.

- Get in the habit of looking at nutrition labels for everything you eat, even if you aren't tracking calories and macros.

- When you check food labels, make sure you look at the portion size. Do you typically wolf down two, three, or even four portions before you feel satisfied?

- For foods that don't come with labels, focus on how you prepare and consume them. Do you cook everything in oil or butter? Do you drown baked potatoes in sour cream? The way you prepare your meals could be adding more calories than you realize.

- Sugary beverages are usually full of unnecessary calories. You can always find a low- or no-calorie option.

- Consider time-restricted feeding. It definitely doesn't work for everyone, but I've found that a moderate intermittent fasting protocol can help some people maintain a caloric deficit. The protocol I've seen the most success with is a sixteen-hour fast followed by an eight-hour eating window.

If your primary goal is muscle gain or body recomposition, here are some nontracking tactics:

- Remember that training is the number one driver of muscle growth. Focus first and foremost on making progress in the gym.

- Use your weekly average body weight as your main metric for progress. If you're gaining too slowly or too quickly, make an effort to adjust your diet by making commonsense food decisions.

- Aim to consume three to five meals per day with about 30 grams of protein in each. Do this by keeping an eye on the nutritional information of what you're eating, even if you aren't tracking it.

- It takes energy to train hard. Being disappointed by your progress could be a sign you're not eating enough. I have some of my best workouts right after a holiday or diet break, when I've eaten more than usual.

- Beware of popular diets. Most are designed to help people eat less. That's especially true for diets that restrict entire categories of food (like keto or vegan) or limit when you can eat (like intermittent fasting). When you're trying to gain weight, you need more options, not fewer.

CONSUMING WATER

Research has shown that a mere 3 percent reduction in hydration status can significantly reduce strength, decrease reps, and make a workout feel harder.[3] So the obvious takeaway is to avoid dehydration.

Fortunately, staying hydrated is easy to accomplish. You don't need to buy sports drinks or lug around a water bottle the size of a surface-to-air missile. Just pay attention to your body, which has highly evolved intricate ways to regulate its fluid levels. Do you feel thirsty? You need to drink something. Don't feel thirsty? You're probably good.

There are some exceptions to what I just described. If you work or train outdoors, for example, your thirst signals may not be able to keep up with the fluids you've lost through perspiration, especially on hot, humid days. You also have a higher dehydration risk if you're older, have diabetes, drink a lot of alcohol, or are recovering from an illness that caused diarrhea or vomiting.

If you're in doubt, check your urine. On a scale of tasty beverages, you want it to look more like lemonade than apple juice. The darker it is, the more likely you are to be dehydrated.

CONSUMING ALCOHOL

I mentioned alcohol as a potential cause of dehydration. That's just one way alcohol makes it harder to reach your goals.

Excessive consumption interferes with your sleep, which subsequently impairs your training performance. It also reduces muscle protein synthesis—an obvious problem for someone trying to gain muscle. It's even worse for someone trying to lose fat. Alcohol has seven calories per gram but no nutritive value. No vitamins, minerals, or fiber. A few drinks can loosen your inhibitions, leading you to eat foods you wouldn't ordinarily touch in quantities you wouldn't ordinarily approach.

Moderate consumption can be a different story. Although no amount of alcohol will help you build muscle or lose fat, an occasional drink is unlikely to negate your efforts or derail your progress. I find an occasional glass of scotch or a beer helps me chill out and might even trigger a temporary release of water weight.

If you don't drink at all, there's no reason to start. If you do, I suggest limiting yourself to a maximum of one or two drinks per day (on days you do drink) and avoiding heavy drinking episodes as much as you can.

I'm not saying you shouldn't enjoy yourself on New Year's Eve or at a wedding reception. But let's be honest: If you're using the "special occasion" excuse to go on a bender every second or third weekend, it's going to affect your gains. Are those celebrations more important than your goals? If the answer is no, you should find ways to limit the damage. Can you skip a few of the celebrations without hurting someone's feelings or damaging relationships? Can you enjoy an event if you stop at one or two drinks? Can you leave early, before the drinking games begin?

MANAGING MICRONUTRIENTS

So far, I've limited the discussion to the "big rocks" of nutrition: calories, macronutrients (protein, fat, and carbohydrates), water, alcohol. Those things will have the greatest effect on your body size and composition. When it comes to health, though, micronutrients are huge.

I won't go into detail about the role of each vitamin or mineral; you can find that information with a couple of clicks, if you're interested.

Fortunately, most of us never need to worry about the specifics. Just follow these simple guidelines:

- Emphasize nutrient-rich whole foods that are minimally processed.

- Aim for at least five servings of fruits and vegetables per day. Seek out produce with a variety of colors.

- Consume fatty fish one or two times per week or consider a fish or algae oil supplement. (I'll discuss supplements later in this chapter.)

- If you decide to avoid entire categories of food—grains, dairy, animal products—you're also avoiding the vitamins and minerals those foods provide. There's a good chance you'll need supplements to avoid deficiencies.

PLANNING MEAL FREQUENCY

When I started lifting, I was told that feeding my body around the clock—six to eight meals per day—was the key to building muscle. The rationale? Muscle tissue builds up and breaks down 24 hours a day. Without food, I'd not only miss an opportunity to add new tissue, I'd *lose* muscle because breakdown would exceed buildup.

A few years later, when I cut down for my first bodybuilding competition, I was once again told that I needed six to eight meals per day. This time, the reason was "to keep the metabolic furnace going."

As it turns out, neither tidbit of gym lore was based on sound evidence.

MEAL FREQUENCY FOR FAT LOSS

For fat loss, the number of meals you eat per day is entirely up to you. That's because the primary driver of fat loss is a *sustained* caloric deficit. Whether you impose that deficit by eating a small number of relatively large meals or a large number of relatively small meals is of no practical consequence, according to a 2020 systematic review on meal frequency.[4]

Some people have success with just one or two large meals per day within a time-restricted window. Limiting your feeding opportunities is an obviously effective way to ensure you eat less. It works best for those who simply don't get hungry until later in the day.

Other people are wired to be hungry in the morning. Skipping breakfast and lunch can feel like torture. The hunger can be so intense it's hard to focus on anything else. For them, four to six relatively smaller meals a day might be the best way to tame their hunger and still maintain an energy deficit.

As the scientific literature shows, the key is to find a meal pattern that allows you to hit your calorie and protein targets while minimizing hunger.[5] The best frequency is the one you can tolerate long enough to reach your fat-loss goal.

MEAL FREQUENCY FOR MUSCLE GAIN

Meal frequency seems to matter a little bit more for muscle gain than fat loss, but the effects are still quite small. Total daily protein intake is far more consequential for hypertrophy than meal frequency.

The sweet spot for maximum muscle growth seems to be three to six meals per day. However, the latest evidence suggests that even one or two ultra-high protein meals per day can be enough to get the job done if you hit your daily protein target.[6] But remember, your workouts are the primary driver of muscle growth. Nothing else comes close.

MANAGING PERI-WORKOUT NUTRITION

Peri-workout nutrition refers to the timing of nutrients before and after a workout. Overall, I think this is an overhyped area of sports nutrition—one that's captured far more attention than it deserves. As long as you hit your calorie and macronutrient targets, the timing is significantly less important.

That doesn't mean you should ignore timing altogether. I recommend following a few simple guidelines.

PRE-WORKOUT NUTRITION

Because the pre-workout meal can impact the quality of your training sessions, I give it more attention than the other peri-workout meals, and I suggest you use the following guidelines:

- **The number one goal of pre-workout nutrition is to prevent you from feeling hungry while training.** A 2020 study from Naharudin and colleagues demonstrated that even a zero-calorie breakfast can boost performance similarly to a carbohydrate-rich breakfast as long as they have a similar volume and consistency.[7] This was supported by a follow-up study by the same group that showed that participants who had a semisolid pre-workout meal completed more reps than a matched group who received a liquid meal, even though both meals contained the same amount of carbohydrate.[8]

- **The pre-workout meal should not cause bloating.** If your pre-workout meal contains a lot of fiber or foods you don't digest well, chances are you'll feel fully satisfied but you won't perform optimally because you'll have a belly full of gas. Most people do well with reliable carb sources like rice, potatoes, oats, and fruit in their pre-workout meal. Fibrous vegetables and legumes are more likely to cause gas and bloating.

- **The pre-workout meal should fit your normal routine.** Just as an athlete believes they perform best when they stick to their pregame ritual, you'll probably get the best results with a consistent routine. However, it only works if those steps are easy and convenient. If your pre-workout meal requires a lot of prep time or expensive ingredients, it's less likely to become part of your routine.

- **The ideal pre-workout meal includes a balanced ratio of carbs, protein, and fat.** If that's too complicated to fit into your routine, prioritize carbs first, protein second, and fat third.

  - For carbs, just 15 grams appears to be enough to fuel a higher-volume workout.[9] That said, I consider 15 grams of pre-workout carbs the *minimum* effective amount. I've found 0.5 to 1 gram of carbs per kilogram of body weight to be a more practical recommendation. So a lifter who weighs 176 pounds (80 kg) would have 40 to 80 grams of carbs in their pre-workout meal (assuming the lifter isn't on a carb-restricted diet).

  - For protein, a 2022 paper suggests consuming 0.3 gram of protein per kilogram of body weight within three hours of your workout.[10] So the 176-pound lifter would have about 24 grams of protein in their pre-workout meal. That sounds reasonable, although I'll once again emphasize that total daily protein is far more important than the timing.

  - Although your body burns some fat, especially between sets, there's no urgent need to get a fresh supply of it from your pre-workout meal. Your body can easily free up fat from existing stores if it needs to. Fat should help with satiety, though. Just be aware that fat can sometimes induce *too much* satiety, leaving you sluggish or even sleepy going into the workout. That's why I usually limit pre-workout fat to about 20 to 25 grams.

- **I recommend eating your pre-workout meal one to three hours before training.** The smaller and lighter the meal, the closer it should be to training. The opposite is true for a bigger and heavier meal. Give yourself plenty of time to digest it.

- **While a pre-workout meal does, on average, seem to enhance performance, habits are probably a greater factor.** If you're a habitual breakfast eater, and you train in the morning, you'll most likely do better with a pre-workout meal. However, if you *never* eat breakfast, you shouldn't have a problem training on an empty stomach. I have one caveat: Fasted training amplifies the importance of post-workout nutrition. I recommend having a protein-rich meal within an hour of leaving the gym. Get your muscle-building machinery up and running without further delay.

INTRA-WORKOUT NUTRITION

If you've eaten something within a few hours of training, you probably don't need more food during your workout. Same with someone who prefers fasted training.

So why am I covering intra-workout nutrition if almost no one needs it? Because there are a few circumstances where a little more energy—

usually 15 to 30 grams of simple liquid carbs—can be helpful:

- If you're doing a high-volume workout that goes beyond 60 to 90 minutes

- If you're extremely lean and nearing the end of a cut

- If you train fasted and find your energy levels crash midway through your workout

Outside of those circumstances, you don't need to worry about intra-workout nutrition.

POST-WORKOUT NUTRITION

For years, bodybuilders obsessed over the post-workout "anabolic window of opportunity." They believed it was absolutely crucial to consume protein as soon as possible after training. To be fair, the idea hasn't been entirely debunked, but we have pretty good evidence that the hype was overblown.

Alan Aragon and Brad Schoenfeld famously pushed back in their 2013 paper, "Nutrient timing revisited: Is there a post-exercise anabolic window?" They argue that the urgency around the post-workout meal is largely unfounded and exaggerated.[11]

Still, there are a few guidelines worth keeping in mind:

- Ideally, you want to separate your pre- and post-workout meals by at least three hours and at most six hours, but the size of the pre-workout meal is also a factor. Larger meals take longer to digest and therefore broaden the window.

- A well-rounded post-workout meal should contain 0.3 to 0.4 gram of protein per kilogram of body weight.[12] The lower number applies to high-quality protein sources (like whey protein), and the higher number is more appropriate for lower-quality types of protein (like nonanimal sources). Rounding up a bit, a 176-pound/80-kg lifter would consume 25 to 35 grams of post-workout protein. (More than that is also fine if it helps you reach your daily total easier.)

- Post-workout carbs usually aren't a huge concern. No matter how hard you train, you probably leave the gym with plenty of glycogen left in your muscles, and then you still have twenty-four hours to replace what you burned before the next workout. A possible exception is if you exercise twice a day, and one of those sessions involves a lot of running (like soccer or basketball) or repetitive efforts (like a combat sport). In that case, you want to get some carbohydrates immediately after the first session so you have the energy you need for the next one.

- Fat is the least important macronutrient following a workout. Some people will tell you to limit fat in your post-workout meal because it slows down protein absorption. If you believe in a limited post-workout anabolic window, any delay in protein absorption is a potential risk to your gains. As you should guess by this point, I believe that concern is overblown. If you hit your daily protein target, your body will figure out the rest. How much fat you include in your post-workout meal is a matter of personal preference and convenience.

DOING CARDIO

Doing regular cardio is generally very beneficial for overall health. An abundance of studies show that cardiorespiratory fitness is a major predictor of all-cause mortality and cardiovascular disease.[13] Having an adequate level of cardiovascular endurance may also indirectly improve your weight training performance, especially in moderate-high rep zones. In this sense, an appropriate amount of cardio may assist your training goals by improving your overall work capacity and recovery between sets.

Despite these important benefits, cardio, in and of itself, doesn't build muscle very effectively and, from a bodybuilding standpoint, should be seen primarily as a fat-loss tool. It's also not a *great* fat-loss tool because your body has ways to limit the calorie-burning effects of endurance-type exercise. If you do too much of it, or at too high an intensity, it could potentially interfere with muscle growth.

I don't want to overstate this risk of interference, though. Most lifters have nothing to fear from cardio, whether they're doing it for health or body composition or because they enjoy it. Some athletes revel in their ability to develop both strength and endurance at a high level, and they compete in both disciplines, separately or together.

To be sure, those athletes are outliers. Those of us with less-than-superhuman abilities quickly realize how hard it is to recover from high volumes of two very different types of exercise. A little cardio can help you recover from resistance training, but a lot of cardio is more likely to wear you down. The same is true in reverse: Some strength training can improve your performance in an endurance sport, but a lot of lifting might do the opposite.

Here are a few ways to get the benefits of cardio without overdoing it:

- There are no strict rules when it comes to cardio. It's neither mandatory nor prohibited.

- The less active you are outside the gym, the more you'll benefit from doing cardio with little risk of it interfering with your muscle and strength development.

- The more active you are at work (if you're a restaurant server, for example, or work in landscaping or construction), the less you need cardio, and the more likely it is to interfere with your training adaptations.

- If you like to warm up on the treadmill or stationary bike before weights, keep it to 10 minutes or less. Otherwise, do cardio after finishing your strength workout or on days you don't lift.

- Low-intensity steady-state cardio (LISS) and high-intensity interval training (HIIT) are similarly effective at stimulating fat loss, assuming you burn the same number of calories.

- You can burn those calories in less time with HIIT, which has the added benefit of improving your cardiovascular fitness more efficiently. But HIIT also requires more time to recover. When muscle and strength gain is your main priority, try to limit HIIT cardio to one to two sessions per week, ideally no longer than thirty minutes per session.

- LISS takes longer to burn the same number of calories, but because it's less taxing, recovery is rarely an issue. If anything, LISS should help you recover from strength training. How much you do is completely up to you. Depending on your goals, you can do two to five sessions per week, with thirty to sixty minutes per session. More is also fine, as long as it isn't negatively impacting your weight training.

- Choose the type of cardio you enjoy most or hate least. You can use cardio machines in the gym; go outside to walk, run, or ride a bike; hike or ruck in a local park; play a sport; or mix and match however you see fit. My only advice is to be more cautious with high-impact activities like running or basketball, which are more likely to interfere with recovery and potentially limit performance in squats and other knee-dominant exercises. That doesn't mean they're off limits, just that you should pay a little closer attention to how they impact your strength output.

- Your body will let you know if you're doing too much. You'll see a drop in strength, energy, and/or motivation in the gym. The solution is simple enough: Just pull back on the cardio and give your body more time to recover.

MANAGING SUPPLEMENTS

As the name implies, supplements are intended to be, and *should* be, supplemental. They're meant to support an intelligent diet and training plan, not become an end in themselves.

The list of supplements that genuinely help you get bigger and stronger is pretty short. Same with the list of products that support your health in other ways.

In the rest of this section, I rank supplements according to their safety, efficacy, and cost. Supplements in the higher tiers are the ones you should consider before wasting your money on the stuff in the lower tiers.

TIER I

We have decades of research showing the supplements in this tier are both safe and effective. Because they've been around so long, they're also affordable.

PROTEIN POWDER

If you only use one supplement, this is the one you want. It's a convenient and affordable way to hit your daily protein target.

Supplement companies give you dozens of options for protein powders, but the choice is usually an easy one: Whey protein is supported by the most research, and you should be able to find a high-quality product for a reasonable price.

The best vegan options are made from soy, pea, or brown rice—although that could change by the time you read this. Vegan proteins are a booming part of the supplement market, and researchers are always working to keep up with all the new options.

You can use a protein powder at any time, either as a meal replacement or to boost the protein content of an otherwise low-protein meal. (You can put some in your morning oatmeal, for example.)

CREATINE

Creatine is a naturally occurring compound used by your muscles for short, maximum-effort bursts of speed or power. It's also one of the supplement industry's few legitimate triumphs.

Your body can synthesize a gram or two of creatine per day, getting most of it from the meat and fish in your diet. That's enough to supply your muscles with the energy they need for just about

any real-life challenge. But it's only about 60 to 80 percent of the muscles' full capacity.[14]

Supplementing with creatine monohydrate helps you fully saturate your muscles, which allows you to work a little harder in the gym. You might get an extra rep or two per set or do the same number of reps with a heavier load. Over time, that boost in performance can help you increase strength and improve body composition, as shown in countless studies over the years.[15] A creatine supplement may be especially useful for vegetarian and vegan athletes, who don't consume natural sources of creatine like seafood or red meat.

There are two methods for supplementing creatine that work equally well over the long term:

- **Loading:** Most creatine studies employ a loading phase of about one week, during which 5 grams of creatine is taken four times per day for a total of 20 grams of creatine per day. The loading phase is followed by a maintenance phase, during which 3 to 5 grams of creatine is taken once per day. The maintenance phase can continue indefinitely. Utilizing a loading phase generally saturates muscle creatine levels faster. However, the larger quantities of creatine during the loading period can lead to stomach discomfort for some and may be more inconvenient than simply starting with the maintenance dose.

- **Standard:** The second approach is to simply start with the 3 to 5 grams-per-day maintenance phase without a loading period. This method may take a week or two longer to reach full saturation levels, but it's simpler, more convenient, and less likely to result in stomach discomfort.

After one month, both strategies will result in fully saturated muscle creatine levels. You can take creatine at any time of day. However, some research suggests that taking it post workout may confer a slight advantage.[16] I typically take my creatine with breakfast for convenience.

Creatine monohydrate has the most research and safety data supporting its use, so it's the only form of creatine I broadly recommend using. There is no need to cycle on and off creatine because your body doesn't develop a tolerance to it. Also, decades of research show no adverse effects with long-term supplementation.[17]

CAFFEINE

Caffeine is worth considering as a pre-workout supplement. It helps you train a little harder with the strength you already have, which subsequently helps you add to that strength over time. That's why it's included in so many sports drinks and pre-workout supplements.

When researchers study the effects of caffeine on performance, they typically give participants 3 to 6 milligrams per kilogram of body weight.[18] For a 176-pound/80-kg lifter, that's 240 to 480 mg. That quantity is equivalent of two to four cups of coffee.

Would that much caffeine get you jacked up for a workout? Absolutely. Is it safe? Maybe, but I wouldn't make a habit of it. For one thing, you don't want to become dependent on a stimulant to get your work done. For another, habitually high caffeine intake blunts its performance-enhancing effects. That's on top of well-known side effects like anxiety and insomnia.

However, consuming caffeine in regular, moderate amounts can be almost magical. It improves your mood, helps you focus, and increases your productivity. My advice: A little caffeine goes a long way. Take the W, and don't try to supercharge it.

TIER 2

I include only two supplements in this category, neither of which is linked to performance. (If they were, they'd be in tier 1.) Whether you use either or both depends on your overall diet. You don't need multivitamins if you eat a diverse diet with a variety of fruits and vegetables every day, and you don't need fish oil if you eat fatty fish at least once or twice a week.

You can think of both tier 2 supplements as a kind of insurance policy. Even with a healthy diet, you may eat the same foods almost every day. There's nothing wrong with that; once you find something that works, it makes sense to stick with it. The downside of consistent food choices is they may be limiting your range of nutrients.

MULTIVITAMINS

Multivitamins, according to research, have virtually no effect on long-term health in the general population. They don't reduce the risk of cardiovascular disease or death from any cause.[19]

So why even consider them? A deficiency in one or more vitamins or minerals might affect some aspect of your performance.[20] And if you're a vegetarian or vegan athlete, there's a good chance you'll need a supplement to get the recommended amounts of vitamins B12 and D3, heme iron, calcium, and zinc.[21]

To be clear, a multivitamin *cannot* make up for a bad diet. That's just as true for omnivores as it is for those with plant-based diets. What it can do is give you an easy and cheap way to make up for potential deficiencies.

If you decide to take a multivitamin, look for something that covers the RDA for most vitamins and minerals. It should come from a reputable brand that uses third-party testing for quality (a site like Labdoor.com gives you an easy way to check this) and costs no more than 25 cents a day.

FISH OIL

In contrast to multivitamins, the research supporting fish oil is robust. For example, a 2019 meta-analysis found that supplementing with marine omega-3 fat appears to reduce the risk of cardiovascular disease, including fatal heart attacks.[22] Fish oil supplements have also been linked to a long list of health benefits, including a potentially lower risk of dementia.

What they don't appear to do (at least not consistently) is boost performance or help with fat loss in healthy individuals.[23]

If you decide to take a fish oil supplement, look for one that provides 1 to 2 grams per day of combined EPA and DHA. Those omega-3 fats are needed everywhere in your body, from your cell membranes to your immune system to your brain. It shouldn't cost more than about 40 cents per day. Vegans can consider algae oil supplementation as a fish oil alternative.

TIER 3

Tier 3 also has two supplements: L-citrulline and melatonin. Both seem to hold some promise but don't exert a strong enough effect to land them in the higher tier.

L-CITRULLINE

L-citrulline is one of the few products to come along in recent years with performance-enhancing claims that seem to hold up under scientific scrutiny. To understand how it works, you first need to understand L-arginine. L-arginine is an amino acid that helps increase nitric oxide. Nitric oxide (not to be confused with *nitrous* oxide, aka laughing gas) has a number of important roles in health and performance. One is vasodilation—relaxing blood vessels to allow higher blood flow. Another is neurotransmission—making it easier for neurons to communicate with each other. And that's just scratching the surface.[24] Both functions could conceivably improve performance.

Interestingly, because of absorption issues with L-arginine, supplementing L-citrulline increases L-arginine more than supplementing L-arginine itself.[25] That's why L-citrulline appears to be a more effective nitric oxide booster.

A 2019 meta-analysis by Trexler and others found small but significant strength improvements after taking an L-citrulline supplement.[26] It's still too early to call L-citrulline a proven performance booster, much less move it to tier 1 with protein and creatine, but it does look promising.

The recommended dose is 6 grams taken about ninety minutes before a workout.[27] It's probably best to use L-citrulline as a stand-alone supplement. Many pre-workout supplements, which often include claims about L-citrulline in their marketing, are notorious for using too small a dose to get the benefits. Of course, you can always check the supplement label yourself to see if they include enough.

MELATONIN

As of now, melatonin is the only sleep-enhancing supplement with a respectable amount of research supporting its safety and efficacy. It falls into tier 3 because the demonstrated benefits are modest, even for those with diagnosed sleep disorders.

Deep inside your brain sits the pineal gland, a tiny organ with a huge responsibility: releasing melatonin, a hormone that helps regulate your body clock. It gives you more melatonin when it's dark outside and you're ready to sleep and less during daylight. That's why researchers have studied melatonin supplementation in relation to sleep since the 1970s.[28]

A 2005 meta-analysis confirmed the safety of melatonin supplements while also showing small but positive effects on sleep quality in those with a primary sleep disorder like insomnia.[29] A 2013 meta-analysis showed an additional benefit: more total sleep.[30] And a 2018 meta-analysis showed that melatonin can also help with secondary sleep disorders, like jet lag and shift work. The supplement improved both sleep onset latency (how fast you fall asleep after turning off the lights) and total sleep time.[31]

As I said, these findings are pretty small. Whether they're clinically meaningful is open to debate. That said, because melatonin is both safe and inexpensive (five cents per dose at the high end), I'd put it into the "can't hurt, might help" category.

The most common dose is 3 to 5 milligrams, taken somewhere between fifteen minutes to two hours before bedtime. Look for a stand-alone melatonin supplement; other ingredients only raise the price without offering a scientifically validated benefit.

WHY DIDN'T YOU MENTION [INSERT SUPPLEMENT HERE]?

My three tiers include just seven supplements, one of which you're more likely to get in coffee or energy drinks than a pill. So why didn't I include some of the most popular supplements, possibly including one or more of your favorites?

Alas, you may not like my answer: If it doesn't appear on my list, it means I don't recommend it. At least not strongly, and certainly not broadly. Remember that supplements are meant to *supplement* what you're already doing with your training and diet. They shouldn't be a major area of focus, which is why I'm going to conclude this chapter here and get back to the stuff that really matters! In the next and final chapter, we'll put our ladder to use and dig into some sample training programs.

PROGRAM TERMINOLOGY

In the following training programs, you may notice a few terms that you aren't familiar with.

- *Early set RPE* simply refers to the RPE on all sets except your last set. So, if the program calls for 3 sets of bench press, sets 1 and 2 would be the early sets. Set 3 is the last set. Reread Chapter 6 (page 187) if you need a refresher on RPE.

- The *last set intensity technique* is to be done on, well, the last set only. There are no intensity techniques in the beginner programs, and a blank cell in other programs means there is no last set intensity technique for that exercise. Refer to Chapter 12 if you aren't sure how to implement the intensity technique given.

- Supersets—performing exercises as a paired circuit by going back and forth with shorter rests in between—are indicated in front of the exercise. If there is just one superset in a workout, the exercises you should pair are labeled as Superset 1; when there are two supersets, the second pair is labeled Superset 2.

I suggest you write down what you do during each workout as you go along. Tracking what you do helps you keep tabs on your progress. You can set up your logbook using the same format the training programs are presented in. I recommend you also add a column for tracking your load and reps for each exercise. The tracking sample shows what this might look like during your first week of training.

The beginner programs emphasize machine-based exercises, which are easier to learn. However, feel free to swap the machine-based exercises for a free weight variation, if you are comfortable with the form, have been training for a few months already, or have a trainer to assist you.

Although the goal is to use the same load and reps for each set, it's normal and expected that you may need to make some adjustments to stay within the rep range and hit the target RPEs, especially when performing an exercise for the first time (or the first time in a while). The number of adjustments needed should decrease as you get more comfortable with each exercise.

TRACKING SAMPLE

Week 1	Exercise	Last Set Intensity Technique	Warm-Up Sets	Working Sets	Reps	Tracking Load and Reps			Early Set RPE	Last Set RPE	Rest	Substitution Option 1	Substitution Option 2	Time Estimate
						Set 1	Set 2	Set 3						
	General warm-up: 5 mins light cardio & dynamic stretching													
Full Body #1	Barbell Back Squat		2–3	2	3–5	185 lb x 4 reps	185 lb x 4 reps		~7	~8	3–4 min	Leg Press	Dumbbell Lunge	15–20 min
	Chest-Supported T-Bar Row		1–2	3	8–10	135 lb x 8 reps	135 lb x 7 reps	125 lb x 10 reps	~7–8	~9	2–3 min	Pendlay Row	Dumbbell Row	10–15 min
	Barbell Romanian Deadlift		1–2	3	6–8	150 lb x 8 reps	150 lb x 8 reps	150 lb x 8 reps	~7	~8	3–4 min	Dumbbell Romanian Deadlift	Hip Thrust	15–20 min
	Incline Dumbbell Press		1–2	3	12–15	50 lb x 12 reps	50 lb x 12 reps	50 lb x 13 reps	~7–8	~9	2–3 min	Incline Machine Chest Press	Incline Barbell Bench Press	10–15 min
	Lat Pulldown		1–2	3	10–12	125 lb x 12 reps	130 lb x 12 reps	130 lb x 12 reps	~7–8	~9	2–3 min	Pull-Up (Optional Assistance)	Chin-Up	10–15 min
	Superset 1: EZ-Bar Biceps Curl		0–1	2	6–8	50 lb x 8 reps	60 lb x 6 reps		~7–8	~10	0–1 min	Standing Barbell Curl	Dumbbell Biceps Curl	3–5 min
	Superset 1: EZ-Bar Skullcrusher		0–1	2	10–12	40 lb x 10 reps	40 lb x 10 reps		~7–8	~10	0–1 min	Dumbbell Skullcrusher	Overhead Triceps Extension	
											Estimated Training Time:			68–95 min

You'll need to do a quick warm-up before starting each workout. From there, the programs should be fairly self-explanatory! If you aren't sure how to perform an exercise, refer to the demo photos and technique checklists in Chapter 4. Train hard, train safe, and have fun!

WARM-UP PROTOCOL

You should complete a general warm-up before starting each workout. You can use the one I've outlined. It should take no more than 5 to 10 minutes. You can save time by doing some of the dynamic stretches as you do warm-up sets for the first exercise.

General Warm-Up	
5 to 10 minutes	Light cardio on your choice of machine (treadmill, stair climber, elliptical, bike, and so on)
10 reps per side	Arm swings
10 reps per side	Arm circles
10 reps per side	Front-to-back leg swings
10 reps per side	Side-to-side leg swings
15 reps per side	Cable external rotation (optional)

After completing the general warm-up, do an exercise-specific warm-up. As I covered in Chapter 2, heavier compound exercises usually need 2 to 4 warm-up sets before you'll feel ready to tackle a real working set. Lighter isolation exercises may need only 1 light warm-up set to get you ready to get started.

Exercise-Specific Warm-Up	
1 warm-up set	Use about 60% of your planned working weight for 6 to 10 reps (or until you feel warm and loose)
2 warm-up sets	Perform a mini warm-up pyramid: Warm-up set #1 = about 50% of planned working weight for 6 to 10 reps Warm-up set #2 = about 70% of planned working weight for 4 to 6 reps
3 warm-up sets	Perform a full warm-up pyramid: Warm-up set #1 = about 45% of planned working weight for 6 to 10 reps Warm-up set #2 = about 65% of planned working weight for 4 to 6 reps Warm-up set #3 = about 85% of planned working weight for 3 to 4 reps
4 warm-up sets	Perform a full warm-up pyramid: Warm-up set #1 = about 45% of planned working weight for 6 to 10 reps Warm-up set #2 = about 60% of planned working weight for 4 to 6 reps Warm-up set #3 = about 75% of planned working weight for 3 to 5 reps Warm-up set #4 = about 85% of planned working weight for 2 to 4 reps

PROGRAM 1: FULL-BODY SPLIT 2X/WEEK

LEVEL: Beginner | **GOAL:** Build muscle and gain strength | **TIME:** 60 to 90 minutes

Week 1	Exercise	Last Set Intensity Technique	Warm-Up Sets	Working Sets	Reps	Early Set RPE	Last Set RPE	Rest	Substitution Option 1	Substitution Option 2	Time Estimate
Full Body #1	*General warm-up: 5 min light cardio & dynamic stretching*										
	Leg Press		2–3	2	6–8	~7	~8	3–4 min	Barbell Back Squat	Dumbbell Lunge	15–20 min
	Chest-Supported T-Bar Row		1–2	3	8–10	~7–8	~9	2–3 min	Pendlay Row	Dumbbell Row	10–15 min
	Barbell Romanian Deadlift		1–2	3	6–8	~7	~8	2–3 min	Dumbbell Romanian Deadlift	Hip Thrust	15–20 min
	Incline Dumbbell Press		1–2	3	12–15	~7–8	~9	2–3 min	Incline Machine Chest Press	Incline Barbell Bench Press	10–15 min
	Lat Pulldown		1–2	3	10–12	~7–8	~9	2–3 min	Pull-Up (Optional Assistance)	Chin-Up	10–15 min
	Superset 1: EZ-Bar Biceps Curl		0–1	2	6–8	~7–8	~10	0–1 min	Standing Barbell Curl	Dumbbell Biceps Curl	3–5 min
	Superset 1: EZ-Bar Skullcrusher		0–1	2	10–12	~7–8	~10	0–1 min	Dumbbell Skullcrusher	Overhead Triceps Extension	
										Estimated Training Time:	68–95 min

Suggested 2–3 Rest Days

Full Body #2	*General warm-up: 5 min light cardio & dynamic stretching*										
	Machine Chest Press		2–3	3	6–8	~7	~8	2–3 min	Bench Press	Flat Dumbbell Press	15–20 min
	Leg Press		1–2	3	6–8	~7	~8	3–4 min	Barbell Front Squat	Dumbbell Lunge	15–20 min
	Lat Pulldown		1–2	3	6–10	~7–8	~9	2–3 min	Pull-Up (optional assistance)	Chin-Up	10–15 min
	Seated Leg Curl		1–2	3	10–12	~7–8	~9	2–3 min	Lying Leg Curl	Nordic Ham Curl	10–15 min
	Cable Lateral Raise		0–1	2	12–15	~9	10	1–2 min	Machine Lateral Raise	Dumbbell Lateral Raise	5–10 min
	Superset 1: Standing Calf Raise		0–1	3	10–12	~9	10	0–1 min	Seated Calf Raise	Leg Press Calf Press	3–5 min
	Superset 1: Cable Crunch		0–1	3	12–15	~9	10	0–1 min	Plate-Weighted Decline Sit-Up	Hanging Leg Raise	
										Estimated Training Time:	63–90 min

Suggested 2–3 Rest Days

PROGRAM 2: FULL-BODY SPLIT 2X/WEEK

LEVEL: All levels | **GOAL:** Time-limited muscle and strength gain | **TIME:** 45 to 60 minutes

Week 1	Exercise	Last Set Intensity Technique	Warm-Up Sets	Working Sets	Reps	Early Set RPE	Last Set RPE	Rest	Substitution Option 1	Substitution Option 2	Time Estimate
Full Body #1	General warm-up: 5 min light cardio & dynamic stretching										
	Superset 1: Leg Press		2–3	3	6–8	~7	~8	30–60 sec	Barbell Front Squat	Dumbbell Lunge	10–12 min
	Superset 1: DB Lateral Raise		0–1	3	8–10	~7–8	~10	30–60 sec	Cable Lateral Raise	Machine Lateral Raise	
	Lat Pulldown		1–2	3	8–10	~7–8	~10	1–2 min	Pull-Up (Optional Assistance)	Chin-Up	8–10 min
	Barbell Romanian Deadlift		2–3	2	8–10	~7	~8	2–3 min	Dumbbell Romanian Deadlift	Hip Thrust	10–12 min
	Superset 2: Machine Chest Press		1–2	3	6–8	~7–8	~10	1–2 min	Bench Press	Flat Dumbbell Press	10–12 min
	Superset 2: Standing Calf Raise		0–1	3	6–8	~7–8	~10	1–2 min	Seated Calf Raise	Leg Press Calf Press	
										Estimated Training Time:	43–51 min

Suggested 2–3 Rest Days

Full Body #2	General warm-up: 5 min light cardio & dynamic stretching										
	Seated Leg Curl		2	3	12–15	~8	~9	1–2 min	Lying Leg Curl	Nordic Ham Curl	5–10 min
	Hack Squat		3–4	3	6–8	~7	~8	3–4 min	Leg Press	Dumbbell Lunge	12–15 min
	Incline Dumbbell Press		1–2	3	8–10	~7–8	~9	2–3 min	Incline Machine Chest Press	Incline Barbell Bench Press	10–12 min
	Chest-Supported T-Bar Row		2–3	3	8–10	~8–9	~10	2–3 min	Pendlay Row	Dumbbell Row	10–12 min
	Superset 1: EZ-Bar Biceps Curl		0–1	2	6–8	~7–8	~10	0–1 min	Standing Barbell Curl	Dumbbell Biceps Curl	3–5 min
	Superset 1: EZ-Bar Skullcrusher		0–1	2	10–12	~7–8	~10	0–1 min	Dumbbell Skullcrusher	Overhead Triceps Extension	
	Cable Crunch		1	3	10–12	~9	10	1–2 min	Plate-Weighted Decline Sit-Up	Hanging Leg Raise	5–6 min
										Estimated Training Time:	50–65 min

Suggested 2–3 Rest Days

PROGRAM 3: FULL-BODY SPLIT 3X/WEEK

LEVEL: Beginner | **GOAL**: Build muscle and gain strength | **TIME**: 60 to 90 minutes

Week 1	Exercise	Last Set Intensity Technique	Warm-Up Sets	Working Sets	Reps	Early Set RPE	Last Set RPE	Rest	Substitution Option 1	Substitution Option 2	Time Estimate
Full Body #1	General warm-up: 5 min light cardio & dynamic stretching										
	Leg Press		2–3	3	6–8	~7	~8	3–4 min	Barbell Back Squat	Dumbbell Lunge	15–20 min
	Chest-Supported T-Bar Row		2–3	3	8–10	~7–8	~9	2–3 min	Dumbbell Row	Cable Row	15–20 min
	Glute Ham Raise		1–2	2	8–10	~7	~8	2–3 min	45° Back Extension	Lying Leg Curl	10–15 min
	Dumbbell Lateral Raise		0–1	3	12–15	~9	10	1–2 min	Cable Lateral Raise	Machine Lateral Raise	5–10 min
	Pec Deck		0–1	2	15–20	~9	10	1–2 min	Dumbbell Fly	Push-Up	5–10 min
	Preacher Curl		0–1	2	12–15	~9	10	1–2 min	EZ-Bar Biceps Curl	Dumbbell Biceps Curl	5–10 min
										Estimated Training Time:	55–85 min

Suggested 1–2 Rest Days

Week 1	Exercise	Last Set Intensity Technique	Warm-Up Sets	Working Sets	Reps	Early Set RPE	Last Set RPE	Rest	Substitution Option 1	Substitution Option 2	Time Estimate
Full Body #2	General warm-up: 5 min light cardio & dynamic stretching										
	Machine Chest Press		2–3	3	6–8	~7–8	~9	2–3 min	Barbell Back Squat	Flat Dumbbell Press	15–20 min
	Leg Press		2–3	3	6–8	~7	~8	3–4 min	Barbell Front Squat	Dumbbell Lunge	15–20 min
	Lat Pulldown		1–2	3	8–10	~7–8	~9	2–3 min	Pull-Up (Optional Assistance)	Chin-Up	10–15 min
	EZ-Bar Skullcrusher		0–1	2	12–15	~9	10	1–2 min	Dumbbell Skullcrusher	Overhead Triceps Extension	5–10 min
	Reverse Pec Deck		0–1	2	15–20	~9	10	1–2 min	Rope Facepull	Reverse Cable Fly	5–10 min
	Seated Calf Raise		0–1	3	10–12	~9	10	1–2 min	Standing Calf Raise	Leg Press Calf Press	5–10 min
										Estimated Training Time:	55–85 min

Suggested 1–2 Rest Days

Week 1	Exercise	Last Set Intensity Technique	Warm-Up Sets	Working Sets	Reps	Early Set RPE	Last Set RPE	Rest	Substitution Option 1	Substitution Option 2	Time Estimate
Full Body #3	General warm-up: 5 min light cardio & dynamic stretching										
	Romanian Deadlift		2–3	3	8–10	~6	~7	2–3 min	Deadlift	Hip Thrust	15–20 min
	Incline Dumbbell Press		2–3	3	8–10	~7–8	~9	2–3 min	Incline Machine Chest Press	Incline Barbell Bench Press	10–15 min
	Seated Leg Curl		1–2	2	10–12	~9	10	1–2 min	Lying Leg Curl	Nordic Ham Curl	5–10 min
	Lat Pulldown		1–2	3	10–12	~7–8	~9	2–3 min	Pull-Up (Optional Assistance)	Chin-Up	10–15 min
	Leg Extension		1–2	2	10–12	~9	10	1–2 min	Goblet Squat	Dumbbell Lunge	5–10 min
	Plate-Weighted Decline Sit-Up		0–1	3	8–10	~9	10	1–2 min	Cable Crunch	Plank	5–10 min
										Estimated Training Time:	50–80 min

Suggested 1–2 Rest Days

PROGRAM 4: FULL-BODY SPLIT 3X/WEEK

LEVEL: Intermediate/advanced | **GOAL:** Build muscle and gain strength | **TIME:** 60 to 90 minutes

Week 1	Exercise	Last Set Intensity Technique	Warm-Up Sets	Working Sets	Reps	Early Set RPE	Last Set RPE	Rest	Substitution Option 1	Substitution Option 2	Time Estimate
Full Body #1	General warm-up: 5 min light cardio & dynamic stretching										
	Barbell Back Squat		2–3	3	3–5	~7	~8	3–4 min	Leg Press	Dumbbell Lunge	20–25 min
	Chest-Supported T-Bar Row		2–3	3	8–10	~7–8	~9	2–3 min	Dumbbell Row	Cable Row	15–20 min
	Glute Ham Raise		1–2	3	8–10	~7	~8	2–3 min	45° Back Extension	Lying Leg Curl	10–15 min
	Dumbbell Lateral Raise	Lengthened Partials (Extended Set)	0–1	2	12–15	~9	10	1–2 min	Cable Lateral Raise	Machine Lateral Raise	5–10 min
	Pec Deck	Dropset	0–1	2	15–20	~9	10	1–2 min	Dumbbell Fly	Push-Up	5–10 min
	Preacher Curl		0–1	3	12–15	~9	10	1–2 min	EZ-Bar Biceps Curl	Dumbbell Biceps Curl	5–10 min
										Estimated Training Time:	60–90 min

Suggested 1–2 Rest Days

Week 1	Exercise	Last Set Intensity Technique	Warm-Up Sets	Working Sets	Reps	Early Set RPE	Last Set RPE	Rest	Substitution Option 1	Substitution Option 2	Time Estimate
Full Body #2	General warm-up: 5 min light cardio & dynamic stretching										
	Bench Press		2–3	3	3–5	~7–8	~9	3–4 min	Machine Chest Press	Flat Dumbbell Press	20–25 min
	Leg Press		2–3	3	6–8	~7	~8	3–4 min	Barbell Front Squat	Dumbbell Lunge	15–20 min
	Pull-Up (Optional Assistance)		1–2	3	8–10	~7–8	~9	2–3 min	Lat Pulldown	Chin-Up	10–15 min
	EZ-Bar Skullcrusher		0–1	3	12–15	~9	10	1–2 min	Dumbbell Skullcrusher	Overhead Triceps Extension	5–10 min
	Reverse Pec Deck		0–1	3	15–20	~9	10	1–2 min	Rope Facepull	Reverse Cable Fly	5–10 min
	Seated Calf Raise		0–1	3	10–12	~9	10	1–2 min	Standing Calf Raise	Leg Press Calf Press	5–10 min
										Estimated Training Time:	60–90 min

Suggested 1–2 Rest Days

Week 1	Exercise	Last Set Intensity Technique	Warm-Up Sets	Working Sets	Reps	Early Set RPE	Last Set RPE	Rest	Substitution Option 1	Substitution Option 2	Time Estimate
Full Body #3	General warm-up: 5 min light cardio & dynamic stretching										
	Deadlift		2–3	3	3–5	~6	~7	3–5 min	Romanian Deadlift	Hip Thrust	20–25 min
	Incline Dumbbell Press		2–3	3	8–10	~7–8	~9	2–3 min	Incline Machine Chest Press	Incline Barbell Bench Press	10–15 min
	Seated Leg Curl	Lengthened Partials (Extended Set)	1–2	2	10–12	~9	10	1–2 min	Lying Leg Curl	Nordic Ham Curl	5–10 min
	Lat Pulldown		1–2	3	10–12	~7–8	~9	2–3 min	Pull-Up (Optional Assistance)	Chin-Up	10–15 min
	Leg Extension	Lengthened Partials (Extended Set)	1–2	2	10–12	~9	10	1–2 min	Goblet Squat	Dumbbell Lunge	5–10 min
	Plate-Weighted Decline Sit-Up		0–1	3	8–10	~9	10	1–2 min	Cable Crunch	Plank	5–10 min
										Estimated Training Time:	55–85 min

Suggested 1–2 Rest Days

PROGRAM 5: FULL-BODY SPLIT 3X/WEEK

LEVEL: All levels | **GOAL:** Time-limited muscle and strength gain | **TIME:** 45 to 60 minutes

Week 1	Exercise	Last Set Intensity Technique	Warm-Up Sets	Working Sets	Reps	Early Set RPE	Last Set RPE	Rest	Substitution Option 1	Substitution Option 2	Time Estimate
Full Body #1											
	General warm-up: 5 min light cardio & dynamic stretching										
	Hack Squat		2–3	3	6–8	~7	~8	2–3 min	Leg Press	Dumbbell Lunge	15–20 min
	Chest-Supported T-Bar Row	Lengthened Partials (Extended Set)	2–3	2	8–10	~9	10	2–3 min	Dumbbell Row	Cable Row	10–15 min
	Superset 1: Glute Ham Raise		1–2	2	8–10	~7	~8	30 sec	45° Back Extension	Lying Leg Curl	5–10 min
	Superset 1: Dumbbell Lateral Raise		0–1	2	12–15	~9	10	30 sec	Cable Lateral Raise	Machine Lateral Raise	
	Superset 2: Pec Deck		0–1	2	15–20	~9	10	30 sec	Dumbbell Fly	Push-Up	5–10 min
	Superset 2: Preacher Curl		0–1	2	12–15	~9	10	30 sec	EZ-Bar Biceps Curl	Dumbbell Biceps Curl	
										Estimated Training Time:	35–55 min

Suggested 1–2 Rest Days

Week 1	Exercise	Last Set Intensity Technique	Warm-Up Sets	Working Sets	Reps	Early Set RPE	Last Set RPE	Rest	Substitution Option 1	Substitution Option 2	Time Estimate
Full Body #2											
	General warm-up: 5 min light cardio & dynamic stretching										
	Machine Chest Press	Dropset	2–3	2	6–8	~9	10	2–3 min	Bench Press	Flat Dumbbell Press	15–20 min
	Leg Press		2–3	3	6–8	~7	~8	2–3 min	Barbell Front Squat	Dumbbell Lunge	15–20 min
	Superset 1: Pull-Up (Optional Assistance)		1–2	3	8–10	~7–8	~9	30 sec	Lat Pulldown	Chin-Up	5–10 min
	Superset 1: Seated Calf Raise		0–1	3	10–12	~9	10	30 sec	Standing Calf Raise	Leg Press Calf Press	
	Superset 2: Reverse Pec Deck		0–1	3	15–20	~9	10	30 sec	Rope Facepull	Reverse Cable Fly	5–10 min
	Superset 2: EZ-Bar Skullcrusher		0–1	3	12–15	~9	10	30 sec	Dumbbell Skullcrusher	Overhead Triceps Extension	
										Estimated Training Time:	40–60 min

Suggested 1–2 Rest Days

Week 1	Exercise	Last Set Intensity Technique	Warm-Up Sets	Working Sets	Reps	Early Set RPE	Last Set RPE	Rest	Substitution Option 1	Substitution Option 2	Time Estimate
Full Body #3											
	General warm-up: 5 min light cardio & dynamic stretching										
	Barbell Romanian Deadlift		2–3	3	8–10	~7	~8	2–3 min	Dumbbell Romanian Deadlift	Hip Thrust	15–20 min
	Incline Dumbbell Press	Lengthened Partials (Extended Set)	2–3	2	8–10	~9	10	2–3 min	Incline Machine Chest Press	Incline Barbell Bench Press	10–15 min
	Superset 1: Seated Leg Curl		1–2	3	10–12	~9	10	30 sec	Lying Leg Curl	Nordic Ham Curl	5–10 min
	Superset 1: Lat Pulldown		1–2	3	10–12	~7–8	~9	30 sec	Pull-Up (Optional Assistance)	Chin-Up	
	Superset 2: Leg Extension		1–2	3	10–12	~9	10	30 sec	Goblet Squat	Dumbbell Lunge	5–10 min
	Superset 2: Plate-Weighted Decline Sit-Up		0–1	3	8–10	~9	10	30 sec	Cable Crunch	Plank	
										Estimated Training Time:	35–55 min

Suggested 1–2 Rest Days

PROGRAM 6: UPPER/LOWER SPLIT 4X/WEEK

LEVEL: Beginner | **GOAL:** Build muscle and gain strength | **TIME:** 60 to 90 minutes

Week 1	Exercise	Last Set Intensity Technique	Warm-Up Sets	Working Sets	Reps	Early Set RPE	Last Set RPE	Rest	Substitution Option 1	Substitution Option 2	Time Estimate
	General warm-up: 5 min light cardio & dynamic stretching										
Upper #1	Machine Chest Press		2–3	3	6–8	~7–8	~9	2–3 min	Bench Press	Flat Dumbbell Press	15–20 min
	Chest-Supported T-Bar Row		2–3	3	8–10	~7–8	~9	2–3 min	Pendlay Row	Dumbbell Row	15–20 min
	Dumbbell Lateral Raise		0–1	3	12–15	~9	10	1–2 min	Cable Lateral Raise	Machine Lateral Raise	5–10 min
	Lat Pulldown		1–2	3	8–10	~7–8	~9	2–3 min	Pull-Up (Optional Assistance)	Chin-Up	10–15 min
	Pec Deck		0–1	2	15–20	~9	10	1–2 min	Dumbbell Fly	Push-Up	5–10 min
	Superset 1: Preacher Curl		0–1	2	12–15	~9	10	30 sec	EZ-Bar Biceps Curl	Dumbbell Biceps Curl	5–10 min
	Superset 1: EZ-Bar Skullcrusher		0–1	2	12–15	~9	10	30 sec	Dumbbell Skullcrusher	Overhead Triceps Extension	
										Estimated Training Time:	55–75 min
	General warm-up: 5 min light cardio & dynamic stretching										
Lower #1	Romanian Deadlift		2–3	3	8–10	~6	~7	2–3 min	Deadlift	Hip Thrust	15–20 min
	Leg Press		2–3	3	6–8	~7	~8	3–4 min	Barbell Front Squat	Dumbbell Lunge	15–20 min
	Glute Ham Raise		1–2	2	8–10	~7	~8	2–3 min	45° Back Extension	Lying Leg Curl	10–15 min
	Seated Calf Raise		0–1	3	10–12	~9	10	1–2 min	Standing Calf Raise	Leg Press Calf Press	5–10 min
	Cable Crunch		0–1	3	10–12	~9	10	1–2 min	Plate-Weighted Decline Sit-Up	Hanging Leg Raise	5–10 min
										Estimated Training Time:	50–75 min

Suggested 1–2 Rest Days

Week 1	Exercise	Last Set Intensity Technique	Warm-Up Sets	Working Sets	Reps	Early Set RPE	Last Set RPE	Rest	Substitution Option 1	Substitution Option 2	Time Estimate
Upper #2	General warm-up: 5 min light cardio & dynamic stretching										
	Lat Pulldown		1–2	3	10–12	~7–8	~9	2–3 min	Pull-Up (Optional Assistance)	Chin-Up	10–15 min
	Dumbbell Shoulder Press (Seated)		2–3	3	6–8	~7–8	~9	2–3 min	Dumbbell Shoulder Press (Standing)	Overhead Barbell Press	15–20 min
	Dumbbell Row		1–2	3	10–12	~7–8	~9	2–3 min	Chest-Supported T-Bar Row	Barbell Row	10–15 min
	Flat Dumbbell Press		1–2	3	8–10	~7–8	~9	2–3 min	Dip	Bench Press	10–15 min
	Reverse Pec Deck		0–1	2	10–12	~9	10	1–2 min	Rope Facepull	Reverse Cable Fly	5–10 min
	Superset 1: Triceps Pressdown		0–1	2	10–12	~9	10	30 sec	Triceps Kickback (Cable)	EZ-Bar Skullcrusher	5–10 min
	Superset 1: Bayesian Cable Curl		0–1	2	10–12	~9	10	30 sec	Incline Dumbbell Curl	Preacher Curl	
										Estimated Training Time:	55–85 min
Lower #2	General warm-up: 5 min light cardio & dynamic stretching										
	Leg Press		2–3	3	6–8	~7	~8	3–4 min	Barbell Back Squat	Dumbbell Lunge	15–20 min
	45° Back Extension		1–2	3	8–10	~7–8	~9	2–3 min	Good Morning	Glute Ham Raise	10–15 min
	Leg Extension		1–2	2	10–12	~9	10	2–3 min	Goblet Squat	Dumbbell Lunge	10–15 min
	Seated Leg Curl		1–2	2	10–12	~9	10	2–3 min	Lying Leg Curl	Nordic Ham Curl	10–15 min
	Standing Calf Raise		0–1	3	12–15	~9	10	1–2 min	Seated Calf Raise	Leg Press Calf Press	5–10 min
	Roman Chair Leg Raise		0–1	3	10–20	~9	10	1–2 min	Hanging Leg Raise	Bent-Knee Leg Raise	5–10 min
										Estimated Training Time:	55–85 min
	**Suggested 1–2 Rest Days**										

LEVEL: Intermediate/advanced | **GOAL:** Build muscle and gain strength | **TIME:** 60 to 90 minutes

Week 1	Exercise	Last Set Intensity Technique	Warm-Up Sets	Working Sets	Reps	Early Set RPE	Last Set RPE	Rest	Substitution Option 1	Substitution Option 2	Time Estimate
Upper #1				General warm-up: 5 min light cardio & dynamic stretching							
	Bench Press		2–3	3	3–5	~7–8	~9	3–4 min	Machine Chest Press	Flat Dumbbell Press	20–25 min
	Barbell Row		2–3	3	8–10	~7–8	~9	2–3 min	Pendlay Row	Dumbbell Row	15–20 min
	Dumbbell Lateral Raise	Lengthened Partials (Extended Set)	0–1	2	12–15	~9	10	1–2 min	Cable Lateral Raise	Machine Lateral Raise	5–10 min
	Pull-Up (Optional Assistance)		1–2	3	8–10	~7–8	~9	2–3 min	Lat Pulldown	Chin-Up	10–15 min
	Pec Deck	Dropset	0–1	2	15–20	~9	10	1–2 min	Dumbbell Fly	Push-Up	5–10 min
	Superset 1: Preacher Curl		0–1	3	12–15	~9	10	30 sec	EZ-Bar Biceps Curl	Dumbbell Biceps Curl	5–10 min
	Superset 1: EZ-Bar Skullcrusher		0–1	3	12–15	~9	10	30 sec	Dumbbell Skullcrusher	Overhead Triceps Extension	
										Estimated Training Time:	60–80 min
Lower #1				General warm-up: 5 min light cardio & dynamic stretching							
	Deadlift		2–3	3	3–5	~6	~7	3–5 min	Romanian Deadlift	Hip Thrust	20–25 min
	Leg Press		2–3	3	6–8	~7	~8	3–4 min	Barbell Front Squat	Dumbbell Lunge	15–20 min
	Glute Ham Raise		1–2	3	8–10	~7	~8	2–3 min	45° Back Extension	Lying Leg Curl	10–15 min
	Seated Calf Raise		0–1	3	10–12	~9	10	1–2 min	Standing Calf Raise	Leg Press Calf Press	5–10 min
	Cable Crunch		0–1	3	10–12	~9	10	1–2 min	Plate-Weighted Decline Sit-Up	Hanging Leg Raise	5–10 min
										Estimated Training Time:	55–80 min

Suggested 1–2 Rest Days

Week 1	Exercise	Last Set Intensity Technique	Warm-Up Sets	Working Sets	Reps	Early Set RPE	Last Set RPE	Rest	Substitution Option 1	Substitution Option 2	Time Estimate
Upper #2											
	General warm-up: 5 min light cardio & dynamic stretching										
	Lat Pulldown		1–2	3	10–12	~7–8	~9	2–3 min	Pull-Up (Optional Assistance)	Chin-Up	10–15 min
	Overhead Barbell Press		2–3	3	6–8	~7–8	~9	3–4 min	Dumbbell Shoulder Press (Standing)	Dumbbell Shoulder Press (Seated)	20–25 min
	Dumbbell Row		1–2	3	10–12	~7–8	~9	2–3 min	Chest-Supported T-Bar Row	Barbell Row	10–15 min
	Flat Dumbbell Press		1–2	3	8–10	~7–8	~9	2–3 min	Dip	Bench Press	10–15 min
	Reverse Pec Deck		0–1	3	10–12	~9	10	1–2 min	Rope Facepull	Reverse Cable Fly	5–10 min
	Superset 1: Triceps Pressdown		0–1	3	10–12	~9	10	30 sec	Triceps Kickback (Cable)	EZ-Bar Skullcrusher	5–10 min
	Superset 1: Bayesian Cable Curl		0–1	3	10–12	~9	10	30 sec	Incline Dumbbell Curl	Preacher Curl	
										Estimated Training Time:	60–90 min
Lower #2											
	General warm-up: 5 min light cardio & dynamic stretching										
	Barbell Back Squat		2–3	3	3–5	~7	~8	3–4 min	Leg Press	Dumbbell Lunge	20–25 min
	45° Back Extension		1–2	3	8–10	~7–8	~9	2–3 min	Good Morning	Glute Ham Raise	10–15 min
	Leg Extension	Lengthened Partials (Extended Set)	1–2	2	10–12	~9	10	2–3 min	Goblet Squat	Dumbbell Lunge	10–15 min
	Seated Leg Curl	Lengthened Partials (Extended Set)	1–2	2	10–12	~9	10	2–3 min	Lying Leg Curl	Nordic Ham Curl	10–15 min
	Standing Calf Raise		0–1	3	12–15	~9	10	1–2 min	Seated Calf Raise	Leg Press Calf Press	5–10 min
	Roman Chair Leg Raise		0–1	3	10–20	~9	10	1–2 min	Hanging Leg Raise	Bent-Knee Leg Raise	5–10 min
										Estimated Training Time:	60–90 min
	Suggested 1–2 Rest Days										

PROGRAM 8: UPPER/LOWER SPLIT 4X/WEEK

LEVEL: All levels | **GOAL:** Time-limited muscle and strength gain | **TIME:** 45 to 60 minutes

Week 1	Exercise	Last Set Intensity Technique	Warm-Up Sets	Working Sets	Reps	Early Set RPE	Last Set RPE	Rest	Substitution Option 1	Substitution Option 2	Time Estimate
Upper #1	General warm-up: 5 min light cardio & dynamic stretching										
	Machine Chest Press	Myo-reps	2–3	2	6–8	~7–8	10	2–3 min	Bench Press	Flat Dumbbell Press	15–20 min
	Dumbbell Row		2–3	3	8–10	~7–8	~9	1–2 min	Pendlay Row	Barbell Row	10–15 min
	Superset 1: Dumbbell Lateral Raise		0–1	3	12–15	~9	10	30 sec	Cable Lateral Raise	Machine Lateral Raise	5–10 min
	Superset 1: Lat Pulldown		1–2	3	8–10	~7–8	~9	30 sec	Pull-Up (Optional Assistance)	Chin-Up	
	Pec Deck		0–1	3	15–20	~9	10	1–2 min	Dumbbell Fly	Push-Up	5–10 min
	Superset 2: Preacher Curl		0–1	3	12–15	~9	10	30 sec	EZ-Bar Biceps Curl	Dumbbell Biceps Curl	5–10 min
	Superset 2: EZ-Bar Skullcrusher		0–1	3	12–15	~9	10	30 sec	Dumbbell Skullcrusher	Overhead Triceps Extension	
										Estimated Training Time:	40–65 min
Lower #1	General warm-up: 5 min light cardio & dynamic stretching										
	Barbell Romanian Deadlift		2–3	3	8–10	~7	~8	2–3 min	Dumbbell Romanian Deadlift	Hip Thrust	15–20 min
	Leg Press	Dropset	2–3	2	6–8	~7–8	10	2–3 min	Dumbbell Lunge	Front Squat	15–20 min
	Glute Ham Raise		1–2	2	8–10	~7	~8	1–2 min	45° Back Extension	Lying Leg Curl	5–10 min
	Superset 1: Seated Calf Raise		0–1	3	10–12	~9	10	30 sec	Standing Calf Raise	Leg Press Calf Press	5–10 min
	Superset 1: Cable Crunch		0–1	3	10–20	~9	10	30 sec	Plate-Weighted Decline Sit-Up	Hanging Leg Raise	
										Estimated Training Time:	40–60 min
Suggested 1–2 Rest Days											

Week 1	Exercise	Last Set Intensity Technique	Warm-Up Sets	Working Sets	Reps	Early Set RPE	Last Set RPE	Rest	Substitution Option 1	Substitution Option 2	Time Estimate
Upper #2											
	General warm-up: 5 min light cardio & dynamic stretching										
	Lat Pulldown	Lengthened Partials (Extended Set)	1–2	2	10–12	~7–8	10	2–3 min	Pull-Up (Optional Assistance)	Chin-Up	10–15 min
	Incline Dumbbell Press		2–3	3	8–10	~7–8	~9	3–4 min	Dumbbell Shoulder Press (Standing)	Dumbbell Shoulder Press (Seated)	10–15 min
	Chest-Supported T-Bar Row	Lengthened Partials (Extended Set)	1–2	2	10–12	~7–8	10	2–3 min	Dumbbell Row	Barbell Row	10–15 min
	Reverse Pec Deck		0–1	3	10–12	~9	10	1–2 min	Rope Facepull	Reverse Cable Fly	5–10 min
	Superset 1: Triceps Pressdown		0–1	3	10–12	~9	10	30 sec	Triceps Kickback (Cable)	EZ-Bar Skullcrusher	5–10 min
	Superset 1: Cable Curl		0–1	3	10–12	~9	10	30 sec	Incline Dumbbell Curl	Preacher Curl	
										Estimated Training Time:	40–65 min
Lower #2											
	General warm-up: 5 min light cardio & dynamic stretching										
	Hack Squat		2–3	3	6–8	~7	~8	2–3 min	Leg Press	Dumbbell Lunge	15–20 min
	45° Back Extension		1–2	2	8–10	~7–8	~9	2–3 min	Good Morning	Glute Ham Raise	10–15 min
	Leg Extension	Lengthened Partials (Extended Set)	1–2	2	10–12	~9	10	1–2 min	Goblet Squat	Dumbbell Lunge	5–10 min
	Seated Leg Curl	Lengthened Partials (Extended Set)	1–2	2	10–12	~9	10	1–2 min	Lying Leg Curl	Nordic Ham Curl	5–10 min
	Superset 1: Standing Calf Raise		0–1	3	12–15	~9	10	30 sec	Seated Calf Raise	Leg Press Calf Press	5–10 min
	Superset 1: Roman Chair Leg Raise		0–1	3	10–20	~9	10	30 sec	Hanging Leg Raise	Bent-Knee Leg Raise	
										Estimated Training Time:	40–65 min

Suggested 1–2 Rest Days

PROGRAM 9: FULL-BODY SPLIT 4X/WEEK

LEVEL: Beginner | **GOAL:** Build muscle and gain strength | **TIME:** 60 to 90 minutes

Week 1	Exercise	Last Set Intensity Technique	Warm-Up Sets	Working Sets	Reps	Early Set RPE	Last Set RPE	Rest	Substitution Option 1	Substitution Option 2	Time Estimate
	General warm-up: 5 min light cardio & dynamic stretching										
Full Body #1	Machine Chest Press		2–3	3	6–8	~7–8	~9	2–3 min	Bench Press	Flat Dumbbell Press	15–20 min
	Leg Press		2–3	3	6–8	~7	~8	3–4 min	Barbell Front Squat	Dumbbell Lunge	15–20 min
	Barbell Row		2–3	3	8–10	~7–8	~9	2–3 min	Pendlay Row	Dumbbell Row	15–20 min
	Dumbbell Lateral Raise		0–1	3	12–15	~9	10	1–2 min	Cable Lateral Raise	Machine Lateral Raise	5–10 min
	Superset 1: Preacher Curl		0–1	2	12–15	~9	10	30 sec	EZ-Bar Biceps Curl	Dumbbell Biceps Curl	5–10 min
	Superset 1: Seated Calf Raise		0–1	2	10–12	~9	10	30 sec	Standing Calf Raise	Leg Press Calf Press	
										Estimated Training Time:	55–80 min
	General warm-up: 5 min light cardio & dynamic stretching										
Full Body #2	Romanian Deadlift		2–3	3	8–10	~6	~7	2–3 min	Deadlift	Hip Thrust	15–20 min
	Lat Pulldown		1–2	3	8–10	~7–8	~9	2–3 min	Pull-Up (Optional Assistance)	Chin-Up	10–15 min
	Glute Ham Raise		1–2	2	8–10	~7	~8	2–3 min	45° Back Extension	Lying Leg Curl	10–15 min
	Pec Deck		0–1	2	15–20	~9	10	1–2 min	Dumbbell Fly	Push-Up	5–10 min
	EZ-Bar Skullcrusher		0–1	2	12–15	~9	10	1–2 min	Dumbbell Skullcrusher	Overhead Triceps Extension	5–10 min
	Cable Crunch		0–1	3	10–12	~9	10	1–2 min	Plate-Weighted Decline Sit-Up	Hanging Leg Raise	5–10 min
										Estimated Training Time:	50–80 min

Suggested 1–2 Rest Days

Week 1	Exercise	Last Set Intensity Technique	Warm-Up Sets	Working Sets	Reps	Early Set RPE	Last Set RPE	Rest	Substitution Option 1	Substitution Option 2	Time Estimate
Full Body #3	General warm-up: 5 min light cardio & dynamic stretching										
	Dumbbell Shoulder Press (Seated)		2–3	3	6–8	~7–8	~9	2–3 min	Dumbbell Shoulder Press (Standing)	Overhead Barbell Press	15–20 min
	45° Back Extension		1–2	3	8–10	~7–8	~9	2–3 min	Good Morning	Glute Ham Raise	10–15 min
	Dumbbell Row		1–2	3	10–12	~7–8	~9	2–3 min	Chest-Supported T-Bar Row	Barbell Row	10–15 min
	Leg Extension		1–2	2	15–20	~9	10	1–2 min	Goblet Squat	Dumbbell Lunge	5–10 min
	Superset 1: Triceps Kickback (Cable)		0–1	2	10–12	~9	10	30 sec	EZ-Bar Skullcrusher	Triceps Pressdown	5–10 min
	Superset 1: Bayesian Cable Curl		0–1	2	10–12	~9	10	30 sec	Incline Dumbbell Curl	Preacher Curl	
	Standing Calf Raise		0–1	3	12–15	~9	10	1–2 min	Seated Calf Raise	Leg Press Calf Press	5–10 min
										Estimated Training Time:	50–80 min
Full Body #4	General warm-up: 5 min light cardio & dynamic stretching										
	Leg Press		2–3	3	6–8	~7	~8	3–4 min	Barbell Back Squat	Dumbbell Lunge	15–20 min
	Flat Dumbbell Press		1–2	3	8–10	~7–8	~9	2–3 min	Dip	Bench Press	10–15 min
	Lat Pulldown		1–2	3	10–12	~7–8	~9	2–3 min	Pull-Up (Optional Assistance)	Chin-Up	10–15 min
	Seated Leg Curl		1–2	2	10–12	~9	10	1–2 min	Lying Leg Curl	Nordic Ham Curl	5–10 min
	Reverse Pec Deck		0–1	2	10–12	~9	10	1–2 min	Rope Facepull	Reverse Cable Fly	5–10 min
	Roman Chair Leg Raise		0–1	3	10–20	~9	10	30 sec	Hanging Leg Raise	Bent-Knee Leg Raise	5–10 min
										Estimated Training Time:	50–80 min
**Suggested 1–2 Rest Days**											

PROGRAM 10: FULL-BODY SPLIT 4X/WEEK

LEVEL: Intermediate/advanced | **GOAL:** Build muscle and gain strength | **TIME:** 60 to 90 minutes

Week 1	Exercise	Last Set Intensity Technique	Warm-Up Sets	Working Sets	Reps	Early Set RPE	Last Set RPE	Rest	Substitution Option 1	Substitution Option 2	Time Estimate
Full Body #1	General warm-up: 5 min light cardio & dynamic stretching										
	Bench Press		2–3	3	3–5	~7–8	~9	3–4 min	Machine Chest Press	Flat Dumbbell Press	20–25 min
	Leg Press		2–3	3	6–8	~7	~8	3–4 min	Barbell Front Squat	Dumbbell Lunge	15–20 min
	Barbell Row		2–3	3	8–10	~7–8	~9	2–3 min	Pendlay Row	Dumbbell Row	15–20 min
	Dumbbell Lateral Raise	Lengthened Partials (Extended Set)	0–1	2	12–15	~9	10	1–2 min	Cable Lateral Raise	Machine Lateral Raise	5–10 min
	Superset 1: Preacher Curl		0–1	3	12–15	~9	10	30 sec	EZ-Bar Biceps Curl	Dumbbell Biceps Curl	5–10 min
	Superset 1: Seated Calf Raise		0–1	3	10–12	~9	10	30 sec	Standing Calf Raise	Leg Press Calf Press	
										Estimated Training Time:	60–85 min
Full Body #2	General warm-up: 5 min light cardio & dynamic stretching										
	Deadlift		2–3	3	3–5	~6	~7	3–5 min	Romanian Deadlift	Hip Thrust	20–25 min
	Pull-Up (Optional Assistance)		1–2	3	8–10	~7–8	~9	2–3 min	Lat Pulldown	Chin-Up	10–15 min
	Glute Ham Raise		1–2	3	8–10	~7	~8	2–3 min	45° Back Extension	Lying Leg Curl	10–15 min
	Pec Deck	Dropset	0–1	2	15–20	~9	10	1–2 min	Dumbbell Fly	Push-up	5–10 min
	EZ-Bar Skullcrusher		0–1	3	12–15	~9	10	1–2 min	Dumbbell Skullcrusher	Overhead Triceps Extension	5–10 min
	Cable Crunch		0–1	3	10–12	~9	10	1–2 min	Plate-Weighted Decline Sit-Up	Hanging Leg Raise	5–10 min
										Estimated Training Time:	55–85 min

Suggested 1–2 Rest Days

Week 1	Exercise	Last Set Intensity Technique	Warm-Up Sets	Working Sets	Reps	Early Set RPE	Last Set RPE	Rest	Substitution Option 1	Substitution Option 2	Time Estimate
Full Body #3	General warm-up: 5 min light cardio & dynamic stretching										
	Overhead Barbell Press		2–3	3	6–8	~7–8	~9	3–4 min	Dumbbell Shoulder Press (Standing)	Dumbbell Shoulder Press (Seated)	20–25 min
	45° Back Extension		1–2	3	8–10	~7–8	~9	2–3 min	Good Morning	Glute Ham Raise	10–15 min
	Dumbbell Row		1–2	3	10–12	~7–8	~9	2–3 min	Chest-Supported T-Bar Row	Barbell Row	10–15 min
	Leg Extension	Lengthened Partials (Extended Set)	1–2	2	15–20	~9	10	1–2 min	Goblet Squat	Dumbbell Lunge	5–10 min
	Superset 1: Triceps Pressdown		0–1	3	10–12	~9	10	30 sec	EZ-Bar Skullcrusher	Triceps Kickback (Cable)	5–10 min
	Superset 1: Bayesian Cable Curl		0–1	3	10–12	~9	10	30 sec	Incline Dumbbell Curl	Preacher Curl	
	Standing Calf Raise		0–1	3	12–15	~9	10	1–2 min	Seated Calf Raise	Leg Press Calf Press	5–10 min
										Estimated Training Time:	55–85 min
Full Body #4	General warm-up: 5 min light cardio & dynamic stretching										
	Barbell Back Squat		2–3	3	3–5	~7	~8	3–4 min	Leg Press	Dumbbell Lunge	20–25 min
	Flat Dumbbell Press		1–2	3	8–10	~7–8	~9	2–3 min	Dip	Bench Press	10–15 min
	Lat Pulldown		1–2	3	10–12	~7–8	~9	2–3 min	Pull-Up (Optional Assistance)	Chin-Up	10–15 min
	Seated Leg Curl	Lengthened Partials (Extended Set)	1–2	2	10–12	~9	10	1–2 min	Lying Leg Curl	Nordic Ham Curl	5–10 min
	Reverse Pec Deck		0–1	3	10–12	~9	10	1–2 min	Rope Facepull	Reverse Cable Fly	5–10 min
	Roman Chair Leg Raise		0–1	3	10–20	~9	10	30 sec	Hanging Leg Raise	Bent-Knee Leg Raise	5–10 min
										Estimated Training Time:	55–85 min
					Suggested 1–2 Rest Days						

PROGRAM 11: FULL-BODY SPLIT 4X/WEEK

LEVEL: All levels | **GOAL:** Time-limited muscle and strength gain | **TIME:** 45 to 60 minutes

Week 1	Exercise	Last Set Intensity Technique	Warm-Up Sets	Working Sets	Reps	Early Set RPE	Last Set RPE	Rest	Substitution Option 1	Substitution Option 2	Time Estimate
Full Body #1	General warm-up: 5 min light cardio & dynamic stretching										
	Machine Chest Press	Myo-reps	2–3	2	6–8	~9	10	2–3 min	Bench Press	Flat Dumbbell Press	15–20 min
	Superset 1: Leg Press		2–3	3	6–8	~7	~8	30–60 sec	Barbell Front Squat	Dumbbell Lunge	10–15 min
	Superset 1: Dumbbell Lateral Raise		0–1	3	12–15	~9	10	30–60 sec	Cable Lateral Raise	Machine Lateral Raise	
	Chest-Supported T-Bar Row	Lengthened Partials (Extended Set)	2–3	2	8–10	~9	10	1–2 min	Pendlay Row	Barbell Row	10–15 min
	Superset 2: Preacher Curl		0–1	2	12–15	~9	10	30 sec	EZ-Bar Biceps Curl	Dumbbell Biceps Curl	5–10 min
	Superset 2: Seated Calf Raise		0–1	2	10–12	~9	10	30 sec	Standing Calf Raise	Leg Press Calf Press	
										Estimated Training Time:	40–60 min
Full Body #2	General warm-up: 5 min light cardio & dynamic stretching										
	Barbell Romanian Deadlift		2–3	3	8–10	~7	~8	2–3 min	Dumbbell Romanian Deadlift	Hip Thrust	15–20 min
	Lat Pulldown		1–2	3	8–10	~7–8	~9	2–3 min	Pull-Up (Optional Assistance)	Chin-Up	10–15 min
	Glute Ham Raise		1–2	2	8–10	~7	~8	1–2 min	45° Back Extension	Lying Leg Curl	5–10 min
	Pec Deck	Lengthened Partials (Extended Set)	0–1	2	15–20	~9	10	1–2 min	Dumbbell Fly	Push-Up	5–10 min
	Superset 1: EZ-Bar Skullcrusher		0–1	2	12–15	~9	10	30 sec	Dumbbell Skullcrusher	Overhead Triceps Extension	5–10 min
	Superset 1: Cable Crunch		0–1	2	10–12	~9	10	30 sec	Plate-Weighted Decline Sit-Up	Hanging Leg Raise	
										Estimated Training Time:	40–65 min

Suggested 1–2 Rest Days

Week 1	Exercise	Last Set Intensity Technique	Warm-Up Sets	Working Sets	Reps	Early Set RPE	Last Set RPE	Rest	Substitution Option 1	Substitution Option 2	Time Estimate
Full Body #3	General warm-up: 5 min light cardio & dynamic stretching										
	Incline Dumbbell Press		2–3	2	8–10	~9	10	3–4 min	Incline Machine Chest Press	Incline Barbell Bench Press	10–15 min
	45° Back Extension		1–2	3	8–10	~7–8	~9	2–3 min	Good Morning	Glute Ham Raise	10–15 min
	Dumbbell Row	Lengthened Partials (Extended Set)	1–2	2	10–12	~9	10	2–3 min	Chest-Supported T-Bar Row	Barbell Row	10–15 min
	Leg Extension		1–2	2	15–20	~9	10	1–2 min	Goblet Squat	Dumbbell Lunge	5–10 min
	Superset 1: Bayesian Cable Curl		0–1	2	10–12	~9	10	30 sec	Incline Dumbbell Curl	Preacher Curl	5–10 min
	Superset 1: Standing Calf Raise		0–1	2	12–15	~9	10	1–2 min	Seated Calf Raise	Leg Press Calf Press	
										Estimated Training Time:	40–65 min
Full Body #4	General warm-up: 5 min light cardio & dynamic stretching										
	Hack Squat		2–3	3	6–8	~7	~8	2–3 min	Leg Press	Dumbbell Lunge	15–20 min
	Lat Pulldown	Lengthened Partials (Extended Set)	1–2	2	10–12	~9	10	2–3 min	Pull-Up (Optional Assistance)	Chin-Up	10–15 min
	Seated Leg Curl	Lengthened Partials (Extended Set)	1–2	2	10–12	~9	10	1–2 min	Lying Leg Curl	Nordic Ham Curl	5–10 min
	Reverse Pec Deck		0–1	2	10–12	~9	10	1–2 min	Rope Facepull	Reverse Cable Fly	5–10 min
	Superset 1: Triceps Pressdown		0–1	2	10–12	~9	10	30 sec	EZ-Bar Skullcrusher	Triceps Kickback (Cable)	5–10 min
	Superset 1: Roman Chair Leg Raise		0–1	2	10–20	~9	10	30 sec	Hanging Leg Raise	Bent-Knee Leg Raise	
										Estimated Training Time:	40–65 min

Suggested 1–2 Rest Days

LEVEL: Advanced | **GOAL:** Build muscle and gain strength | **TIME:** 60 to 90 minutes

Week 1	Exercise	Last Set Intensity Technique	Warm-Up Sets	Working Sets	Reps	Early Set RPE	Last Set RPE	Rest	Substitution Option 1	Substitution Option 2	Time Estimate
Full Body #1	General warm-up: 5 min light cardio & dynamic stretching										
	Bench Press		2–3	3	3–5	~7–8	~9	3–4 min	Machine Chest Press	Flat Dumbbell Press	20–25 min
	Leg Press		2–3	3	6–8	~7	~8	3–4 min	Barbell Front Squat	Dumbbell Lunge	15–20 min
	Lat Pulldown		1–2	3	8–10	~7–8	~9	2–3 min	Pull-Up (Optional Assistance)	Chin-Up	10–15 min
	Dumbbell Lateral Raise	Lengthened Partials (Extended Set)	0–1	2	12–15	~9	10	1–2 min	Cable Lateral Raise	Machine Lateral Raise	5–10 min
	Preacher Curl		0–1	3	12–15	~9	10	1–2 min	EZ-Bar Biceps Curl	Dumbbell Biceps Curl	5–10 min
	Seated Calf Raise		0–1	3	10–12	~9	10	1–2 min	Standing Calf Raise	Leg Press Calf Press	5–10 min
										Estimated Training Time:	60–90 min
Full Body #2	General warm-up: 5 min light cardio & dynamic stretching										
	Deadlift		2–3	3	3–5	~7	~8	3–5 min	Romanian Deadlift	Hip Thrust	20–25 min
	Overhead Barbell Press		1–2	3	8–10	~7–8	~9	2–3 min	Dumbbell Shoulder Press (Seated)	Barbell Upright Row	10–15 min
	Cable Lat Pullover	Lengthened Partials (Extended Set)	0–1	2	12–15	~9	10	1–2 min	Dumbbell Lat Pullover	Cable Lat Pull-In	5–10 min
	Pec Deck	Dropset	0–1	2	12–15	~9	10	1–2 min	Dumbbell Fly	Push-Up	5–10 min
	Cable Crunch		0–1	3	10–12	~9	10	1–2 min	Plate-Weighted Decline Sit-Up	Hanging Leg Raise	5–10 min
	EZ-Bar Skullcrusher		0–1	3	12–15	~9	10	1–2 min	Dumbbell Skullcrusher	Overhead Triceps Extension	5–10 min
										Estimated Training Time:	50–80 min
Full Body #3	General warm-up: 5 min light cardio & dynamic stretching										
	Barbell Row		2–3	3	8–10	~7–8	~9	2–3 min	Pendlay Row	Dumbbell Row	15–20 min
	Glute Ham Raise		1–2	3	8–10	~7	~8	2–3 min	45° Back Extension	Lying Leg Curl	10–15 min
	Barbell Shrug	Cheat Reps	0–1	2	10–12	~9	10	1–2 min	Dumbbell Shrug	Trap Bar Shrug	5–10 min
	Reverse Pec Deck		0–1	3	10–12	~9	10	1–2 min	Rope Facepull	Reverse Cable Fly	5–10 min
	Triceps Pressdown		0–1	3	12–15	~9	10	1–2 min	Triceps Kickback (Cable)	EZ-Bar Skullcrusher	5–10 min
	Dumbbell Biceps Curl		0–1	3	12–15	~9	10	1–2 min	EZ-Bar Biceps Curl	Standing Barbell Curl	5–10 min
	Roman Chair Leg Raise		0–1	3	10–20	~9	10	30 sec	Hanging Leg Raise	Bent-Knee Leg Raise	5–10 min
										Estimated Training Time:	50–85 min
	Suggested Rest Day										

Week 1	Exercise	Last Set Intensity Technique	Warm-Up Sets	Working Sets	Reps	Early Set RPE	Last Set RPE	Rest	Substitution Option 1	Substitution Option 2	Time Estimate
Full Body #4	colspan general											
	General warm-up: 5 min light cardio & dynamic stretching										
	Barbell Back Squat		2–3	3	3–5	~7	~8	3–4 min	Leg Press	Dumbbell Lunge	20–25 min
	Flat Dumbbell Press		1–2	3	8–10	~7–8	~9	2–3 min	Dip	Bench Press	10–15 min
	Lat Pulldown		1–2	3	10–12	~7–8	~9	2–3 min	Pull-Up (Optional Assistance)	Chin-Up	10–15 min
	Cable Lateral Raise		0–1	3	10–12	~9	10	1–2 min	Machine Lateral Raise	Dumbbell Lateral Raise	5–10 min
	Cable Lat Pull-In		0–1	3	10–12	~9	10	1–2 min	Cable Lat Pullover	Dumbbell Lat Pullover	5–10 min
	Overhead Triceps Extension		0–1	3	10–12	~9	10	1–2 min	EZ-Bar Skullcrusher	Dumbbell Skullcrusher	5–10 min
										Estimated Training Time:	55–85 min
Full Body #5	General warm-up: 5 min light cardio & dynamic stretching										
	Overhead Barbell Press		2–3	3	6–8	~7–8	~9	3–4 min	Dumbbell Shoulder Press (Standing)	Dumbbell Shoulder Press (Seated)	20–25 min
	Dumbbell Row		1–2	3	10–12	~7–8	~9	2–3 min	Chest-Supported T-Bar Row	Barbell Row	10–15 min
	Leg Extension	Lengthened Partials (Extended Set)	1–2	2	15–20	~9	10	2–3 min	Goblet Squat	Dumbbell Lunge	10–15 min
	Seated Leg Curl	Lengthened Partials (Extended Set)	1–2	2	10–12	~9	10	2–3 min	Lying Leg Curl	Nordic Ham Curl	10–15 min
	Cable Fly	Myo-reps	0–1	2	10–12	~9	10	1–2 min	Dumbbell Fly	Pec Deck	5–10 min
	Bayesian Cable Curl		0–1	3	10–12	~9	10	1–2 min	Incline Dumbbell Curl	Preacher Curl	5–10 min
										Estimated Training Time:	60–90 min

Suggested Rest Day

PROGRAM 13: FULL-BODY SPLIT 5X/WEEK

LEVEL: Advanced | **GOAL:** Time-limited muscle and strength gain | **TIME:** 45 to 60 minutes

Week 1	Exercise	Last Set Intensity Technique	Warm-Up Sets	Working Sets	Reps	Early Set RPE	Last Set RPE	Rest	Substitution Option 1	Substitution Option 2	Time Estimate
	General warm-up: 5 min light cardio & dynamic stretching										
Full Body #1	Machine Chest Press	Myo-reps	1–2	2	6–8	~9	10	2–3 min	Flat Dumbbell Press	Bench Press	15–20 min
	Superset 1: Leg Press		2–3	3	6–8	~7	~8	30–60 sec	Barbell Front Squat	Dumbbell Lunge	10–15 min
	Superset 1: Dumbbell Lateral Raise	Lengthened Partials (Extended Set)	0–1	2	12–15	~9	10	30–60 sec	Cable Lateral Raise	Machine Lateral Raise	
	Lat Pulldown		1–2	3	8–10	~7–8	~9	2–3 min	Pull-Up (Optional Assistance)	Chin-Up	10–15 min
	Superset 2: Preacher Curl		0–1	3	12–15	~9	10	30 sec	EZ-Bar Biceps Curl	Dumbbell Biceps Curl	5–10 min
	Superset 2: Seated Calf Raise		0–1	3	10–12	~9	10	30 sec	Standing Calf Raise	Leg Press Calf Press	
										Estimated Training Time:	40–60 min
	General warm-up: 5 min light cardio & dynamic stretching										
Full Body #2	Barbell Romanian Deadlift		2–3	3	8–10	~7	~8	2–3 min	Dumbbell Romanian Deadlift	Hip Thrust	15–20 min
	Dumbbell Shoulder Press (Seated)		1–2	3	8–10	~7–8	~9	2–3 min	Overhead Barbell Press	Barbell Upright Row	10–15 min
	Superset 1: Cable Lat Pullover	Lengthened Partials (Extended Set)	0–1	2	12–15	~9	10	30 sec	Dumbbell Lat Pullover	Cable Lat Pull-In	5–10 min
	Superset 1: Pec Deck	Dropset	0–1	2	12–15	~9	10	30 sec	Dumbbell Fly	Push-up	
	Superset 2: Cable Crunch		0–1	3	10–12	~9	10	30 sec	Plate-Weighted Decline Sit-Up	Hanging Leg Raise	5–10 min
	Superset 2: EZ-Bar Skullcrusher		0–1	3	12–15	~9	10	30 sec	Dumbbell Skullcrusher	Overhead Triceps Extension	
										Estimated Training Time:	35–55 min
	General warm-up: 5 min light cardio & dynamic stretching										
Full Body #3	Chest-Supported T-Bar Row		1–2	3	8–10	~7–8	~9	2–3 min	Pendlay Row	Dumbbell Row	15–20 min
	Glute Ham Raise		1–2	3	8–10	~7	~8	2–3 min	45° Back Extension	Lying Leg Curl	10–15 min
	Barbell Shrug	Cheat Reps	0–1	2	10–12	~9	10	1–2 min	Dumbbell Shrug	Trap Bar Shrug	5–10 min
	Superset 1: Reverse Pec Deck		0–1	3	10–12	~9	10	30 sec	Rope Facepull	Reverse Cable Fly	5–10 min
	Superset 1: Triceps Pressdown		0–1	3	12–15	~9	10	30 sec	Triceps Kickback (Cable)	EZ-Bar Skullcrusher	
	Superset 2: Dumbbell Biceps Curl		0–1	3	12–15	~9	10	30 sec	EZ-Bar Biceps Curl	Standing Barbell Curl	5–10 min
	Superset 2: Roman Chair Leg Raise		0–1	3	10–20	~9	10	30 sec	Hanging Leg Raise	Bent-Knee Leg Raise	
										Estimated Training Time:	40–65 min
	Suggested Rest Day										

Week 1	Exercise	Last Set Intensity Technique	Warm-Up Sets	Working Sets	Reps	Early Set RPE	Last Set RPE	Rest	Substitution Option 1	Substitution Option 2	Time Estimate
Full Body #4		General warm-up: 5 min light cardio & dynamic stretching									
	Hack Squat		2–3	3	6–8	~7	~8	2–3 min	Leg Press	Dumbbell Lunge	15–20 min
	Flat Dumbbell Press		1–2	3	8–10	~7–8	~9	2–3 min	Dip	Bench Press	10–15 min
	Lat Pulldown	Lengthened Partials (Extended Set)	1–2	2	10–12	~9	10	2–3 min	Pull-Up (Optional Assistance)	Chin-Up	10–15 min
	Superset 1: Cable Lateral Raise		0–1	3	10–12	~9	10	30 sec	Machine Lateral Raise	Dumbbell Lateral Raise	10–15 min
	Superset 1: Cable Seated Row		0–1	3	10–12	~9	10	30 sec	Dumbbell Row	Chest-Supported T-Bar Row	
	Superset 1: Overhead Triceps Extension		0–1	3	10–12	~9	10	30 sec	EZ-Bar Skullcrusher	Dumbbell Skullcrusher	
										Estimated Training Time:	45–65 min
Full Body #5		General warm-up: 5 min light cardio & dynamic stretching									
	Cable Upright Row		1–2	3	6–8	~7–8	~9	1–2 min	Dumbbell Lateral Raise	Dumbbell Shoulder Press (Standing)	10–15 min
	Dumbbell Row		1–2	3	10–12	~7–8	~9	2–3 min	Chest-Supported T-Bar Row	Barbell Row	10–15 min
	Superset 1: Leg Extension	Lengthened Partials (Extended Set)	1–2	2	10–12	~9	10	30 sec	Goblet Squat	Dumbbell Lunge	5–10 min
	Superset 1: Seated Leg Curl	Lengthened Partials (Extended Set)	1–2	2	10–12	~9	10	30 sec	Lying Leg Curl	Nordic Ham Curl	
	Superset 2: Cable Fly	Myo-reps	0–1	2	10–12	~9	10	30 sec	Dumbbell Fly	Pec Deck	5–10 min
	Superset 2: Bayesian Cable Curl		0–1	2	10–12	~9	10	30 sec	Incline Dumbbell Curl	Preacher Curl	
										Estimated Training Time:	30–50 min
						Suggested Rest Day					

PROGRAM 14: UPPER/LOWER/PUSH/PULL/LEGS 5X/WEEK

LEVEL: Intermediate/advanced | **GOAL:** Build muscle and gain strength | **TIME:** 60 to 90 minutes

Week 1	Exercise	Last Set Intensity Technique	Warm-Up Sets	Working Sets	Reps	Early Set RPE	Last Set RPE	Rest	Substitution Option 1	Substitution Option 2	Time Estimate
	General warm-up: 5 min light cardio & dynamic stretching									
Upper #1 (Strength Focus)	Bench Press		2–3	3	3–5	~7–8	~9	3–4 min	Machine Chest Press	Flat Dumbbell Press	20–25 min
	Barbell Row		2–3	3	6–8	~7–8	~9	2–3 min	Pendlay Row	Dumbbell Row	15–20 min
	Dumbbell Lateral Raise	Lengthened Partials (Extended Set)	0–1	2	8–10	~9	10	1–2 min	Cable Lateral Raise	Machine Lateral Raise	5–10 min
	Pull-Up (Optional Assistance)		1–2	3	8–10	~7–8	~9	2–3 min	Lat Pulldown	Chin-Up	10–15 min
	Pec Deck	Dropset	0–1	2	8–10	~9	10	1–2 min	Dumbbell Fly	Push-Up	5–10 min
	Superset 1: Preacher Curl		0–1	3	8–10	~9	10	30 sec	EZ-Bar Biceps Curl	Dumbbell Biceps Curl	5–10 min
	Superset 1: EZ-Bar Skullcrusher		0–1	3	8–10	~9	10	30 sec	Dumbbell Skullcrusher	Overhead Triceps Extension	
										Estimated Training Time:	60–80 min
	General warm-up: 5 min light cardio & dynamic stretching									
Lower #1 (Strength Focus)	Deadlift		2–3	3	3–5	~6	~7	3–5 min	Romanian Deadlift	Hip Thrust	20–25 min
	Leg Press		2–3	3	6–8	~7	~8	3–4 min	Barbell Front Squat	Dumbbell Lunge	15–20 min
	Glute Ham Raise		1–2	3	8–10	~7	~8	2–3 min	45° Back Extension	Lying Leg Curl	10–15 min
	Seated Calf Raise		0–1	3	8–10	~9	10	1–2 min	Standing Calf Raise	Leg Press Calf Press	5–10 min
	Cable Crunch		0–1	3	10–12	~9	10	1–2 min	Plate-Weighted Decline Sit-Up	Hanging Leg Raise	5–10 min
										Estimated Training Time:	55–80 min
	Suggested Rest Day									

Week 1	Exercise	Last Set Intensity Technique	Warm-Up Sets	Working Sets	Reps	Early Set RPE	Last Set RPE	Rest	Substitution Option 1	Substitution Option 2	Time Estimate
Push #1 (Hypertrophy Focus)	General warm-up: 5 min light cardio & dynamic stretching										
	Overhead Barbell Press		2–3	3	8–10	~7–8	~9	3–4 min	Dumbbell Shoulder Press (Standing)	Dumbbell Shoulder Press (Seated)	20–25 min
	Flat Dumbbell Press		1–2	3	10–12	~7–8	~9	2–3 min	Dip	Bench Press	10–15 min
	Cable Lateral Raise		0–1	3	12–15	~9	10	1–2 min	Machine Lateral Raise	Dumbbell Lateral Raise	5–10 min
	Cable Fly	Myo-reps	0–1	2	12–15	~9	10	1–2 min	Dumbbell Fly	Pec Deck	5–10 min
	Triceps Kickback (Cable)		0–1	3	12–15	~9	10	1–2 min	EZ-Bar Skullcrusher	Triceps Pressdown	5–10 min
	Overhead Triceps Extension		0–1	3	15–20	~9	10	1–2 min	EZ-Bar Skullcrusher	Dumbbell Skullcrusher	5–10 min
										Estimated Training Time:	50–80 min
Pull #1 (Hypertrophy Focus)	General warm-up: 5 min light cardio & dynamic stretching										
	Lat Pulldown		1–2	3	10–12	~7–8	~9	2–3 min	Pull-Up (Optional Assistance)	Chin-Up	10–15 min
	Dumbbell Row		1–2	3	10–12	~7–8	~9	2–3 min	Chest-Supported T-Bar Row	Barbell Row	10–15 min
	Cable Lat Pull-In		0–1	3	12–15	~9	10	1–2 min	Cable Lat Pullover	Dumbbell Lat Pullover	5–10 min
	Reverse Pec Deck		0–1	3	12–15	~9	10	1–2 min	Rope Facepull	Reverse Cable Fly	5–10 min
	Barbell Shrug	Cheat Reps	0–1	2	12–15	~9	10	1–2 min	Dumbbell Shrug	Trap Bar Shrug	5–10 min
	Hammer Curl		0–1	3	12–15	~9	10	1–2 min	Dumbbell Biceps Curl	EZ-Bar Biceps Curl	5–10 min
	Bayesian Cable Curl		0–1	3	15–20	~9	10	1–2 min	Incline Dumbbell Curl	Preacher Curl	5–10 min
										Estimated Training Time:	45–80 min
Legs #1 (Hypertrophy Focus)	General warm-up: 5 min light cardio & dynamic stretching										
	Barbell Back Squat		2–3	3	3–5	~7	~8	3–4 min	Leg Press	Dumbbell Lunge	20–25 min
	45° Back Extension		1–2	3	10–12	~7–8	~9	2–3 min	Good Morning	Glute Ham Raise	10–15 min
	Leg Extension	Lengthened Partials (Extended Set)	1–2	2	12–15	~9	10	2–3 min	Goblet Squat	Dumbbell Lunge	10–15 min
	Seated Leg Curl	Lengthened Partials (Extended Set)	1–2	2	12–15	~9	10	2–3 min	Lying Leg Curl	Nordic Ham Curl	10–15 min
	Standing Calf Raise		0–1	3	15–20	~9	10	1–2 min	Seated Calf Raise	Leg Press Calf Press	5–10 min
	Roman Chair Leg Raise		0–1	3	10–20	~9	10	30 sec	Hanging Leg Raise	Bent-Knee Leg Raise	5–10 min
										Estimated Training Time:	60–90 min
	**Suggested Rest Day**										

Week 1	Exercise	Last Set Intensity Technique	Warm-Up Sets	Working Sets	Reps	Early Set RPE	Last Set RPE	Rest	Substitution Option 1	Substitution Option 2	Time Estimate
	General warm-up: 5 min light cardio & dynamic stretching										
Upper #1 (Strength Focus)	Machine Chest Press	Myo-reps	2–3	2	6–8	~9	10	2–3 min	Bench Press	Flat Dumbbell Press	10–15 min
	Chest-Supported T-Bar Row		2–3	2	6–8	~7–8	~9	2–3 min	Barbell Row	Dumbbell Row	10–15 min
	Superset 1: Dumbbell Lateral Raise	Lengthened Partials (Extended Set)	0–1	2	8–10	~9	10	30 sec	Cable Lateral Raise	Machine Lateral Raise	5–10 min
	Superset 1: Lat Pulldown		1–2	2	8–10	~7–8	~9	30 sec	Pull-Up (Optional Assistance)	Chin-Up	
	Pec Deck	Dropset	0–1	2	8–10	~9	10	1–2 min	Dumbbell Fly	Push-Up	5–10 min
	Superset 2: Preacher Curl		0–1	2	8–10	~9	10	30 sec	EZ-Bar Biceps Curl	Dumbbell Biceps Curl	5–10 min
	Superset 2: EZ-Bar Skullcrusher		0–1	2	8–10	~9	10	30 sec	Dumbbell Skullcrusher	Overhead Triceps Extension	
										Estimated Training Time:	40–65 min
	General warm-up: 5 min light cardio & dynamic stretching										
Lower #1 (Strength Focus)	Barbell Romanian Deadlift		2–3	3	8–10	~6	~7	2–3 min	Dumbbell Romanian Deadlift	Hip Thrust	15–20 min
	Leg Press		2–3	3	6–8	~7	~8	2–3 min	Barbell Front Squat	Dumbbell Lunge	15–20 min
	Glute Ham Raise		1–2	2	8–10	~7	~8	2–3 min	45° Back Extension	Lying Leg Curl	5–10 min
	Superset 1: Seated Calf Raise		0–1	3	8–10	~9	10	30 sec	Standing Calf Raise	Leg Press Calf Press	5–10 min
	Superset 1: Cable Crunch		0–1	3	10–12	~9	10	30 sec	Plate-Weighted Decline Sit-Up	Hanging Leg Raise	
										Estimated Training Time:	40–60 min

Suggested Rest Day

Week 1	Exercise	Last Set Intensity Technique	Warm-Up Sets	Working Sets	Reps	Early Set RPE	Last Set RPE	Rest	Substitution Option 1	Substitution Option 2	Time Estimate
Push #1 (Hypertrophy Focus)	General warm-up: 5 min light cardio & dynamic stretching										
	Cable Upright Row		2–3	3	8–10	~7–8	~9	1–2 min	Dumbbell Lateral Raise	Dumbbell Shoulder Press (Standing)	10–15 min
	Flat Dumbbell Press		1–2	3	10–12	~7–8	~9	2–3 min	Dip	Bench Press	10–15 min
	Cable Lateral Raise		0–1	3	12–15	~9	10	1–2 min	Machine Lateral Raise	Dumbbell Lateral Raise	5–10 min
	Cable Fly	Myo–reps	0–1	2	12–15	~9	10	1–2 min	Dumbbell Fly	Pec Deck	5–10 min
	Overhead Triceps Extension		0–1	3	15–20	~9	10	1–2 min	EZ-Bar Skullcrusher	Dumbbell Skullcrusher	5–10 min
										Estimated Training Time:	35–60 min
Pull #1 (Hypertrophy Focus)	General warm-up: 5 min light cardio & dynamic stretching										
	Lat Pulldown	Lengthened Partials (Extended Set)	1–2	3	10–12	~9	10	2–3 min	Pull-Up (Optional Assistance)	Chin-Up	10–15 min
	Dumbbell Row		1–2	3	10–12	~7–8	~9	2–3 min	Chest-Supported T-Bar Row	Barbell Row	10–15 min
	Cable Lat Pull-In		0–1	3	12–15	~9	10	1–2 min	Cable Lat Pullover	Dumbbell Lat Pullover	5–10 min
	Reverse Pec Deck		0–1	3	12–15	~9	10	1–2 min	Rope Facepull	Reverse Cable Fly	5–10 min
	Bayesian Cable Curl		0–1	3	15–20	~9	10	1–2 min	Incline Dumbbell Curl	Preacher Curl	5–10 min
										Estimated Training Time:	35–60 min
Legs #1 (Hypertrophy Focus)	General warm-up: 5 min light cardio & dynamic stretching										
	Hack Squat		2–3	3	8–10	~7	~8	2–3 min	Leg Press	Dumbbell Lunge	15–20 min
	45° Back Extension		1–2	3	10–12	~7–8	~9	2–3 min	Good Morning	Glute Ham Raise	10–15 min
	Leg Extension	Lengthened Partials (Extended Set)	1–2	2	12–15	~9	10	1–2 min	Goblet Squat	Dumbbell Lunge	5–10 min
	Seated Leg Curl	Lengthened Partials (Extended Set)	1–2	2	12–15	~9	10	1–2 min	Lying Leg Curl	Nordic Ham Curl	5–10 min
	Superset 1: Standing Calf Raise		0–1	2	15–20	~9	10	30 sec	Seated Calf Raise	Leg Press Calf Press	5–10 min
	Superset 1: Roman Chair Leg Raise		0–1	2	10–20	~9	10	30 sec	Hanging Leg Raise	Bent-Knee Leg Raise	
										Estimated Training Time:	40–65 min
**Suggested Rest Day**											

PROGRAM 16: UPPER/LOWER 6X/WEEK

LEVEL: Intermediate/advanced | **GOAL:** Build muscle and gain strength | **TIME:** 60 to 90 minutes

Week 1	Exercise	Last Set Intensity Technique	Warm-Up Sets	Working Sets	Reps	Early Set RPE	Last Set RPE	Rest	Substitution Option 1	Substitution Option 2	Time Estimate
	General warm-up: 5 min light cardio & dynamic stretching										
Upper #1 (Strength Focus)	Bench Press		2–3	3	3–5	~7–8	~9	3–4 min	Machine Chest Press	Flat Dumbbell Press	20–25 min
	Pull-Up (Optional Assistance)		1–2	3	8–10	~7–8	~9	2–3 min	Lat Pulldown	Chin-Up	10–15 min
	Dumbbell Lateral Raise	Lengthened Partials (Extended Set)	0–1	2	8–10	~9	10	1–2 min	Cable Lateral Raise	Machine Lateral Raise	5–10 min
	Rope Facepull		0–1	3	8–10	~9	10	1–2 min	Reverse Pec Deck	Reverse Cable Fly	5–10 min
	EZ-Bar Skullcrusher		0–1	3	8–10	~9	10	1–2 min	Dumbbell Skullcrusher	Overhead Triceps Extension	5–10 min
	Preacher Curl		0–1	3	8–10	~9	10	1–2 min	EZ-Bar Biceps Curl	Dumbbell Biceps Curl	5–10 min
										Estimated Training Time:	50–80 min
	General warm-up: 5 min light cardio & dynamic stretching										
Lower #1 (Strength Focus)	Deadlift		2–3	3	3–5	~7	~8	3–5 min	Romanian Deadlift	Hip Thrust	20–25 min
	Leg Press		2–3	3	6–8	~7	~8	3–4 min	Barbell Front Squat	Dumbbell Lunge	15–20 min
	Glute Ham Raise		1–2	3	8–10	~7	~8	2–3 min	45° Back Extension	Lying Leg Curl	10–15 min
	Seated Calf Raise		0–1	3	8–10	~9	10	1–2 min	Standing Calf Raise	Leg Press Calf Press	5–10 min
	Cable Crunch		0–1	3	10–12	~9	10	1–2 min	Plate-Weighted Decline Sit-Up	Hanging Leg Raise	5–10 min
										Estimated Training Time:	55–80 min
	General warm-up: 5 min light cardio & dynamic stretching										
Upper #2 (Hypertrophy Focus)	Barbell Row		2–3	3	8–10	~7–8	~9	2–3 min	Pendlay Row	Dumbbell Row	15–20 min
	Overhead Barbell Press		2–3	3	6–8	~7–8	~9	3–4 min	Dumbbell Shoulder Press (Standing)	Dumbbell Shoulder Press (Seated)	20–25 min
	Cable Lat Pullover	Lengthened Partials (Extended Set)	0–1	2	10–12	~9	10	1–2 min	Dumbbell Lat Pullover	Cable Lat Pull-In	5–10 min
	Cable Fly	Myo-reps	0–1	2	10–12	~9	10	1–2 min	Dumbbell Fly	Pec Deck	5–10 min
	Hammer Curl		0–1	3	12–15	~9	10	1–2 min	Dumbbell Biceps Curl	EZ-Bar Biceps Curl	5–10 min
	Triceps Kickback (Cable)		0–1	3	12–15	~9	10	1–2 min	EZ-Bar Skullcrusher	Triceps Pressdown	5–10 min
										Estimated Training Time:	55–85 min

Week 1	Exercise	Last Set Intensity Technique	Warm-Up Sets	Working Sets	Reps	Early Set RPE	Last Set RPE	Rest	Substitution Option 1	Substitution Option 2	Time Estimate
Lower #2 (Hypertrophy Focus)											
	General warm-up: 5 min light cardio & dynamic stretching										
	Barbell Back Squat		2–3	3	3–5	~7	~8	3–4 min	Leg Press	Dumbbell Lunge	20–25 min
	45° Back Extension		1–2	3	8–10	~7–8	~9	2–3 min	Good Morning	Glute Ham Raise	10–15 min
	Leg Extension		1–2	3	10–12	~9	10	2–3 min	Goblet Squat	Lunge (Barbell)	10–15 min
	Seated Leg Curl	Lengthened Partials (Extended Set)	1–2	2	10–12	~9	10	2–3 min	Lying Leg Curl	Nordic Ham Curl	10–15 min
	Standing Calf Raise		0–1	3	12–15	~9	10	1–2 min	Seated Calf Raise	Leg Press Calf Press	5–10 min
	Roman Chair Leg Raise		0–1	3	10–20	~9	10	30 sec	Hanging Leg Raise	Bent-Knee Leg Raise	5–10 min
										Estimated Training Time:	60–90 min
Upper #3 (Muscle Endurance Focus)											
	General warm-up: 5 min light cardio & dynamic stretching										
	Flat Dumbbell Press		1–2	3	10–12	~7–8	~9	2–3 min	Dip	Bench Press	10–15 min
	Lat Pulldown		1–2	3	10–12	~7–8	~9	2–3 min	Pull-Up (Optional Assistance)	Chin-Up	10–15 min
	Cable Lateral Raise		0–1	3	12–15	~9	10	1–2 min	Machine Lateral Raise	Dumbbell Lateral Raise	5–10 min
	Dumbbell Row		1–2	3	12–15	~7–8	~9	2–3 min	Chest-Supported T-Bar Row	Barbell Row	10–15 min
	Overhead Triceps Extension		0–1	3	15–20	~9	10	1–2 min	EZ-Bar Skullcrusher	Dumbbell Skullcrusher	5–10 min
	Bayesian Cable Curl		0–1	3	15–20	~9	10	1–2 min	Incline Dumbbell Curl	Preacher Curl	5–10 min
										Estimated Training Time:	45–75 min
Lower #3 (Muscle Endurance Focus)											
	General warm-up: 5 min light cardio & dynamic stretching										
	Lunge (Barbell)		2–3	3	6–8	~7	~8	2–3 min	Dumbbell Lunge	Leg Press	15–20 min
	Good Morning		1–2	3	10–12	~7–8	~9	2–3 min	45° Back Extension	Glute Ham Raise	10–15 min
	Goblet Squat		1–2	3	12–15	~9	10	2–3 min	Leg Extension	Front Squat	10–15 min
	Cable Hip Abduction		0–1	3	12–15	~9	10	1–2 min	Machine Hip Abduction	Weighted Hip Abduction	5–10 min
	Standing Calf Raise		0–1	3	15–20	~9	10	1–2 min	Seated Calf Raise	Leg Press Calf Press	5–10 min
	Plank		0–1	3	30–60s	~9	10	1–2 min	LLPT Plank	Cable Crunch	5–10 min
										Estimated Training Time:	50–80 min
	Suggested Rest Day										

PROGRAM 17: UPPER/LOWER 6X/WEEK

LEVEL: All levels | **GOAL:** Time-limited muscle and strength gain | **TIME:** 45 to 60 minutes

Week 1	Exercise	Last Set Intensity Technique	Warm-Up Sets	Working Sets	Reps	Early Set RPE	Last Set RPE	Rest	Substitution Option 1	Substitution Option 2	Time Estimate
Upper #1 (Strength Focus)	General warm-up: 5 min light cardio & dynamic stretching										
	Machine Chest Press	Myo-reps	1–2	2	6–8	~7–8	~9	2–3 min	Flat Dumbbell Press	Bench Press	15–20 min
	Lat Pulldown		1–2	3	8–10	~7–8	~9	2–3 min	Pull-Up (Optional Assistance)	Chin-Up	10–15 min
	Superset 1: Dumbbell Lateral Raise	Lengthened Partials (Extended Set)	0–1	2	8–10	~9	10	30 sec	Cable Lateral Raise	Machine Lateral Raise	5–10 min
	Superset 1: Rope Facepull		0–1	2	8–10	~9	10	30 sec	Reverse Pec Deck	Reverse Cable Fly	
	Superset 2: EZ-Bar Skullcrusher		0–1	3	8–10	~9	10	30 sec	Dumbbell Skullcrusher	Overhead Triceps Extension	5–10 min
	Superset 2: Preacher Curl		0–1	3	8–10	~9	10	30 sec	EZ-Bar Biceps Curl	Dumbbell Biceps Curl	
										Estimated Training Time:	35–55 min
Lower #1 (Strength Focus)	General warm-up: 5 min light cardio & dynamic stretching										
	Barbell Romanian Deadlift		2–3	3	8–10	~7	~8	2–3 min	Dumbbell Romanian Deadlift	Hip Thrust	15–20 min
	Leg Press		2–3	3	6–8	~7	~8	2–3 min	Dumbbell Lunge	Front Squat	15–20 min
	Glute Ham Raise		1–2	2	8–10	~7	~8	1–2 min	45° Back Extension	Lying Leg Curl	5–10 min
	Superset 1: Seated Calf Raise		0–1	3	8–10	~9	10	30 sec	Standing Calf Raise	Leg Press Calf Press	5–10 min
	Superset 1: Cable Crunch		0–1	3	10–12	~9	10	30 sec	Plate-Weighted Decline Sit-Up	Hanging Leg Raise	
										Estimated Training Time:	40–60 min
Upper #2 (Hypertrophy Focus)	General warm-up: 5 min light cardio & dynamic stretching										
	Chest-Supported T-Bar Row	Lengthened Partials (Extended Set)	2–3	2	8–10	~7–8	~9	2–3 min	Pendlay Row	Dumbbell Row	15–20 min
	Dumbbell Shoulder Press (Seated)		1–2	3	10–12	~7–8	~9	1–2 min	Dumbbell Shoulder Press (Standing)	Cable Upright Row	10–15 min
	Cable Lat Pullover	Lengthened Partials (Extended Set)	0–1	2	10–12	~9	10	1–2 min	Dumbbell Lat Pullover	Cable Lat Pull-In	5–10 min
	Cable Fly	Myo-reps	0–1	2	10–12	~9	10	1–2 min	Dumbbell Fly	Pec Deck	5–10 min
	Superset 1: Hammer Curl		0–1	3	12–15	~9	10	30 sec	Dumbbell Biceps Curl	EZ-Bar Biceps Curl	5–10 min
	Superset 1: Triceps Pressdown		0–1	3	12–15	~9	10	30 sec	EZ-Bar Skullcrusher	Triceps Kickback (Cable)	
										Estimated Training Time:	40–65 min

Week 1	Exercise	Last Set Intensity Technique	Warm-Up Sets	Working Sets	Reps	Early Set RPE	Last Set RPE	Rest	Substitution Option 1	Substitution Option 2	Time Estimate
Lower #2 (Hypertrophy Focus)											
	colspan general	General warm-up: 5 min light cardio & dynamic stretching									
	Hack Squat		2–3	3	6–8	~7	~8	2–3 min	Leg Press	Dumbbell Lunge	15–20 min
	45° Back Extension		1–2	3	10–12	~7–8	~9	2–3 min	Good Morning	Glute Ham Raise	10–15 min
	Leg Extension	Lengthened Partials (Extended Set)	1–2	2	10–12	~9	10	1–2 min	Goblet Squat	Dumbbell Lunge	5–10 min
	Seated Leg Curl	Lengthened Partials (Extended Set)	1–2	2	10–12	~9	10	1–2 min	Lying Leg Curl	Nordic Ham Curl	5–10 min
	Superset 1: Standing Calf Raise		0–1	3	12–15	~9	10	30 sec	Seated Calf Raise	Leg Press Calf Press	5–10 min
	Superset 1: Plate-Weighted Decline Sit-Up		0–1	3	10–12	~9	10	30 sec	Cable Crunch	Plank	
										Estimated Training Time:	40–65 min
Upper #3 (Muscle Endurance Focus)											
		General warm-up: 5 min light cardio & dynamic stretching									
	Flat Dumbbell Press		1–2	3	10–12	~7–8	~9	2–3 min	Dip	Bench Press	10–15 min
	Lat Pulldown	Lengthened Partials (Extended Set)	1–2	2	10–12	~7–8	~9	2–3 min	Pull-Up (Optional Assistance)	Chin-Up	10–15 min
	Cable Lateral Raise		0–1	3	12–15	~9	10	1–2 min	Machine Lateral Raise	Dumbbell Lateral Raise	5–10 min
	Dumbbell Row		1–2	3	12–15	~7–8	~9	2–3 min	Chest-Supported T-Bar Row	Barbell Row	10–15 min
	Superset 1: Overhead Triceps Extension		0–1	3	15–20	~9	10	30 sec	EZ-Bar Skullcrusher	Dumbbell Skullcrusher	5–10 min
	Superset 1: Bayesian Cable Curl		0–1	3	15–20	~9	10	30 sec	Incline Dumbbell Curl	Preacher Curl	
										Estimated Training Time:	40–65 min
Lower #3 (Muscle Endurance Focus)											
		General warm-up: 5 min light cardio & dynamic stretching									
	Dumbbell Lunge		1–2	2	8–10	~7	~8	2–3 min	Lunge (Barbell)	Leg Press	10–15 min
	Good Morning		1–2	3	10–12	~7–8	~9	2–3 min	45° Back Extension	Glute Ham Raise	10–15 min
	Goblet Squat		1–2	2	12–15	~9	10	1–2 min	Leg Extension	Leg Press	5–10 min
	Cable Hip Abduction		0–1	2	12–15	~9	10	1–2 min	Machine Hip Abduction	Weighted Hip Abduction	5–10 min
	Superset 1: Standing Calf Raise		0–1	2	15–20	~9	10	30 sec	Seated Calf Raise	Leg Press Calf Press	5–10 min
	Superset 1: Roman Chair Leg Raise		0–1	2	10–20	~9	10	30 sec	Hanging Leg Raise	Bent-Knee Leg Raise	
										Estimated Training Time:	40–65 min
					Suggested Rest Day						

PROGRAM 18: PUSH/PULL/LEGS SPLIT 6X/WEEK

LEVEL: Beginner | **GOAL:** Build muscle and gain strength | **TIME:** 60 to 90 minutes

Week 1	Exercise	Last Set Intensity Technique	Warm-Up Sets	Working Sets	Reps	Early Set RPE	Last Set RPE	Rest	Substitution Option 1	Substitution Option 2	Time Estimate
Push #1 (Strength Focus)	General warm-up: 5 min light cardio & dynamic stretching										
	Machine Chest Press		2–3	3	6–8	~7–8	~9	2–3 min	Bench Press	Flat Dumbbell Press	15–20 min
	Dumbbell Shoulder Press (Seated)		1–2	3	8–10	~7–8	~9	2–3 min	Overhead Barbell Press	Barbell Upright Row	10–15 min
	Pec Deck		0–1	3	8–10	~9	10	1–2 min	Dumbbell Fly	Push-Up	5–10 min
	Dumbbell Lateral Raise		0–1	3	8–10	~9	10	1–2 min	Cable Lateral Raise	Machine Lateral Raise	5–10 min
	EZ-Bar Skullcrusher		0–1	2	8–10	~9	10	1–2 min	Dumbbell Skullcrusher	Overhead Triceps Extension	5–10 min
	Triceps Pressdown		0–1	2	8–10	~9	10	1–2 min	Triceps Kickback (Cable)	EZ-Bar Skullcrusher	5–10 min
										Estimated Training Time:	45–75 min
Pull #1 (Strength Focus)	General warm-up: 5 min light cardio & dynamic stretching										
	Chest-Supported T-Bar Row		2–3	3	8–10	~7–8	~9	2–3 min	Pendlay Row	Dumbbell Row	15–20 min
	Lat Pulldown		1–2	3	8–10	~7–8	~9	2–3 min	Pull-Up (Optional Assistance)	Chin-Up	10–15 min
	Rope Facepull		0–1	3	8–10	~9	10	1–2 min	Reverse Pec Deck	Reverse Cable Fly	5–10 min
	Cable Lat Pullover		0–1	3	8–10	~9	10	1–2 min	Dumbbell Lat Pullover	Cable Lat Pull-In	5–10 min
	Preacher Curl		0–1	2	8–10	~9	10	1–2 min	EZ-Bar Biceps Curl	Dumbbell Biceps Curl	5–10 min
	EZ-Bar Biceps Curl		0–1	2	8–10	~9	10	1–2 min	Standing Barbell Curl	Dumbbell Biceps Curl	5–10 min
										Estimated Training Time:	45–75 min
Legs #1 (Strength Focus)	General warm-up: 5 min light cardio & dynamic stretching										
	Romanian Deadlift		2–3	3	8–10	~6	~7	2–3 min	Deadlift	Hip Thrust	15–20 min
	Leg Press		2–3	3	6–8	~7	~8	3–4 min	Barbell Front Squat	Dumbbell Lunge	15–20 min
	Glute Ham Raise		1–2	2	8–10	~7	~8	2–3 min	45° Back Extension	Lying Leg Curl	10–15 min
	Seated Calf Raise		0–1	3	8–10	~9	10	1–2 min	Standing Calf Raise	Leg Press Calf Press	5–10 min
	Cable Crunch		0–1	3	10–12	~9	10	1–2 min	Plate-Weighted Decline Sit-Up	Hanging Leg Raise	5–10 min
										Estimated Training Time:	50–75 min

Week 1	Exercise	Last Set Intensity Technique	Warm-Up Sets	Working Sets	Reps	Early Set RPE	Last Set RPE	Rest	Substitution Option 1	Substitution Option 2	Time Estimate
Push #2 (Hypertrophy Focus)	General warm-up: 5 min light cardio & dynamic stretching										
	Dumbbell Shoulder Press (Seated)		2–3	3	10–12	~7–8	~9	2–3 min	Dumbbell Shoulder Press (Standing)	Overhead Barbell Press	15–20 min
	Flat Dumbbell Press		1–2	3	10–12	~7–8	~9	2–3 min	Dip	Bench Press	10–15 min
	Cable Lateral Raise		0–1	3	12–15	~9	10	1–2 min	Machine Lateral Raise	Dumbbell Lateral Raise	5–10 min
	Cable Fly		0–1	3	15–20	~9	10	1–2 min	Dumbbell Fly	Pec Deck	5–10 min
	Triceps Kickback (Cable)		0–1	2	12–15	~9	10	1–2 min	EZ-Bar Skullcrusher	Triceps Pressdown	5–10 min
	Overhead Triceps Extension		0–1	2	12–15	~9	10	1–2 min	EZ-Bar Skullcrusher	Dumbbell Skullcrusher	5–10 min
										Estimated Training Time:	45–75 min
Pull #2 (Hypertrophy Focus)	General warm-up: 5 min light cardio & dynamic stretching										
	Lat Pulldown		1–2	3	10–12	~7–8	~9	2–3 min	Pull-Up (Optional Assistance)	Chin-Up	10–15 min
	Dumbbell Row		1–2	3	10–12	~7–8	~9	2–3 min	Chest-Supported T-Bar Row	Barbell Row	10–15 min
	Cable Lat Pull-In		0–1	3	10–12	~9	10	1–2 min	Cable Lat Pullover	Dumbbell Lat Pullover	5–10 min
	Reverse Pec Deck		0–1	2	15–20	~9	10	1–2 min	Rope Facepull	Reverse Cable Fly	5–10 min
	Barbell Shrug		0–1	2	12–15	~9	10	1–2 min	Dumbbell Shrug	Trap Bar Shrug	5–10 min
	Hammer Curl		0–1	2	12–15	~9	10	1–2 min	Dumbbell Biceps Curl	EZ-Bar Biceps Curl	5–10 min
	Bayesian Cable Curl		0–1	2	12–15	~9	10	1–2 min	Incline Dumbbell Curl	Preacher Curl	5–10 min
										Estimated Training Time:	45–80 min
Legs #2 (Hypertrophy Focus)	General warm-up: 5 min light cardio & dynamic stretching										
	Leg Press		2–3	3	8–10	~7	~8	3–4 min	Barbell Back Squat	Dumbbell Lunge	15–20 min
	45° Back Extension		1–2	3	10–12	~7–8	~9	2–3 min	Good Morning	Glute Ham Raise	10–15 min
	Leg Extension		1–2	2	12–15	~9	10	2–3 min	Goblet Squat	Dumbbell Lunge	10–15 min
	Seated Leg Curl		1–2	2	12–15	~9	10	2–3 min	Lying Leg Curl	Nordic Ham Curl	10–15 min
	Standing Calf Raise		0–1	3	15–20	~9	10	1–2 min	Seated Calf Raise	Leg Press Calf Press	5–10 min
	Roman Chair Leg Raise		0–1	3	10–20	~9	10	1–2 min	Hanging Leg Raise	Bent-Knee Leg Raise	5–10 min
										Estimated Training Time:	55–85 min

Suggested Rest Day

PROGRAM 19: PUSH/PULL/LEGS SPLIT 6X/WEEK

LEVEL: Intermediate/Advanced | **GOAL:** Build muscle and gain strength | **TIME:** 60 to 90 minutes

Week 1	Exercise	Last Set Intensity Technique	Warm-Up Sets	Working Sets	Reps	Early Set RPE	Last Set RPE	Rest	Substitution Option 1	Substitution Option 2	Time Estimate
Push #1 (Strength Focus)	General warm-up: 5 min light cardio & dynamic stretching										
	Bench Press		2–3	3	3–5	~7–8	~9	3–4 min	Machine Chest Press	Flat Dumbbell Press	20–25 min
	Dumbbell Shoulder Press (Seated)		1–2	3	8–10	~7–8	~9	2–3 min	Overhead Barbell Press	Barbell Upright Row	10–15 min
	Pec Deck	Dropset	0–1	2	8–10	~9	10	1–2 min	Dumbbell Fly	Push-Up	5–10 min
	Dumbbell Lateral Raise	Lengthened Partials (Extended Set)	0–1	2	8–10	~9	10	1–2 min	Cable Lateral Raise	Machine Lateral Raise	5–10 min
	EZ-Bar Skullcrusher		0–1	3	8–10	~9	10	1–2 min	Dumbbell Skullcrusher	Overhead Triceps Extension	5–10 min
	Triceps Pressdown		0–1	3	8–10	~9	10	1–2 min	Triceps Kickback (Cable)	EZ-Bar Skullcrusher	5–10 min
										Estimated Training Time:	50–80 min
Pull #1 (Strength Focus)	General warm-up: 5 min light cardio & dynamic stretching										
	Barbell Row		2–3	3	8–10	~7–8	~9	2–3 min	Pendlay Row	Dumbbell Row	15–20 min
	Pull-Up (Optional Assistance)		1–2	3	8–10	~7–8	~9	2–3 min	Lat Pulldown	Chin-Up	10–15 min
	Rope Facepull		0–1	3	8–10	~9	10	1–2 min	Reverse Pec Deck	Reverse Cable Fly	5–10 min
	Cable Lat Pullover	Lengthened Partials (Extended Set)	0–1	2	8–10	~9	10	1–2 min	Dumbbell Lat Pullover	Cable Lat Pull-In	5–10 min
	Preacher Curl		0–1	3	8–10	~9	10	1–2 min	EZ-Bar Biceps Curl	Dumbbell Biceps Curl	5–10 min
	EZ-Bar Biceps Curl		0–1	3	8–10	~9	10	1–2 min	Standing Barbell Curl	Dumbbell Biceps Curl	5–10 min
										Estimated Training Time:	45–75 min
Legs #1 (Strength Focus)	General warm-up: 5 min light cardio & dynamic stretching										
	Deadlift		2–3	3	3–5	~7	~8	3–5 min	Romanian Deadlift	Hip Thrust	20–25 min
	Leg Press		2–3	3	6–8	~7	~8	3–4 min	Barbell Front Squat	Dumbbell Lunge	15–20 min
	Glute Ham Raise		1–2	3	8–10	~7	~8	2–3 min	45° Back Extension	Lying Leg Curl	10–15 min
	Seated Calf Raise		0–1	3	8–10	~9	10	1–2 min	Standing Calf Raise	Leg Press Calf Press	5–10 min
	Cable Crunch		0–1	3	10–12	~9	10	1–2 min	Plate-Weighted Decline Sit-Up	Hanging Leg Raise	5–10 min
										Estimated Training Time:	55–80 min

Week 1	Exercise	Last Set Intensity Technique	Warm-Up Sets	Working Sets	Reps	Early Set RPE	Last Set RPE	Rest	Substitution Option 1	Substitution Option 2	Time Estimate
Push #2 (Hypertrophy Focus)	General warm-up: 5 min light cardio & dynamic stretching										
	Overhead Barbell Press		2–3	3	6–8	~7–8	~9	3–4 min	Dumbbell Shoulder Press (Standing)	Dumbbell Shoulder Press (Seated)	20–25 min
	Flat Dumbbell Press		1–2	3	10–12	~7–8	~9	2–3 min	Dip	Bench Press	10–15 min
	Cable Lateral Raise		0–1	3	12–15	~9	10	1–2 min	Machine Lateral Raise	Dumbbell Lateral Raise	5–10 min
	Cable Fly	Myo-reps	0–1	2	15–20	~9	10	1–2 min	Cable Lateral Raise	Pec Deck	5–10 min
	Triceps Kickback (Cable)		0–1	3	12–15	~9	10	1–2 min	EZ-Bar Skullcrusher	Triceps Pressdown	5–10 min
	Overhead Triceps Extension		0–1	3	12–15	~9	10	1–2 min	EZ-Bar Skullcrusher	Dumbbell Skullcrusher	5–10 min
										Estimated Training Time:	50–80 min
Pull #2 (Hypertrophy Focus)	General warm-up: 5 min light cardio & dynamic stretching										
	Lat Pulldown		1–2	3	10–12	~7–8	~9	2–3 min	Pull-Up (Optional Assistance)	Chin-Up	10–15 min
	Dumbbell Row		1–2	3	10–12	~7–8	~9	2–3 min	Chest-Supported T-Bar Row	Barbell Row	10–15 min
	Cable Lat Pull-In		0–1	3	10–12	~9	10	1–2 min	Cable Lat Pullover	Dumbbell Lat Pullover	5–10 min
	Reverse Pec Deck		0–1	3	15–20	~9	10	1–2 min	Rope Facepull	Reverse Cable Fly	5–10 min
	Barbell Shrug	Cheat Reps	0–1	2	12–15	~9	10	1–2 min	Dumbbell Shrug	Trap Bar Shrug	5–10 min
	Hammer Curl		0–1	3	12–15	~9	10	1–2 min	Dumbbell Biceps Curl	EZ-Bar Biceps Curl	5–10 min
	Bayesian Cable Curl		0–1	3	12–15	~9	10	1–2 min	Incline Dumbbell Curl	Preacher Curl	5–10 min
										Estimated Training Time:	45–80 min
Legs #2 (Hypertrophy Focus)	General warm-up: 5 min light cardio & dynamic stretching										
	Barbell Back Squat		2–3	3	3–5	~7	~8	3–4 min	Leg Press	Dumbbell Lunge	20–25 min
	45° Back Extension		1–2	3	10–12	~7–8	~9	2–3 min	Good Morning	Glute Ham Raise	10–15 min
	Leg Extension	Lengthened Partials (Extended Set)	1–2	2	12–15	~9	10	2–3 min	Goblet Squat	Dumbbell Lunge	10–15 min
	Seated Leg Curl	Lengthened Partials (Extended Set)	1–2	2	12–15	~9	10	2–3 min	Lying Leg Curl	Nordic Ham Curl	10–15 min
	Standing Calf Raise		0–1	3	15–20	~9	10	1–2 min	Seated Calf Raise	Leg Press Calf Press	5–10 min
	Roman Chair Leg Raise		0–1	3	10–20	~9	10	1–2 min	Hanging Leg Raise	Bent-Knee Leg Raise	5–10 min
										Estimated Training Time:	60–90 min
Suggested Rest Day											

PROGRAM 20: PUSH/PULL/LEGS SPLIT 6X/WEEK

LEVEL: All levels | **GOAL:** Time-limited muscle and strength gain | **TIME:** 45 to 60 minutes

Week 1	Exercise	Last Set Intensity Technique	Warm-Up Sets	Working Sets	Reps	Early Set RPE	Last Set RPE	Rest	Substitution Option 1	Substitution Option 2	Time Estimate
Push #1 (Strength Focus)	General warm-up: 5 min light cardio & dynamic stretching										
	Machine Chest Press	Myo-reps	1–2	2	6–8	~7–8	~9	2–3 min	Flat Dumbbell Press	Bench Press	15–20 min
	Dumbbell Shoulder Press (Seated)		1–2	3	8–10	~7–8	~9	1–2 min	Dumbbell Shoulder Press (Standing)	Cable Upright Row	10–15 min
	Pec Deck	Dropset	0–1	2	8–10	~9	10	1–2 min	Dumbbell Fly	Push-up	5–10 min
	Superset 1: Dumbbell Lateral Raise	Lengthened Partials (Extended Set)	0–1	2	8–10	~9	10	30 sec	Cable Lateral Raise	Machine Lateral Raise	5–10 min
	Superset 1: Triceps Pressdown		0–1	2	8–10	~9	10	30 sec	Triceps Kickback (Cable)	EZ-Bar Skullcrusher	
										Estimated Training Time:	35–55 min
Pull #1 (Strength Focus)	General warm-up: 5 min light cardio & dynamic stretching										
	Chest-Supported T-Bar Row	Lengthened Partials (Extended Set)	1–2	2	8–10	~7–8	~9	2–3 min	Pendlay Row	Dumbbell Row	15–20 min
	Lat Pulldown		1–2	3	8–10	~7–8	~9	1–2 min	Pull-Up (Optional Assistance)	Chin-Up	10–15 min
	Rope Facepull		0–1	3	8–10	~9	10	1–2 min	Reverse Pec Deck	Reverse Cable Fly	5–10 min
	Superset 1: Cable Lat Pullover	Lengthened Partials (Extended Set)	0–1	2	8–10	~9	10	30 sec	Dumbbell Lat Pullover	Cable Lat Pull-In	5–10 min
	Superset 1: Preacher Curl		0–1	3	8–10	~9	10	30 sec	EZ-Bar Biceps Curl	Dumbbell Biceps Curl	
										Estimated Training Time:	35–55 min
Legs #1 (Strength Focus)	General warm-up: 5 min light cardio & dynamic stretching										
	Barbell Romanian Deadlift		2–3	3	8–10	~7	~8	2–3 min	Dumbbell Romanian Deadlift	Hip Thrust	15–20 min
	Leg Press		2–3	3	6–8	~7	~8	2–3 min	Dumbbell Lunge	Front Squat	15–20 min
	Glute Ham Raise		1–2	2	8–10	~7	~8	1–2 min	45° Back Extension	Lying Leg Curl	5–10 min
	Superset 1: Seated Calf Raise		0–1	3	8–10	~9	10	30 sec	Standing Calf Raise	Leg Press Calf Press	5–10 min
	Superset 1: Cable Crunch		0–1	3	10–12	~9	10	30 sec	Plate-Weighted Decline Sit-Up	Hanging Leg Raise	
										Estimated Training Time:	40–60 min

Week 1	Exercise	Last Set Intensity Technique	Warm-Up Sets	Working Sets	Reps	Early Set RPE	Last Set RPE	Rest	Substitution Option 1	Substitution Option 2	Time Estimate
Push #2 (Hypertrophy Focus)	General warm-up: 5 min light cardio & dynamic stretching										
	Cable Upright Row		1–2	3	10–12	~7–8	~9	1–2 min	Dumbbell Lateral Raise	Dumbbell Shoulder Press (Standing)	10–15 min
	Flat Dumbbell Press		1–2	3	10–12	~7–8	~9	2–3 min	Dip	Bench Press	10–15 min
	Cable Lateral Raise		0–1	3	12–15	~9	10	1–2 min	Machine Lateral Raise	Dumbbell Lateral Raise	5–10 min
	Cable Fly	Myo-reps	0–1	2	15–20	~9	10	1–2 min	Dumbbell Fly	Pec Deck	5–10 min
	Overhead Triceps Extension		0–1	3	12–15	~9	10	1–2 min	EZ-Bar Skullcrusher	Dumbbell Skullcrusher	5–10 min
										Estimated Training Time:	35–60 min
Pull #2 (Hypertrophy Focus)	General warm-up: 5 min light cardio & dynamic stretching										
	Lat Pulldown	Lengthened Partials (Extended Set)	1–2	2	10–12	~7–8	~9	2–3 min	Pull-Up (Optional Assistance)	Chin-Up	10–15 min
	Dumbbell Row		1–2	3	10–12	~7–8	~9	2–3 min	Chest-Supported T-Bar Row	Barbell Row	10–15 min
	Cable Lat Pull-In		0–1	3	12–15	~9	10	1–2 min	Cable Lat Pullover	Dumbbell Lat Pullover	5–10 min
	Reverse Pec Deck		0–1	3	15–20	~9	10	1–2 min	Rope Facepull	Reverse Cable Fly	5–10 min
	Bayesian Cable Curl		0–1	3	12–15	~9	10	1–2 min	Incline Dumbbell Curl	Preacher Curl	5–10 min
										Estimated Training Time:	35–60 min
Legs #2 (Hypertrophy Focus)	General warm-up: 5 min light cardio & dynamic stretching										
	Hack Squat		2–3	3	6–8	~7	~8	2–3 min	Leg Press	Dumbbell Lunge	15–20 min
	45° Back Extension		1–2	3	10–12	~7–8	~9	2–3 min	Good Morning	Glute Ham Raise	10–15 min
	Leg Extension	Lengthened Partials (Extended Set)	1–2	2	12–15	~9	10	1–2 min	Goblet Squat	Dumbbell Lunge	5–10 min
	Seated Leg Curl	Lengthened Partials (Extended Set)	1–2	2	12–15	~9	10	1–2 min	Lying Leg Curl	Nordic Ham Curl	5–10 min
	Superset 1: Standing Calf Raise		0–1	2	15–20	~9	10	30 sec	Seated Calf Raise	Leg Press Calf Press	5–10 min
	Superset 1: Roman Chair Leg Raise		0–1	2	10–20	~9	10	30 sec	Hanging Leg Raise	Bent-Knee Leg Raise	
										Estimated Training Time:	40–65 min
Suggested Rest Day											

ACKNOWLEDGMENTS

I began this project seven years ago with the goal of making it the only book anyone ever needs to read to understand training to build muscle and gain strength. I hope I've come close to achieving that objective.

This project could not have happened without the help and support from a small army of people who provided contributions of time, knowledge, inspiration, and encouragement.

My father, William, helped me come up with the idea of using a ladder to organize all my ideas about training in an ordered hierarchy.

Thanks to Dr. Eric Helms for his invaluable contributions to the field of exercise science. Without inspiration from his *Muscle & Strength Pyramid* books, *The Muscle Ladder* wouldn't exist.

I'd also like to thank my research assistant, Max Edsey, for helping me tremendously through all seven years of writing this book. Fitness writing legend, Lou Schuler, was another rock in helping me make the final product easy to read and digestible for trainees at every level. My partner, Stephanie, is my round-the-clock soundboard for ideas. She always provides the best constructive criticism and guidance. Matt Dziadecki came through with the cover shot and all the exercise demonstration photos. I think they add a lot of value to the text.

I owe immense appreciation to anyone who has done research in the field of exercise science. We're all extremely grateful for your work.

And I'm very thankful for my community on YouTube, who continually motivates me to get better at learning and communicating.

Thanks to my publisher, Victory Belt, for believing in the project and being patient with me through the entire writing process. They truly helped me mold this book into the piece of work that I wanted it to be.

Lastly, thank you to all the readers who share my passion for learning how to get jacked and strong. I hope you enjoy reading the book as much as I've enjoyed writing it!

GLOSSARY

accentuated eccentric training: Training that involves overloading the negative/eccentric portion of the lift—for example, a training partner manually adding resistance to the negative.

AMRAP: As many reps as possible (with good form). AMRAP sets are a useful way to track your strength progress over time without actually testing your 1RM.

body recomposition: The process of losing fat and gaining muscle at the same time.

caloric deficit: When you burn more calories than you consume, your body gets the energy it needs from the reserves you have in your fat cells.

caloric surplus: When you consume more calories than you burn, your body stores the excess in your tissues, primarily in your muscles and fat cells.

cheat reps: Repetitions that involve a significant deviation from the standard technique of an exercise to achieve more reps or use more weight.

compound exercises: Exercises that target multiple muscle groups and involve movement at more than one joint. Examples include squats, deadlifts, presses, and rows.

concentric: Also known as the "positive," this is the lifting phase of an exercise, when the targeted muscles contract.

daily undulating periodization: This is characterized by changing up the reps, sets, and/or load each workout within a given week.

deload: A period of training when you reduce your volume and/or intensity with the goal of allowing more complete recovery.

dirty bulk: A caloric surplus characterized by a lack of restrictions, meaning that individuals often eat lots of high-calorie foods with little nutritional value, resulting in rapid weight gain.

drop set: After reaching failure on a set (or coming close to it), you reduce the weight and continue until you reach failure with the lighter load.

early set RPE: The RPE you should aim to hit on all but the last set of an exercise. This should put you on track to hit the last set RPE.

eccentric: Also known as the "negative," this is the lowering phase of an exercise, when the targeted muscles lengthen.

effort: How hard you push a set relative to failure. It can be measured with RPE or RIR.

failure training: Training to failure means not ending a set until you can't do another repetition. There are two variations: muscular failure, in which you couldn't lift the weight again if your life depended on it, and technical failure, in which you stop a set because you couldn't do another rep without deviating significantly from proper form.

forced reps: A training partner helps you grind out a few additional reps after you reach failure on a set.

genetic muscular limit: Theoretically, there's a point beyond which a drug-free lifter can no longer build new muscle while staying relatively lean. (You can always pack on a combination of muscle and fat.) It's not clear if there's a true limit or if progress slows to the point that it's hard to detect.

hypertrophy: When muscles get larger as an adaptation to resistance training. The opposite is atrophy—when muscles get smaller due to training less, eating less, illness, injury, or some combination of factors.

intensity: Casually, it's a synonym for effort. But technically, it refers to your load as a percentage of your 1RM. The higher the percentage, the higher the intensity.

iso-hold: Holding a position for an amount of time where the muscle is under tension but you are not moving—for example, holding dumbbells at the bottom of a bench press for thirty seconds. Also known as a static hold.

isolation exercises: Exercises that target one muscle group and involve movement at a single joint. Examples include biceps curls, leg extensions, and calf raises.

last set intensity technique: An intensity technique that is to be performed on the last set only (for example, drop set, lengthened partials, and so on).

last set RPE: The RPE you should aim to hit on the last set of an exercise.

linear periodization: When intensity (load) goes up while volume goes down. This is achieved by increasing the weight and decreasing the reps each week.

load: A synonym for the weight you're lifting, aka the amount of external resistance.

macrocycle: A big picture look at how you might organize training across an entire year to reach a certain goal.

mesocycle: The layer below a macrocycle that focuses on how training is organized within a period of a few months.

microcycle: The layer below a mesocycle that focuses on how training is organized within a single week.

mind-muscle connection: This is the ability to consciously focus on and engage specific muscles during an exercise.

multijoint muscle: A muscle that acts on more than one joint and contributes to multiple movement patterns. The trapezius, for example, contributes to exercises that target the shoulders (shoulder press), upper and middle back (row and pulldown), and lower back (deadlift).

myo-reps: After reaching or approaching failure on a set, you stop and recover for about three seconds. Then you perform three reps, rest for another three seconds, perform three more reps, and continue until you can no longer complete all three reps.

one-rep max (1RM): On any given exercise, your 1RM is the most weight you can lift for a single repetition. Some training programs prescribe workout intensity with a percentage of your 1RM.

overtraining: Training at a volume, intensity, and/or frequency that exceeds your body's ability to recover. The first signs of overtraining could be stalled progress and reduced energy for your workouts. Over time, they could include chronic exhaustion, poor sleep, and constant, nagging injuries.

partial reps: Repetitions that don't use the entire range of motion of an exercise. The most effective use of these is with lengthened partials, which focus on performing the half of the range of motion where the muscle is lengthened—for example, the bottom half of a lying leg curl or the bottom half of a preacher curl.

periodization: A way to organize your training over time. An athlete, for example, typically has a defined offseason, preseason, competitive season, and postseason. A periodized training program focuses on different goals in different parts of that training cycle. In a muscle and strength context, periodization mainly refers to how you organize your training over time.

primary exercises: These are the heavy, compound movements that you should generally prioritize in your training program by doing them first, when you have the most energy and focus. They typically involve the most muscle mass and create the most fatigue.

progressive overload: In training, your goal is to gradually increase the challenge to your muscles and joints, starting with relatively little stress and building up over time to relatively high stress. The increased challenge will usually come from heavier weights and/or higher volume. It works best when you focus on one or two parameters at a time, rather than trying to build up everything at once.

rate of perceived exertion (RPE): A measure of how difficult a set was on a scale of 1 to 10. RPE 10 means you reached failure. RPE 9 means you could have gotten one more rep, RPE 8 means you had two more in the tank, and so on.

recovery: This can refer to the rest period between sets, when your breathing and heart rate return to normal, or the time between workouts, when your muscles repair themselves and restore their energy supplies.

reps in reserve (RIR): Another way to describe how hard you're working. At RPE 10, you have zero RIR. At RPE 9, you have 1 RIR, and so on.

reverse linear periodization: When intensity (load) goes down while volume goes up. This is achieved by decreasing the weight and increasing the reps each week.

secondary exercises: These are compound exercises that are less fatiguing than your primary exercises, even if they involve a similar amount of muscle mass. Examples include lunges, hip thrusts, and machine-based compound exercises.

tempo: The speed of your repetitions. When a bodybuilding program prescribes tempo, it usually tells you how fast to lift (usually one or two seconds) and lower (usually one to four seconds) the weight. It might also specify transition time between lifting and lowering.

tertiary exercises: These are usually isolation movements like biceps curls and triceps pressdowns, which aim to target a single muscle.

training split: This is the organizing principle for your training throughout the week, including which muscles you train on which days.

volume: The amount of work performed in a single training session or series of sessions. It's usually defined as the total number of hard sets—non-warm-up sets in which you challenge and fatigue your muscles.

weekly undulating periodization: Training characterized by changing the reps, sets, and/or load each week.

work capacity: This combination of strength, muscular endurance, and aerobic conditioning determines how much you can accomplish in your workouts. More experienced lifters should develop a higher work capacity over time, allowing them to perform more volume and recover better.

REFERENCES

CHAPTER 2

1. Haruki Momma et al., "Muscle-Strengthening Activities Are Associated with Lower Risk and Mortality in Major Non-Communicable Diseases: A Systematic Review and Meta-Analysis of Cohort Studies," *British Journal of Sports Medicine* 55 (2022): 755–763, https://bjsm.bmj.com/content/56/13/755.info.

2. Brad J. Schoenfeld et al., "Strength and Hypertrophy Adaptations Between Low- vs. High-Load Resistance Training: A Systematic Review and Meta-Analysis," *Journal of Strength and Conditioning Research* 31, no. 12 (December 2017): 3508–3523, https://pubmed.ncbi.nlm.nih.gov/28834797/; Brad J. Schoenfeld et al., "Loading Recommendations for Muscle Strength, Hypertrophy, and Local Endurance: A Re-Examination of the Repetition Continuum," *Sports* (Basel) 9, no. 2 (February 2021): 32, https://www.ncbi.nlm.nih.gov/pmc/articles/PMC7927075/.

3. Anna Christakou et al., "Re-Injury Worry, Confidence and Attention as Predictors of a Sport Re-Injury During a Competitive Season," *Research in Sports Medicine* 30, no. 1 (January-February 2022): 19–29; https://pubmed.ncbi.nlm.nih.gov/33256461/; Mark V. Paterno, Kaitlyn Flynn, Staci Thomas, and Laura C. Schmitt, "Self-Reported Fear Predicts Functional Performance and Second ACL Injury After ACL Reconstruction and Return to Sport: A Pilot Study," *Sports Health* 10, no. 3 (May/June 2018): 228–233: https://pubmed.ncbi.nlm.nih.gov/29272209/.

4. Justin W. L. Keogh and Paul W. Winwood, "The Epidemiology of Injuries Across the Weight-Training Sports," *Sports Medicine* (Auckland, New Zealand) 47, no. 3 (March 2017): 479–501, https://pubmed.ncbi.nlm.nih.gov/27328853/.

5. Albert Sánchez Pastor et al., "Influence of Strength Training Variables on Neuromuscular and Morphological Adaptations in Prepubertal Children: A Systematic Review," *International Journal of Environmental Research and Public Health* 20, no. 6 (March 2023): 4833, https://pubmed.ncbi.nlm.nih.gov/36981742/.

6. Matteo Ponzano et al., "Progressive Resistance Training for Improving Health-Related Outcomes in People at Risk of Fracture: A Systematic Review and Meta-Analysis of Randomized Controlled Trials," *Physical Therapy* 101, no. 2 (February 4, 2021): pzaa221, https://pubmed.ncbi.nlm.nih.gov/33367736/; Daniel Souza et al., "High and Low-Load Resistance Training Produce Similar Effects on Bone Mineral Density of Middle-Aged and Older People: A Systematic Review with Meta-Analysis of Randomized Clinical Trials," *Experimental Gerontology* 138 (September 2020): 110973, https://pubmed.ncbi.nlm.nih.gov/32454079/; Nan Chen et al., "Effects of Resistance Training in Healthy Older People with Sarcopenia: A Systematic Review and Meta-Analysis of Randomized Controlled Trials," *European Review of Aging and Physical Activity: Official Journal of the European Group for Research into Elderly and Physical Activity* 18, no. 1 (November 11, 2021): 23, https://pubmed.ncbi.nlm.nih.gov/34763651/.

7. Consensus Conference Panel et al., "Joint Consensus Statement of the American Academy of Sleep Medicine and Sleep Research Society on the Recommended Amount of Sleep for a Healthy Adult: Methodology and Discussion," *Sleep* 38, no. 8 (August 1, 2015): 1161–83, https://pubmed.ncbi.nlm.nih.gov/26194576/.

8. Daniel Bonnar et al., "Sleep Interventions Designed to Improve Athletic Performance and Recovery: A Systematic Review of Current Approaches," *Sports Medicine* (Auckland, New Zealand) 48, no. 3 (March 2018): 683–703, https://pubmed.ncbi.nlm.nih.gov/29352373/.

9. T. Reilly and M. Piercy, "The Effect of Partial Sleep Deprivation on Weightlifting Performance," *Ergonomics* 37, no. 1 (January 1994): 107–15, https://pubmed.ncbi.nlm.nih.gov/8112265/.

10. Jennifer Schwartz and Richard D. Simon, Jr., "Sleep Extension Improves Serving Accuracy: A Study with College Varsity Tennis Players," *Physiology & Behavior* 151 (November 2015):541–4, https://pubmed.ncbi.nlm.nih.gov/26325012/.

11. Cheri D. Mah et al., "The Effects of Sleep Extension on the Athletic Performance of Collegiate Basketball Players," *Sleep* 34, no. 7 (July 1, 2011): 943–50, https://pubmed.ncbi.nlm.nih.gov/21731144/.

12. Neil P. Walsh et al., "Sleep and the Athlete: Narrative Review and 2021 Expert Consensus Recommendations," *British Journal of Sports Medicine* (November 3, 2020): bjsports-2020-102025, https://pubmed.ncbi.nlm.nih.gov/33144349/.

13. Catherine E. Milner and Kimberly A. Cote, "Benefits of Napping in Healthy Adults: Impact of Nap Length, Time of Day, Age, and Experience with Napping," *Journal of Sleep Research* 18, no. 2 (June 2009): 272–81, https://pubmed.ncbi.nlm.nih.gov/19645971/.

14. Julia M. Malowany et al., "Protein to Maximize Whole-Body Anabolism in Resistance-Trained Females After Exercise," *Medicine and Science in Sports and Exercise* 51, no. 4 (April 2019): 798–804, https://pubmed.ncbi.nlm.nih.gov/30395050/.

15. Michael Kellmann et al., "Recovery and Performance in Sport: Consensus Statement," *International Journal of Sports Physiology and Performance* 13, no. 2 (February 1, 2018): 240–5, https://pubmed.ncbi.nlm.nih.gov/29345524/.

16. Jonathan M. Peake et al., "The Effects of Cold Water Immersion and Active Recovery on Molecular Factors That Regulate Growth and Remodeling of Skeletal Muscle After Resistance Exercise," *Frontiers in Physiology* 11 (June 30, 2020): 737, https://pubmed.ncbi.nlm.nih.gov/32695024/; Jackson J. Fyfe et al., "Cold Water Immersion Attenuates Anabolic Signaling and Skeletal Muscle Fiber Hypertrophy, but Not Strength Gain, Following Whole-Body Resistance Training," *Journal of Applied Physiology* (Bethesda, MD: 1985) 127, no. 5 (November 1, 2019): 1403–18, https://pubmed.ncbi.nlm.nih.gov/31513450/.

17. Patroklos Androulakis Korakakis et al., "Optimizing Resistance Training Technique to Maximize Muscle Hypertrophy: A Narrative Review," *Journal of Functional Morphology and Kinesiology* 9, no. 1 (March 2024): 9, https://www.ncbi.nlm.nih.gov/pmc/articles/PMC10801605/.

18. Katherine Herman et al., "The Effectiveness of Neuromuscular Warm-Up Strategies, That Require No Additional Equipment, for Preventing Lower Limb Injuries During Sports Participation: A Systematic Review," *BMC Medicine* 10 (July 2012): 75, https://bmcmedicine.biomedcentral.com/articles/10.1186/1741-7015-10-75.

CHAPTER 3

1. Pedro J. Benito et al., "A Systematic Review with Meta-Analysis of the Effect of Resistance Training on Whole-Body Muscle Growth in Healthy Adult Males," *International Journal of Environmental Research and Public Health* 17, no. 4 (February 17, 2020): 1285, https://pubmed.ncbi.nlm.nih.gov/32079265/; E. M. Kouri et al., "Fat-Free Mass Index in Users and Nonusers of Anabolic-Androgenic Steroids," *Clinical Journal of Sport Medicine: Official Journal of the Canadian Academy of Sport Medicine* 5, no. 4 (October 1995): 223–8, https://pubmed.ncbi.nlm.nih.gov/7496846/.

2. I. Janssen et al., "Skeletal Muscle Mass and Distribution in 468 Men and Women Aged 18–88 Yr," *Journal of Applied Physiology* (Bethesda, MD: 1985) 89, no. 1 (July 2000): 81–8, https://pubmed.ncbi.nlm.nih.gov/10904038/; Brandon M. Roberts, Greg Nuckols, and James W. Krieger, "Sex Differences in Resistance Training: A Systematic Review and Meta-Analysis," *Journal of Strength and Conditioning Research* 34, no. 5 (May 2020): 1448–60, https://pubmed.ncbi.nlm.nih.gov/32218059/.

3. Bettina Höchli, Adrian Brügger, and Claude Messner, "How Focusing on Superordinate Goals Motivates Broad, Long-Term Goal Pursuit: A Theoretical Perspective," *Frontiers in Psychology* 9 (October 1, 2018): 1879, https://www.frontiersin.org/journals/psychology/articles/10.3389/fpsyg.2018.01879/full.

4. Katherine L. Milkman, Julia A. Minson, and Kevin G. M. Volpp, "Holding the Hunger Games Hostage at the Gym: An Evaluation of Temptation Bundling," *Management Science* 60, no. 2 (February 2014): 283–99, https://www.ncbi.nlm.nih.gov/pmc/articles/PMC4381662/.

5. J. Westenhoefer, A. J. Stunkard, and V. Pudel, "Validation of the Flexible and Rigid Control Dimensions of Dietary Restraint," *The International Journal of Eating Disorders* 26, no. 1 (July 1999): 53–64, https://pubmed.ncbi.nlm.nih.gov/10349584/.

6. J. Westenhoefer et al., "Behavioural Correlates of Successful Weight Reduction over 3 y. Results from the Lean Habits Study," *International Journal of Obesity and Related Metabolic Disorders: Journal of the International Association for the Study of Obesity* 28, no. 2 (February 2004): 334–5: https://pubmed.ncbi.nlm.nih.gov/14647175/.

CHAPTER 4

1. Shigeru Sato et al., "Comparison Between Concentric-Only, Eccentric-Only, and Concentric-Eccentric Resistance Training of the Elbow Flexors for Their Effects on Muscle Strength and Hypertrophy," *European Journal of Applied Physiology* 122, no. 12 (December 2022): 2608–14, https://pubmed.ncbi.nlm.nih.gov/36107233/; Omar Valdes et al., "Contralateral Effects of Eccentric Resistance Training on Immobilized Arm," *Scandinavian Journal of Medicine & Science in Sports* 31, no. 1 (January 2021): 76–90, https://pubmed.ncbi.nlm.nih.gov/32897568/.

2. Patroklos Androulakis Korakakis et al., "Optimizing Resistance Training Technique to Maximize Muscle Hypertrophy: A Narrative Review," *Journal of Functional Morphology and Kinesiology* 9, no. 1 (March 2024): 9, https://www.ncbi.nlm.nih.gov/pmc/articles/PMC10801605/.

3. Milo Wolf et al., "Partial vs Full Range of Motion Resistance Training: A Systematic Review and Meta-Analysis," *International Journal of Strength and Conditioning* 3, no. 1 (2023), https://journal.iusca.org/index.php/Journal/article/view/182.

4. Adam S. Lepley and Brian M. Hatzel, "Effects of Weightlifting and Breathing Technique on Blood Pressure and Heart Rate," *Journal of Strength and Conditioning Research* 24, no. 8 (August 2010): 2179–83, https://pubmed.ncbi.nlm.nih.gov/20634749/.

CHAPTER 5

1. Neil T. Roach et al., "Elastic Energy Storage in the Shoulder and the Evolution of High-Speed Throwing in *Homo*," *Nature* 498 (June 26, 2013): 483–6: www.nature.com/articles/nature12267.

2. J. M. M. Brown et al., "Muscles Within Muscles: Coordination of 19 Muscle Segments Within Three Shoulder Muscles During Isometric Motor Tasks," *Journal of Electromyography and Kinesiology* 17, no. 1 (February 2007): 57–73, https://pubmed.ncbi.nlm.nih.gov/16458022/.

3. Yuri A. C. Campos et al., "Different Shoulder Exercises Affect the Activation of Deltoid Portions in Resistance-Trained Individuals," *Journal of Human Kinetics* 75 (October 2020): 5–14, www.ncbi.nlm.nih.gov/pmc/articles/PMC7706677/.

4. Atle H. Saeterbakken and Marius S. Fimland, "Effects of Body Position and Loading Modality on Muscle Activity and Strength in Shoulder Presses," *Journal of Strength and Conditioning Research* 27, no. 7 (July 2013): 1824–31, https://pubmed.ncbi.nlm.nih.gov/23096062/.

5. Andrew D. Vigotsky et al., "Longing for a Longitudinal Proxy: Acutely Measured Surface EMG Amplitude Is Not a Validated Predictor of Muscle Hypertrophy," *Sports Medicine* 52, no. 2 (February 2022): 193–99, https://pubmed.ncbi.nlm.nih.gov/35006527/.

6. See note 3 above.

7. Paulo Gentil, Saulo Soares, and Martim Bottaro, "Single vs. Multi-Joint Resistance Exercises: Effects on Muscle Strength and Hypertrophy," *Asian Journal of Sports Medicine* 6, no. 2 (June 2015): e24057, www.ncbi.nlm.nih.gov/pmc/articles/PMC4592763/.

8. Pietro Mannarino et al., "Single-Joint Exercise Results in Higher Hypertrophy of Elbow Flexors Than Multijoint Exercise," *Journal of Strength and Conditioning Research* 35, no. 10 (October 2021): 2677–81, https://pubmed.ncbi.nlm.nih.gov/31268995/.

9. Sumiaki Maeo et al., "Triceps Brachii Hypertrophy Is Substantially Greater After Elbow Extension Training Performed in the Overhead Versus Neutral Arm Position," *European Journal of Sport Science* 23, no. 7 (July 2023): 1240–50: https://pubmed.ncbi.nlm.nih.gov/35819335/.

10. Michael S. Conley et al., "Specificity of Resistance Training Responses in Neck Muscle Size and Strength," *European Journal of Applied Physiology and Occupational Physiology* 75 (May 1997): 443–8, https://link.springer.com/article/10.1007/s004210050186.

11. K. Grob et al., "A Newly Discovered Muscle: The Tensor of the Vastus Intermedius," *Clinical Anatomy* (NewYork, NY) 29, no. 2 (March 2016): 256–63, https://pubmed.ncbi.nlm.nih.gov/26732825/.

12. Kevin E. Wilk et al., "Consideration with Open Kinetic Chain Knee Extension Exercise Following ACL Reconstruction," *International Journal of Sports Physical Therapy* 16, no. 1 (2021): 282–4, https://www.ncbi.nlm.nih.gov/pmc/articles/PMC8341750/; Brian Noehren and Lynn Snyder-Mackler, "Who's Afraid of the Big Bad Wolf? Open-Chain Exercises After Anterior Cruciate Ligament Reconstruction," *The Journal of Orthopaedic and Sports Physical Therapy* 50, no. 9 (September 2020), 473–5, https://pubmed.ncbi.nlm.nih.gov/32867579/.

13. Sumiaki Maeo et al., "Greater Hamstrings Muscle Hypertophy but Similar Damage Protection After Training at Long Versus Short Muscle Lengths," *Medicine and Science in Sports and Exercise* 53, no. 4 (April 1, 2021): 825–37, https://pubmed.ncbi.nlm.nih.gov/33009197/.

14. Milo Wolf et al., "Partial vs. Full Range of Motion Resistance Training: A Systematic Review and Meta-Analysis," *International Journal of Strength and Conditioning* 3, no. 1 (March 2, 2023), https://journal.iusca.org/index.php/Journal/article/view/182.

15. T. W. Worrell et al., "Influence of Joint Position on Electromyographic and Torque Generation During Maximal Voluntary Isometric Contractions of the Hamstrings and Gluteus Maximus Muscles," *The Journal of Orthopaedic and Sports Physical Therapy* 31, no. 12 (December 2001): 730–40, https://pubmed.ncbi.nlm.nih.gov/11767248/.

16. Rodrigo R. Aspe and Paul A. Swinton, "Electromyographic and Kinetic Comparison of the Back Squat and Overhead Squat," *Journal of Strength and Conditioning Research* 28, no. 10 (October 2014): 2827–36, https://pubmed.ncbi.nlm.nih.gov/24662228.

17. Rodrigo M. Fonseca et al., "Changes in Exercises Are More Effective Than in Loading Schemes to Improve Muscle Strength," *Journal of Strength and Conditioning Research* 28, no. 11 (November 2014): 3085–92, https://pubmed.ncbi.nlm.nih.gov/24832974/.

18. Bruna Daniella de Vasconcelos Costa et al., "Does Performing Different Resistance Exercises for the Same Muscle Group Induce Non-Homogenous Hypertrophy?" *International Journal of Sports Medicine* 42, no. 9 (July 2021): 803–11, https://pubmed.ncbi.nlm.nih.gov/33440446/.

19. Dirk Aerenhouts and Eva D'Hondt, "Using Machines or Free Weights for Resistance Training in Novice Males? A Randomized Parallel Trial," *International Journal of Environmental Research and Public Health* 17, no. 21 (October 26, 2020): 7848, https://pubmed.ncbi.nlm.nih.gov/33114782/; Shane R. Schwanbeck et al., "Effects of Training with Free Weights Versus Machines on Muscle Mass, Strength, Free Testosterone, and Free Cortisol Levels," *The Journal of Strength and Conditioning Research* 34, no. 7 (July 2020): 1851–9, https://pubmed.ncbi.nlm.nih.gov/32358310/.

20. João Pedro Nunes et al., "What Influence Does Resistance Exercise Order Have on Muscular Strength Gains and Muscle Hypertrophy? A Systematic Review and Meta-Analysis," *European Journal of Sports Science* 21, no. 2 (February 2021): 149–57, https://pubmed.ncbi.nlm.nih.gov/32077380/; Gary A. Sforzo and Paul R. Touey, "Manipulating Exercise Order Affects Muscular Performance During a Resistance Exercise Training Session," *The Journal of Strength and Conditioning Research* 10, no. 1 (February 1996): 20–4, https://journals.lww.com/nsca-jscr/abstract/1996/02000/manipulating_exercise_order_affects_muscular.4.aspx.

CHAPTER 6

1. Sebastião Barbosa-Netto, Obanshe S. d'Acelino-E-Porto, and Marcos B. Almeida, "Self-Selected Resistance Exercise Load: Implications for Research and Prescription," *Journal of Strength and Conditioning Research* 35, no. suppl. 1 (February 2021): S166–72, https://pubmed.ncbi.nlm.nih.gov/29112055/.

2. Henning Wackerhage et al., "Stimuli and Sensors That Initiate Skeletal Muscle Hypertrophy Following Resistance Exercise," *Journal of Applied Physiology* 126, no. 1 (January

9, 2019): 30–43, https://journals.physiology.org/doi/full/10.1152/japplphysiol.00685.2018.

3. Felipe Damas, Cleiton A. Libardi, and Carlos Ugrinowitsch, "The Development of Skeletal Muscle Hypertrophy Through Resistance Training: The Role of Muscle Damage and Muscle Protein Synthesis," *European Journal of Applied Physiology* 118, no. 3 (March 2018): 485–500, https://pubmed.ncbi.nlm.nih.gov/29282529/

4. See note 2 above.

5. See note 2 above.

6. James P. Fisher, James Steele, and Dave Smith, "Intensity of Effort and Momentary Failure in Resistance Training: Are We Asking a Binary Question for a Continuous Variable?" *Journal of Sport and Health Science* 11, no. 6 (March 6, 2022): 644–7, www.ncbi.nlm.nih.gov/pmc/articles/PMC9729922/.

7. Daniel Varela-Olalla et al., "Rating of Perceived Exertion and Velocity Loss as Variables for Controlling the Level of Effort in the Bench Press Exercise," *Sports Biomechanics* 21, no. 1 (July 29, 2019): 41–55, www.tandfonline.com/doi/full/10.1080/14763141.2019.1640278.

8. Alexandra F. Vieria et al., "Effects of Resistance Training Performed to Failure or Not to Failure on Muscle Strength, Hypertrophy, and Power Output: A Systematic Review with Meta-Analysis," *Journal of Strength and Conditioning Research* 35, no. 4 (April 2021): 1165–75, https://pubmed.ncbi.nlm.nih.gov/33555822/.

9. Jozo Grgic et al., "Effects of Resistance Training Performed to Repetition Failure or Non-Failure on Muscular Strength and Hypertrophy: A Systematic Review and Meta-Analysis," *Journal of Sport and Health Science* 11, no. 2 (March 2022): 202–11, https://pubmed.ncbi.nlm.nih.gov/33497853/; Martin C. Refalo et al., "Influence of Resistance Training Proximity-to-Failure on Skeletal Muscle Hypertrophy: A Systematic Review with Meta-Analysis," *Sports Medicine* (Auckland, NZ) 53, no. 3 (March 2023): 649–65, https://pubmed.ncbi.nlm.nih.gov/36334240/; Martin C. Refalo et al., "Similar Muscle Hypertrophy Following Eight Weeks of Resistance Training to Momentary Muscular Failure or with Repetitions-in-Reserve in Resistance-Trained Individuals," *Journal of Sports Sciences* 42, no. 1 (January 2024): 85–101, https://pubmed.ncbi.nlm.nih.gov/38393985/.

10. Martin C. Refalo et al., "Similar Muscle Hypertrophy…"

11. Ricardo Morán-Navarro et al., "Time Course of Recovery Following Resistance Training Leading or Not to Failure," *European Journal of Applied Physiology* 117, no. 12 (December 2017): 2382–99, https://pubmed.ncbi.nlm.nih.gov/28965198/.

12. James Krieger, "Set Volume for Muscle Size: The Ultimate Evidence Based Bible," *Weightology: The Science of Body Metamorphosis* (website), accessed May 16, 2024, https://weightology.net/the-members-area/evidence-based-guides/set-volume-for-muscle-size-the-ultimate-evidence-based-bible/.

13. Vidar Andersen et al., "Resistance Training with Different Velocity Loss Thresholds Induce Similar Changes in Strength and Hypertrophy," *Journal of Strength and Conditioning Research* 38, no. 3 (March 2024): e135–42, https://pubmed.ncbi.nlm.nih.gov/34100789/.

14. See note 1 above.

15. Michael C. Zourdos et al., "Novel Resistance Training-Specific Rating of Perceived Exertion Scale Measuring Repetitions in Reserve," *Journal of Strength and Conditioning Research* 30, no. 1 (January 2016): 267–75, https://pubmed.ncbi.nlm.nih.gov/26049792/.

CHAPTER 7

1. William J. Kraemer and Nicholas A. Ratamess, "Fundamentals of Resistance Training: Progression and Exercise Prescription," *Medicine and Science in Sports and Exercise* 36, no. 4 (2004): 674–88, https://pubmed.ncbi.nlm.nih.gov/15064596/.

2. Joaquin Calatayud et al., "Importance of Mind-Muscle Connection During Progressive Resistance Training," *European Journal of Applied Physiology* 116, no. 3 (March 2016): 527–33, https://pubmed.ncbi.nlm.nih.gov/26700744/; Brad Jon Schoenfeld et al., "Differential Effects of Attentional Focus Strategies During Long-Term Resistance Training," *European Journal of Sport Science* 18, no. 5 (June 2018): 705–12, https://pubmed.ncbi.nlm.nih.gov/29533715/.

3. Brad J. Schoenfeld et al., "Longer Interset Rest Periods Enhance Muscle Strength and Hypertrophy in Resistance-Trained Men," *Journal of Strength and Conditioning Research* 30, no. 7 (July 2016): 1805–12, https://pubmed.ncbi.nlm.nih.gov/26605807/; Jozo Grgic et al., "The Effects of Short Versus Long Inter-Set Rest Intervals in Resistance Training on Measures of Muscle Hypertrophy: A Systematic Review," *European Journal of Sports Science* 17, no. 8 (September 2017): 983–93, https://pubmed.ncbi.nlm.nih.gov/28641044/.

CHAPTER 8

1. Mathias Wernbom, Jesper Augustsson, and Roland Thomeé, "The Influence of Frequency, Intensity, Volume and Mode of Strength Training on Whole Muscle Cross-Sectional Area in Humans," *Sports Medicine* (Auckland, NZ) 37, no. 3 (2007): 225–64, https://pubmed.ncbi.nlm.nih.gov/17326698/.

2. Brad J. Schoenfeld, Dan Ogborn, and James W. Krieger, "Dose-Response Relationship Between Weekly Resistance Training Volume and Increases in Muscle Mass: A Systematic Review and Meta-Analysis," *Journal of Sports Sciences* 35, no. 11 (June 2017): 1073–82, https://pubmed.ncbi.nlm.nih.gov/27433992/.

3. James Krieger, "Set Volume for Muscle Size: The Ultimate Evidence Based Bible," *Weightology: The Science of Body Metamorphosis* (website), accessed June 21, 2024, https://weightology.net/the-members-area/evidence-based-guides/set-volume-for-muscle-size-the-ultimate-evidence-based-bible/#Radaelli.

4. Alysson Enes, Eduardo O DE Souza, and Tácito P Souza-Junior, "Effects of Different Weekly Set Progressions on Muscular Adaptations in Trained Males: Is There a Dose-Response Effect?" *Medicine and Science in Sports and Exercise* 56, no. 3 (March 1, 2024): 553–63, https://pubmed.ncbi.nlm.nih.gov/37796222/.

5. Maíra C. Scarpelli et al., "Muscle Hypertrophy Response Is Affected by Previous Resistance Training Volume in Trained Individuals," *Journal of Strength and Conditioning Research* 36, no. 4 (April 1, 2022): 1153–7, https://pubmed.ncbi.nlm.nih.gov/32108724/.

6. See note 2 above.

7. Matthew R. Rhea et al., "Three Sets of Weight Training Superior to 1 Set with Equal Intensity for Eliciting Strength," *Journal of Strength and Conditioning Research* 16, no. 4 (November 2002): 525–9, https://pubmed.ncbi.nlm.nih.gov/12423180.

8. Karl J. Ostrowski et al., "The Effect of Weight Training Volume on Hormonal Output and Muscular Size and Function," *Journal of Strength and Conditioning Research* 11, no. 3 (August 1997): 148–54, https://journals.lww.com/

nsca-jscr/abstract/1997/08000/the_effect_of_weight_training_volume_on_hormonal.3.aspx.

CHAPTER 9

1. Benjamin F. Miller et al., "Coordinated Collagen and Muscle Protein Synthesis in Human Patella Tendon and Quadriceps Muscle After Exercise," *The Journal of Physiology* 567, pt. 3 (September 15, 2005): 1021–33, https://www.ncbi.nlm.nih.gov/pmc/articles/PMC1474228/.

2. Brad Jon Schoenfeld, Jozo Grgic, and James Krieger, "How Many Times per Week Should a Muscle Be Trained to Maximize Muscle Hypertrophy? A Systematic Review and Meta-Analysis of Studies Examining the Effects of Resistance Training Frequency," *Journal of Sports Science* 37, no. 11 (June 2019): 1286–95, https://pubmed.ncbi.nlm.nih.gov/30558493/.

3. See note 2 above.

4. See note 2 above.

5. Daniel A. Corrêa et al., "Twice-Daily Sessions Result in a Greater Muscle Strength and a Similar Muscle Hypertrophy Compared to Once-Daily Session in Resistance-Trained Men," *The Journal of Sports Medicine and Physical Fitness* 62, no. 3 (March 2022): 324–36, https://pubmed.ncbi.nlm.nih.gov/33634677/; Helene Pedersen et al., "Effects of One Long vs. Two Short Resistance Training Sessions on Training Volume and Affective Responses in Resistance-Trained Women," *Frontiers in Psychology* 13 (September 29, 2022): 1010596, https://pubmed.ncbi.nlm.nih.gov/36248475/.

6. Daniel A. Hackett, Nathan A. Johnson, Chin-Moi Chow, "Training Practices and Ergogenic Aids Used by Male Bodybuilders," *Journal of Strength and Conditioning Research* 27, no. 6

(June 2013): 1609–17, https://pubmed.ncbi.nlm.nih.gov/22990567/.

7. See note 2 above.

CHAPTER 10

1. Robert W. Morton et al., "Neither Load nor Systemic Hormones Determine Resistance Training-Mediated Hypertrophy or Strength Gains in Resistance-Trained Young Men," *Journal of Applied Physiology* (Bethesda, MD: 1985) 121, no. 1 (July 2016): 129–38, https://pubmed.ncbi.nlm.nih.gov/27174923/.

2. Julius Fink et al., "Impact of High Versus Low Fixed Loads and Non-Linear Training Loads on Muscle Hypertrophy, Strength and Force Development," *SpringerPlus* 5 (2016): 698, https://springerplus.springeropen.com/articles/10.1186/s40064-016-2333-z.

3. J. Schoenfeld et al., "Effects of Varied Versus Constant Loading Zones on Muscular Adaptations in Trained Men," *International Journal of Sports Medicine* 37, no. 6 (2016): 442–7, https://www.thieme-connect.com/products/ejournals/abstract/10.1055/s-0035-1569369.

4. Thiago Lasevicius et al., "Effects of Different Intensities of Resistance Training with Equated Volume Load on Muscle Strength and Hypertrophy," *European Journal of Sports Science* 18, no. 6 (July 2018): 772–80, https://pubmed.ncbi.nlm.nih.gov/29564973/.

5. Brad J. Schoenfeld et al., "Effects of Different Volume-Equated Resistance Training Loading Strategies on Muscular Adaptations in Well-Trained Men," *Journal of Strength and Conditioning Research* 28, no. 10 (October 2014): 2909–18, https://pubmed.ncbi.nlm.nih.gov/24714538/.

6. David Rodríguez-Rosell et al., "Relationship Between Velocity Loss and Repetitions in Reserve in the Bench Press and Back Squat Exercises," *Journal of Strength and Conditioning Research* 34, no. 9 (September 2020): 2537–47, https://pubmed.ncbi.nlm.nih.gov/31045753/.

CHAPTER 11

1. Henning Wackerhage et al., "Stimuli and Sensors That Initiate Skeletal Muscle Hypertrophy Following Resistance Exercise," *Journal of Applied Physiology* 126, no. 1 (January 9, 2019): 30–43, https://journals.physiology.org/doi/full/10.1152/japplphysiol.00685.2018.

2. Nicholas A. Ratamess et al., "The Effect of Rest Interval Length on Metabolic Responses to the Bench Press Exercise," *European Journal of Applied Physiology* 100, no. 1 (May 2007): 1–17, https://pubmed.ncbi.nlm.nih.gov/17237951/.

3. Alec Singer et al., "Give It a Rest: A Systematic Review with Bayesian Meta-Analysis on the Effect of Inter-Set Rest Interval Duration on Muscle Hypertrophy," *SportRxiv* (2024), https://rgu-repository.worktribe.com/output/2344312.

4. "Jonathon J. S. Weakley et al., "The Effects of Superset Configuration on Kinetic, Kinematic, and Perceived Exertion in the Barbell Bench Press," *Journal of Strength and Conditioning Research* 34, no. 1 (January 2020): 65–72, https://pubmed.ncbi.nlm.nih.gov/28796130/.

5. James Krieger, "Set Volume for Muscle Size: The Ultimate Evidence Based Bible," *Weightology: The Science of Body Metamorphosis* (website), accessed May 16, 2024, https://weightology.net/the-members-area/evidence-based-guides/set-volume-for-muscle-size-the-ultimate-evidence-based-bible/.

6. Tácito P de Souza Jr. et al., "Comparison Between Constant and Decreasing Rest Intervals: Influence on Maximal Strength and Hypertrophy," *Journal of Strength and Conditioning Research* 24, no. 7 (July 2010): 1843–50, https://pubmed.ncbi.nlm.nih.gov/20543741/; Tácito P. Souza-Junior et al., "Strength and Hypertrophy Responses to Constant and Decreasing Rest Intervals in Trained Men Using Creatine Supplementation," *Journal of the International Society of Sports Nutrition* 8, no. 1 (October 2011), https://pubmed.ncbi.nlm.nih.gov/22032491/.

CHAPTER 12

1. Witalo Kassiano et al., "Greater Gastrocnemius Muscle Hypertrophy After Partial Range of Motion Training Performed at Long Muscle Lengths," *Journal of Strength and Conditioning Research* 37, no. 9 (September 1, 2023): 1746–53, https://pubmed.ncbi.nlm.nih.gov/37015016/; Gustavo F. Pedrosa et al., "Training in the Initial Range of Motion Promotes Greater Muscle Adaptations Than at Final in the Arm Curl," *Sports* (Basel, Switzerland) 11, no. 2 (February 6, 2023): 39, https://pubmed.ncbi.nlm.nih.gov/36828324/; Sumiaki Maeo et al., "Triceps Brachii Hypertrophy Is Substantially Greater After Elbow Extension Training Performed in the Overhead Versus Neutral Arm Position," *European Journal of Sports Science* 23, no. 7 (July 2023): 1240–50, https://pubmed.ncbi.nlm.nih.gov/35819335/.

2. Witalo Kassian et al., "Greater Gastrocnemius Muscle Hypertrophy"; Gustavo F. Pedrosa et al., "Training in the Initial Range"; Masahiro Goto et al., "Partial Range of Motion Exercise Is Effective for Facilitating Muscle Hypertrophy and Function Through Sustained Intramuscular Hypoxia

in Young Trained Men," *Journal of Strength and Conditioning Research* 33, no. 5 (May 2019): 1286–94, https://pubmed.ncbi.nlm.nih.gov/31034463/.

3. Lena Krstiansen Sødal et al., "Effects of Drop Sets on Skeleatal Muscle Hypertrophy: A Systematic Review and Meta-Analysis," *Sports Medicine-Open* 9 (December 2023): 66, https://www.ncbi.nlm.nih.gov/pmc/articles/PMC10390395/.

4. Fabian Arntz et al., "Chronic Effects of Static Stretch Exercises on Muscle Strength and Power in Healthy Individuals Across the Lifespan: A Systematic Review with Multi-Level Meta-Analysis," *Sports Medicine* (Auckland, N.Z.) 53, no. 3 (March 2023): 723–45, https://pubmed.ncbi.nlm.nih.gov/36719536/.

5. Brad J. Schoenfeld, Henning Wackerhage, and Eduardo De Souza, "Inter-Set Stretch: A Potential Time-Efficient Strategy for Enhancing Skeletal Muscle Adaptations," *Frontiers in Sports and Active Living* 4 (2022): 1035190, https://www.ncbi.nlm.nih.gov/pmc/articles/PMC9706104/.

6. João Pedro Nunes et al., "Does Stretch Training Induce Muscle Hypertrophy in Humans? A Review of the Literature," *Clinical Physiology and Functional Imaging* 40, no. 3 (May 2020): 148–56, https://pubmed.ncbi.nlm.nih.gov/31984621/.

7. Tanuj Wadhi et al., "Loaded Inter-Set Stretching for Muscular Adaptations in Trained Males: Is the Hype Real?" *International Journal of Sports Medicine* 43, no. 2 (February 2022): 168–76, https://pubmed.ncbi.nlm.nih.gov/34375990/.

8. Guilherme Borsett Businari et al., "Chronic Effects of Inter-Set Static Stretching on Morphofunctional Outcomes in Recreationally Resistance-Trained Male and Female," *Research Quarterly for Exercise and Sport* 95, no. 1 (March 2024): 10–23, https://pubmed.ncbi.nlm.nih.gov/36638500.

9. Alexandre L. Evangelista et al., "Interset Stretching vs. Traditional Strength Training: Effects on Muscle Strength and Size in Untrained Individuals," *Journal of Strength and Conditioning Research* 33 supplement (July 2019): S159–66, https://pubmed.ncbi.nlm.nih.gov/30688865/; Derrick W. Van Every et al., "Loaded Inter-Set Stretch May Selectively Enhance Muscular Adaptations of the Plantar Flexors," *PLoS One* 17, no. 9 (September 1, 2022): e0273451, https://pubmed.ncbi.nlm.nih.gov/36048793/.

10. Helmi Chaabene et al., "Acute Effects of Static Stretching on Muscle Strength and Power: An Attempt to Clarify Previous Caveats," *Frontiers in Physiology* 10, (November 2019): 1468, https://www.ncbi.nlm.nih.gov/pmc/articles/PMC6895680/.

11. Shigeru Sato et al., "Comparison Between Concentric-Only, Eccentric-Only, and Concentric-Eccentric Resistance Training of the Elbow Flexors for Their Effects on Muscle Strength and Hypertrophy," *European Journal of Applied Physiology* 122, no. 12 (December 2022): 2607–14, https://pubmed.ncbi.nlm.nih.gov/36107233/; Pawel Pakosz et al., "Comparison of Concentric and Eccentric Resistance Training in Terms of Changes in the Muscle Contractile Properties," *Journal of Electromyography and Kinesiology* 73 (December 2023): 102824, https://pubmed.ncbi.nlm.nih.gov/37696055/#:~:text=Eccentric%20training%20causes%20greater%20changes,be%20more%20effective%20in%20training.

12. Jamie Douglas et al., "Effects of Accentuated Eccentric Loading on Muscle Properties, Strength, Power, and Speed in Resistance-Trained Rugby Players," *Journal of Strength and Conditioning Research* 32, no. 10 (October

2018): 2750–61, https://pubmed.ncbi.nlm.nih.gov/30113915/; Christian J. Cook, C. Martyn Beaven, and Liam P. Kilduff, "Three Weeks of Eccentric Training Combined with Overspeed Exercises Enhances Power and Running Speed Performance Gains in Trained Athletes," *Journal of Strength and Conditioning Research* 27, no. 5 (May 2013): 1280–6, https://pubmed.ncbi.nlm.nih.gov/22820207/.

13. Simon Walker et al., "Acute Elevations in Serum Hormones Are Attenuated After Chronic Training with Traditional Isoinertial but Not Accentuated Eccentric Loads in Strength-Trained Men," *Physiological Reports* 5, no. 7 (April 2017): e13241, https://pubmed.ncbi.nlm.nih.gov/28400506/; Jason P. Brandenburg and David Docherty, "The Effects of Accentuated Eccentric Loading on Strength, Muscle Hypertrophy, and Neural Adaptations in Trained Individuals," *Journal of Strength and Conditioning* 16, no. 1 (February 2002): 25–32, https://pubmed.ncbi.nlm.nih.gov/11834103/; Birgit Friedmann-Bette et al., "Effects of Strength Training with Eccentric Overload on Muscle Adaptation in Male Athletes," *European Journal of Applied Physiology* 108, no. 4 (March 2010): 821–36, https://pubmed.ncbi.nlm.nih.gov/19937450/.

CHAPTER 13

1. Riki Ogasawara et al., "Effects of Periodic and Continued Resistance Training on Muscle CSA and Strength in Previously Untrained Men," *Clinical Physiology and Functional Imaging* 31, no. 5 (September 2011): 399–404, https://pubmed.ncbi.nlm.nih.gov/21771261/; Paul S. Hwang et al., "Resistance Training–Induced Elevations in Muscular Strength in Trained Men Are Maintained After 2 Weeks of Detraining and Not Differentially Affected by Whey Protein Supplementation," *Journal of Strength*

and Conditioning Research 31, no. 4 (April 2017): 869–81, https://pubmed.ncbi.nlm.nih.gov/28328712/.

2. John Kiely, "Periodization Paradigms in the 21st Century: Evidence-Led or Tradition-Driven?" *International Journal of Sports Physiology and Performance* 7, no. 3 (September 2012): 242–50, https://pubmed.ncbi.nlm.nih.gov/22356774/.

CHAPTER 14

1. Gary John Slater et al., "Is an Energy Surplus Required to Maximize Skeletal Muscle Hypertrophy Associated with Resistance Training," *Frontiers in Nutrition* 6 (2019): 131, https://www.ncbi.nlm.nih.gov/pmc/articles/PMC6710320/.

2. Fatemeh Ramezani et al., "Dietary Fiber Intake and All-Cause and Cause-Specific Mortality: An Updated Systematic Review and Meta-Analysis of Prospective Cohort Studies," *Clinical Nutrition* (Edinburgh, Scotland) 43, no. 1 (January 2024): 65–83, https://pubmed.ncbi.nlm.nih.gov/38011755/.

2. Justin A. Kraft et al., "Impact of Dehydration on a Full Body Resistance Exercise Protocol," *European Journal of Applied Physiology* 109, no. 2 (May 2010): 259–67, https://pubmed.ncbi.nlm.nih.gov/20066432/.

3. Lukas Schwingshackl et al., "Impact of Meal Frequency on Anthropometric Outcomes: A Systematic Review and Network Meta-Analysis of Randomized Controlled Trials," *Advances in Nutrition* 11, no. 5 (September 2020): 1108–22, https://www.ncbi.nlm.nih.gov/pmc/articles/PMC7490164/.

4. Brad Jon Schoenfeld, Alan Albert Aragon, and James W. Krieger, "Effects of Meal Frequency on Weight Loss and Body Composition: A Meta-Analysis," *Nutrition Reviews* 73, no. 2 (February

2015): 69–82, https://pubmed.ncbi.nlm.nih.gov/26024494/.

5. Jorn Trommelen et al., "The Anabolic Response to Protein Ingestion During Recovery from Exercise Has No Upper Limit in Magnitude and Duration *in vivo* in Humans," *Cell Reports Medicine* 4, no. 12 (December 19, 2023): 101324, https://www.ncbi.nlm.nih.gov/pmc/articles/PMC10772463/.

6. M. N. Naharudin et al., "Viscous Placebo and Carbohydrate Breakfasts Similarly Decrease Appetite and Increase Resistance Exercise Performance Compared with a Control Breakfast in Trained Males," *The British Journal of Nutrition* (March 16, 2020): 1–9, https://pubmed.ncbi.nlm.nih.gov/32174286/.

7. Mohamed Nashrudin Naharudin et al., "Starving Your Performance? Reduced Preexercise Hunger Increases Resistance Exercise Performance," *International Journal of Sports Physiology and Performance* 17, no. 3 (March 1, 2022): 458–64, https://pubmed.ncbi.nlm.nih.gov/34872065/.

8. Menno Henselmans et al., "The Effect of Carbohydrate Intake on Strength and Resistance Training Performance: A Systematic Review," *Nutrients* 14, no. 4 (February 18, 2022): 856, https://pubmed.ncbi.nlm.nih.gov/35215506/.

9. See note 8 above.

10. Alan Albert Aragon and Brad Jon Schoenfeld, "Nutrient Timing Revisited: Is There a Post-Exercise Anabolic Window?" *Journal of the International Society of Sports Nutrition* 10, no. 5 (2013), https://jissn.biomedcentral.com/articles/10.1186/1550-2783-10-5.

11. Daniel R. Moore, "Maximizing Post-Exercise Anabolism: The Case for Relative Protein Intakes," *Frontiers in Nutrition*, 6 (September 10, 2019), https://www.frontiersin.org/articles/10.3389/fnut.2019.00147/full?_ga=2.16317685.299115439.1620641505-750103269.1609867861.

12. Justin J. Lang et al., "Cardiorespiratory Fitness Is a Strong and Consistent Predictor of Morbidity and Mortality Among Adults: An Overview of Meta-Analyses Representing over 20.9 Million Observations from 199 Unique Cohort Studies," *The British Journal of Sports Medicine* 58, no. 10 (May 2, 2024), https://pubmed.ncbi.nlm.nih.gov/38599681/.

13. Richard B. Kreider et al., "International Society of Sports Nutrition Position Stand: Safety and Efficacy of Creatine Supplementation in Exercise, Sport, and Medicine," *Journal of the International Society of Sports Nutrition* 14 (2017): 18, https://www.ncbi.nlm.nih.gov/pmc/articles/PMC5469049/.

14. See note 13 above.

15. Darren G. Candow et al., "Strategic Creatine Supplementation and Resistance Training in Healthy Older Adults," *Applied Physiology, Nutrition, and Metabolism* 40, no. 7 (July 2015): 689–94, https://pubmed.ncbi.nlm.nih.gov/25993883/.

16. See note 13 above.

17. Nanci S. Guest et al., "International Society of Sports Nutrition Position Stand: Caffeine and Exercise Performance," *Journal of the International Society of Sports Nutrition* 18 (2021): 1, https://www.ncbi.nlm.nih.gov/pmc/articles/PMC7777221/.

18. Joonseok Kim et al., "Association of Multivitamin and Mineral Supplementation and Risk of Cardiovascular Disease: A Systematic Review and Meta-Analysis," *Circulation: Cardiovascular Quality and Outcomes* 11, no. 7 (July 2018): e004224, https://pubmed.ncbi.nlm.nih.gov/29991644/.

19. Chad M. Kerksick et al., "ISSN Exercise & Sports Nutrition Review Update: Research & Recommendations," *Journal of the International Society of Sports Nutrition* 15, no. 1 (August 1, 2018): 38, https://pubmed.ncbi.nlm.nih.gov/30068354/.

20. David Rogerson, "Vegan Diets: Practical Advice for Athletes and Exercises," *Journal of the International Society of Sports Nutrition* 14 (September 13, 2017): 36, https://pubmed.ncbi.nlm.nih.gov/28924423/.

21. Yang Hu, Frank B. Hu, and JoAnn E. Manson, "Marine Omega-3 Supplementation and Cardiovascular Disease: An Updated Meta-Analysis of 13 Randomized Controlled Trials Involving 127 477 Participants," *Journal of the American Heart Association* 8, no. 19 (October 2019): e013543, https://pubmed.ncbi.nlm.nih.gov/31567003/.

22. Felipe Mendes Delpino, Lílian Munhoz Figueiredo, and Bruna Gonçalves Cordeiro da Silva, "Effects of Omega-3 Supplementation on Body Weight and Body Fat Mass: A Systematic Review," *Clinical Nutrition ESPEN* 44 (August 2021): 122–9, https://pubmed.ncbi.nlm.nih.gov/34330455/.

23. Stephen J. Bailey et al., "The Nitrate-Nitrite-Nitric Oxide Pathway: Its Role in Human Exercise Physiology," *European Journal of Sport Science* 12, no. 4 (2012): 309–20, https://www.tandfonline.com/doi/abs/10.1080/17461391.2011.635705.

24. Umang Agarwal et al., "Supplemental Citrulline Is More Efficient Than Arginine in Increasing Systemic Arginine Availability in Mice," *The Journal of Nutrition* 147, no. 4 (April 2017): 496–602, https://pubmed.ncbi.nlm.nih.gov/28179487/.

25. Eric T. Trexler et al., "Acute Effects of Citrulline Supplementation on High-Intensity Strength and Power Performance: A Systematic Review and Meta-Analysis," *Sports Medicine* (Auckland, NZ): 49, no. 5 (May 2019): 707–18, https://pubmed.ncbi.nlm.nih.gov/30895562/.

26. Adam M. Gonzalez and Eric T. Trexler, "Effects of Citrulline Supplementation on Exercise Performance in Humans: A Review of the Current Literature," *Journal of Strength and Conditioning Research* 34, no. 5 (May 2020): 1480–95, https://pubmed.ncbi.nlm.nih.gov/31977835/.

27. F. Antón-Tay, J. L. Díaz, and A. Fernández-Guardiola, "On the Effect of Melatonin upon Human Brain. Its Possible Therapeutic Implications," *Life Sciences Pt. 1: Physiology and Pharmacology* 10, no. 15 (August 1, 1971) 841–50, https://pubmed.ncbi.nlm.nih.gov/5566131/.

28. Nina Buscemi et al., "The Efficacy and Safety of Exogenous Melatonin for Primary Sleep Disorders. A Meta-Analysis," *Journal of General Internal Medicine* 20, no. 12 (December 2005): 1151–8, https://pubmed.ncbi.nlm.nih.gov/16423108/.

29. Eduardo Ferracioli-Oda, Ahmad Qawasmi, and Michael H. Bloch, "Meta-Analysis: Melatonin for the Treatment of Primary Sleep Disorders," *PLoS ONE* 8, no. 5 (May 17, 2013): e63773, https://pubmed.ncbi.nlm.nih.gov/23691095/.

30. Tian Li et al., "Exogenous Melatonin as a Treatment for Secondary Sleep Disorders: A Systematic Review and Meta-Analysis," *Frontiers in Neuroendocrinology* 52 (January 2019): 22–8, https://pubmed.ncbi.nlm.nih.gov/29908879/.

INDEX

A

abdominals
    about, 166–167
    adjusting volume for, 212, 213
    Cable Crunch for, 139
    exercises for, 139–143
    Hanging Leg Raise for, 140–141
    Long-Lever Pelvic Tilt (LLPT) Plank for, 143
    Plank for, 142
    Plate-Loaded Decline Sit-Up for, 140
    progress photos for, 40
absolute failure, 182
accentuated eccentric training, 266–267, 355
acceptance, self-trust and, 56–57
adding sets
    mesocycle and, 279
    as a strategy for progressive overload, 200
adductors
    Barbell Back Squat for, 65–66
    Barbell Front Squat for, 67–68
    Goblet Squat for, 69
    Hip Adduction for, 82
    squat-type movements and, 149, 155
    Sumo Deadlift for, 77–78
advanced progressions
    about, 279
    linear periodization, 279–280
    reverse linear periodization, 280–281
    weekly undulating periodization, 281–283
advanced techniques
    about, 256–257
    accentuated eccentric training, 266–267
    cheat reps, 263–264
    drop sets, 259–260
    forced reps, 262
    myo-reps, 260–261
    partial reps, 257–259
    as a rung of the Muscle Ladder, 9
    stretching, 264–265
advanced training status, 5

aerobic exercise, 249
agonist-antagonist superset, 252
alcohol, consuming, 305
alternate-peripheral superset, 252
AMRAP, 244, 355
anaerobic exercise, 249
anchoring sets, as a strategy for estimating RPE, 187
anterior delts, 157
Aragon, Alan, 309
Atomic Habits (Clear), 54
audiobooks, listening to, 17

B

back
    about, 159
    adjusting volume for, 212, 213
    exercises for, 92–101
ball-and-socket hip joint, 164
ball-and-socket shoulder joint, 156
Band Pull-Apart, 123
Banded Push-Up, 115
Barbell Back Squat, 65–66, 194–195, 196, 197
Barbell Front Squat, 67–68
Barbell Lunge, 70
Barbell Overhead Press, 116–117
Barbell Row, 96
    in body-part split for advanced, 222
    in body-part split for beginners, 221–222
    in body-part split for intermediates, 222
    in four-day-per-week upper/lower split, 223
    in six-day-per-week upper/lower split, 224
Barbell Shrug, 134–135
Barbell Standing Curl, 124–127
Barbell Upright Row, 120
beginner training status (newbie), 5
Bench Press, 102–106
    double progression on, 278
    for high-frequency, full-body training, 226

Bench Press *(continued)*
  hypertrophy focus using, 282
  linear progression on, 278
  for progressive overload, 197
  strength focus using, 282
biarticular muscle, 160, 163
biceps
  about, 159–160
  adjusting volume for, 212, 213
  Barbell Row for, 96
  Barbell Standing Curl for, 124–125
  Chin-Ups for, 94
  exercises for, 124–127
  horizonal pulling movements and, 154, 155
  Pendlay Row for, 97
  Pull-Ups for, 92–93
  vertical pulling movements and, 153, 155
Biceps Curl, for progressive overload, 203
biceps femoris muscle, 163
Big Six
  about, 149
  hip-hinge movements, 150, 155
  horizontal pulling movements, 154, 155
  horizontal pushing movements, 152, 155
  squat-type movements, 149, 155
  vertical pulling movements, 153, 155
  vertical pushing movements, 151, 155
bioelectrical impedance analysis (BIA) devices, 48
BodPod, 48
body fat assessment, 48–49
body recomposition
  about, 35, 45, 47
  calories for, 296–297
  defined, 355
  protein for, 299
body weight, for measuring progress, 43–44
bodybuilding, macrocycle for, 270–271
body parts
  adjusting volume according to, 212–214
  measurements, 48
  splits, 221–222
brachialis muscle, 160
brachioradialis muscle, 160

breathing, 62–63
bulking phase
  calories for, 296–297
  protein for, 299
"the burn," 254

C
Cable Crossover, for high-frequency, full-body training, 226
Cable Crunch, 139
  for progressive overload, 203
Cable Fly, 113
Cable Lat Pull-In, 101
Cable Lateral Raise, 120
Cable Pec Fly, for progressive overload, 203
Cable Pullover
  in body-part split for advanced, 222
  in body-part split for beginners, 221–222
  in body-part split for intermediates, 222
  in four-day-per-week upper/lower split, 223
  in six-day-per-week upper/lower split, 224
Cable Triceps Kickback, 131
Cable Upright Row, 121
caffeine, 313
calculated deload, 285
caloric deficit, 355
caloric surplus, 291, 294, 355
calories
  about, 293, 294
  for body recomposition, 35, 296–297
  bulking, 296–297
  cutting, 296–297
  for fat loss, 35
  maintenance, 294–296
  requirements for, 23
calories-in, calories-out (CICO), 291–293
calves
  about, 165–166
  adjusting volume for, 212, 213
  calf insertions, 165
  exercises for, 90–91
  Seated Calf Raise for, 91
  Standing Calf Raise for, 90–91

carbohydrates, setting up, 300–301

cardio, 310–311

catastrophizing, avoiding, 26

cheat reps, 263–264, 355

chest
>about, 158
>adjusting volume for, 212, 213
>exercises for, 102–115

Chest-Supported T-Bar Row, 99, 232

Chin-Up, 94

clavicular head, of pectorals, 158

Clear, James, Atomic Habits, 54

Close-Grip Bench Press, 107, 281

comfort with failure, as a strategy for estimating RPE, 186

communities, supportive, 52

comparisons, to others, 36

compound exercises
>about, 15–16
>defined, 355
>incorporating RPE and RIR in training with, 189
>isolation exercises vs., 145–148
>pros and cons of, 147
>rest period recommendations for, 250–251
>systemic fatigue from, 21

concentric, 355

Conventional Deadlift, 74–76

core
>about, 166–167
>exercises for, 139–143

core muscles, genetics and, 167

creatine, 312–313

creatine kinase, 184

creatine monohydrate, 313

cutting phase
>calories for, 296–297
>fats for, 300
>protein for, 299

D

daily undulating periodization (DUP), 281, 287–288, 355

Decline Bench Press, 108

Deficit Push-Up, 115

dehydration, 304

delayed-onset muscle soreness (DOMS), 281

deloads
>about, 20, 284
>calculated, 285
>defined, 355
>full training break, 284–285
>instinctive, 285

deltoids
>about, 156–158
>anterior, 157
>Band Pull-Apart for, 123
>Banded Push-Up for, 115
>Barbell and Overhead Press for, 116–117
>Barbell Row for, 96
>Barbell Upright Row for, 120
>Bench Press for, 102–106
>Cable Fly for, 113
>Cable Lateral Raise for, 120
>Cable Upright Row for, 121
>Chest-Supported T-Bar Row for, 99
>Close-Grip Bench Press for, 107
>Decline Bench Press for, 108
>Deficit Push-Up for, 115
>Dip for, 111
>Dumbbell Bench Press for, 109
>Dumbbell Bent-Over Reverse Fly for, 121–122
>Dumbbell Incline Press for, 110
>Dumbbell Lateral Raise for, 119
>Dumbbell Row for, 98
>Dumbbell Seated Shoulder Press for, 118
>Dumbbell Standing Shoulder Press for, 117
>horizontal pulling movements and, 154, 155
>horizontal pushing movements and, 152, 155
>Incline Bench Press for, 107
>Lat Pulldown for, 94–95
>Pec Deck for, 114
>Pendlay Row for, 97
>Pull-Ups for, 92–93
>Push-Up for, 114
>Reverse Pec Deck for, 122
>Rope Face Pull for, 123
>vertical pulling movements and, 153, 155
>vertical pushing movements and, 151, 155

DEXA, 48

diet
as a factor influencing rate of muscle gain, 31, 32
nontracking approaches to, 303–304
recovery and, 23–24

digital scale, 43–44

Dip, 111

dirty bulk, 355

double progression
on Bench Press, 278
as a strategy for progressive overload, 197–199

double-split routines, 232

drop sets, 259–260, 355

Dumbbell Bench Press, 109

Dumbbell Bent-Over Reverse Fly, 121–122

Dumbbell Fly, 112

Dumbbell Incline Press, 110

Dumbbell Lateral Raise, 119
in double-split routines, 232
for progressive overload, 198–199

Dumbbell Lunge, 71

Dumbbell Row, 98

Dumbbell Seated Shoulder Press, 118

Dumbbell Shrug, 135–136

Dumbbell Standing Shoulder Press, 117

Dumbbell Wrist Curl, 132

Dumbbell Wrist Extension, 133

E

early set RPE, 317, 355

eccentric, 355

effective reps, 260

effectiveness, efficiency vs., 14–15

effectiveness-first approach, 16

efficiency, effectiveness vs., 14–15

efficiency-first approach, 16

effort
about, 178–179
defined, 355
defining failure, 182–183
how far to push, 184–186
rating of perceived exertion (RPE), 186–190

reasons for muscle growth, 179–182
relationship with volume and frequency, 219
reps in reserve (RIR), 186–190
as a rung of the Muscle Ladder, 8

electromyography (EMG), 157–158

elite training status, 5

endurance, combining with hypertrophy, 274

enjoyment
about, 13–14
approach and, 16
frequency and, 16
generating more, 17–18
training minimalism and, 14–15
workout length and, 15–16

entry point, 26

environments, modifying, 51–52

"An Evidence-Based Approach to Goal Setting and Behavior Change," 54

exercise activity thermogenesis (EAT), 291, 292, 293

exercises. *See also specific exercises*
about, 144–145
Big Six, 149–155
compound vs. isolation exercises, 145–148
exercise order, 176
free weights vs. machines, 170–174
high-tension, 175
muscle isolation, 156–167
optimizing, 175
order of, 176
primary, 146
prioritizing ones you enjoy, 17
rotating, 205
as a rung of the Muscle Ladder, 8
secondary, 146–147
technique for, 64–143
tertiary, 147
variation and, 168–170, 289
weak point prioritization, 176

exercise-specific warm-up, 27

extending sets, as a strategy for progressive overload, 204

EZ-Bar Biceps Curl, in double-split routines, 232

F

Fagerli, Børge, 260

failure
defining, 182–183
true, 236

failure training, 355

fat loss
with excess muscle loss, 46, 47
meal frequency for, 306
with muscle maintenance, 45, 47

fatigue, 184

fats, setting up, 300

fatty fish, 306

feedback, as a strategy for estimating RPE, 187

fiber, 301

fish oil, 314

Fisher, James, 182

Flat Dumbbell Press, in double-split routines, 232

flexibility
importance of, 53–54
importance of having, 302

foam rolling, 24

food labels, 303

forced reps, 262, 355

forearms
about, 161
adjusting volume for, 212, 213–214
Barbell Row for, 96
exercises for, 132–133
Pendlay Row for, 97
Pull-Ups for, 92–93

45-Degree Back Extension, 80

free weights
machines compared with, 170–174
machines vs., 15
pros and cons of, 171

frequency
of meals, 306–307
relationship with effort and volume, 219
training, 16, 220, 233

front delts. *See* deltoids

front double biceps, progress photos for, 41

front lat spread, progress photos for, 40

front relaxed, progress photos for, 41

Full Body Split
2x/week, 319–320
3x/week, 321–323
4x/week, 330–335
5x/week, 336–339

full ROM, 59–60

full training break, 284–285

full-body splits, 225

"fuzzy" goals, 37

G

general warm-up, 26–27

genetic muscular limit, 355–356

genetics
core muscles and, 167
as a factor influencing rate of muscle gain, 31, 32

glute exercises, 74–82

Glute-Ham Raise, 88

glutes
about, 164–165
adjusting volume for, 212, 213
Barbell Back Squat for, 65–66
Barbell Front Squat for, 67–68
Barbell Lunge for, 70
Conventional Deadlift for, 74–76
Dumbbell Lunge for, 71
45-Degree Back Extension for, 80
Glute-Ham Raise for, 88
Goblet Squat for, 69
Good Morning for, 84–85
Hip Thrust for, 79
hip-hinge movements and, 150, 155
Leg Press for, 71–72
Nordic Ham Curl for, 89
Romanian Deadlift (RDL) for, 83–84
squat-type movements and, 149, 155
Sumo Deadlift for, 77–78

gluteus maximus, 164

gluteus medius, 81, 164

gluteus minimus, 164

goals, setting, 36–39

Goblet Squat, 69

Good Morning, 84–85

guess-and-check model, 241, 295–296

H

habit stacking, 51

habits and routines, building, 50–54

hamstrings
    about, 163
    adjusting volume for, 212, 213
    Conventional Deadlift for, 74–76
    exercises for, 83–89
    45-Degree Back Extension for, 80
    Glute-Ham Raise for, 88
    Good Morning for, 84–85
    hip-hinge movements and, 150, 155
    Lying Leg Curl for, 86
    Nordic Ham Curl for, 89
    Romanian Deadlift (RDL) for, 83–84
    Seated Leg Curl for, 87
    Sumo Deadlift for, 77–78

Hanging Leg Raise, 140–141

hard sets, 207–208

Head Harness Neck Extension, 138

healthy, staying, 18

high-frequency, full-body training, 226–227

high-intensity training (HIT), 206

high-rep realities, 236

high-tension exercises, 175

Hip Abduction, 81

Hip Adduction, 82

hip flexors
    Hanging Leg Raise for, 140–141
    Plate-Loaded Decline Sit-Up for, 140

Hip Thrust, 79

hip-hinge movements, 150, 155, 164

horizonal pulling movements, 154, 155

horizontal pushing movements, 152

hormonal signals, for triggering muscle growth, 180–182

hybrid splits, 231

hypertrophy
    combining with endurance, 274
    defined, 356
    as a nonspecific adaptation, 240
    partial reps and, 60–61
    practical hypertrophy rep range, 238–239
    reverse linear periodization for focus on, 281
    strength vs., 224
    weekly undulating periodization for focus on, 282

hypertrophy-oriented training, 179–180

I–J

ice baths, 24

Incline Bench Press, 107

Incline Dumbbell Press, for high-frequency, full-body training, 226

increasing load, as a strategy for progressive overload, 194–196

increasing reps, as a strategy for progressive overload, 196

individualizing volume, 214–215

injuries
    handling, 25–26
    risk of from lifting, 19–20

instinctive deload, 285

intensity, 356

intermediate goals, 37

intermediate training status, 5

interset stretching, 264–265

intra-workout nutrition, 308–309

iso-hold, 356

isolation exercises
    about, 15
    compound exercises vs., 145–148
    defined, 356
    incorporating RPE and RIR in training with, 190
    pros and cons of, 148
    rest period recommendations for, 250–251

K

Kiely, John, 287

Krieger, James, 185, 253

L

L-arginine, 314

last set intensity technique, 317, 356

last set RPE, 356

Lat Pulldown, 94–95

    in body-part splits, 221–222

    in double-split routines, 232

    in four-day-per-week upper/lower split, 223

    for progressive overload, 203

    in six-day-per-week upper/lower split, 224

lateral head, of triceps, 160–161

Lateral Raise, for progressive overload, 203

lats

    about, 159

    Barbell Row for, 96

    Cable Lat Pull-In for, 101

    Chest-Supported T-Bar Row for, 99

    Chin-Ups for, 94

    Dumbbell Row for, 98

    horizonal pulling movements and, 154, 155

    Lat Pulldown for, 94–95

    Pendlay Row for, 97

    Pull-Ups for, 92–93

    Straight-Arm Lat Pullover for, 100

    vertical pulling movements and, 153, 155

L-citrulline, 314

lean muscle gain, 44, 47

Leg Curl, for progressive overload, 203

Leg Extension, 73, 203

Leg Press, 71–72

length

    of rest periods, 253

    of workouts, 15–16

lengthened partial, 61

levator scapulae

    Barbell Shrug for, 134–135

    Dumbbell Shrug for, 135–136

lifestyle

    affecting recovery, 21

    as a factor influencing rate of muscle gain, 31, 32

lifting

    experience, as a strategy for estimating RPE, 186

    risk of injury from, 19–20

linear periodization, 279–280, 356

linear progression

    on Bench Press, 278

    as a strategy for progressive overload, 194–196

load

    defined, 356

    increasing, as a strategy for progressive overload, 194–196

load and rep ranges. See also reps

    about, 234

    logbook, 246

    practical hypertrophy rep range, 238–239

    prioritizing ones you enjoy, 17

    realities of high-reps, 236

    realities of low-reps, 237–238

    research on, 235

    as a rung of the Muscle Ladder, 9

    strength, 240

    weight of lift, 241–246

loading phase, for creatine, 312

local recovery, 21

logbook, 246

long head, of triceps, 160–161

Long-Level Pelvic Tilt (LLPT) Plank, 143

low-rep realities, 237–238

Lying Leg Curl, 86

M

machines

    free weights compared with, 170–174

    free weights vs., 15

    pros and cons of, 172

macrocycle

    about, 269, 270

    bodybuilding, 270–271

    combining hypertrophy and endurance, 274

    defined, 356

    noncompetitive lifter, 276

    plateaued, advanced trainee (specialization phases), 275

    powerbuilding, 273

    powerlifting, 272

maintenance calories, 294–296

maintenance phase, for creatine, 312

massage, 24

meal frequency, planning, 306–307

measuring progress, 39–49

mechanical tension, 180

medial head, of triceps, 160–161

melatonin, 315

mental state, 17, 33–34

Mentzer, Mike, 206

mesocycle

    about, 269, 277, 283–284

    advanced progressions, 279–283

    basic progressions, 277–279

    defined, 356

    deloads, 284–285

metabolic adaptation, 293

metabolic stress, 180

microcycle

    about, 269, 286

    defined, 356

    prioritization, 286–287

    variation, 287–289

micronutrients, managing, 305–306

mid-traps

    horizonal pulling movements and, 154, 155

    vertical pulling movements and, 153, 155

Mifflin-St. Jeor equation, 294–295

military press, 151

mind-muscle connection

    defined, 356

    overloading via, as a strategy for progressive overload, 202–203

mindset

    about, 30, 57

    building habits and routines, 50–54

    comparing yourself to others, 36

    factors influencing rate of muscle gain, 31–35

    measuring progress, 39–49

    no pain, no gain, 55–56

    self-trust and acceptance, 56–57

    setting science-based goals for building muscle, 36–39

    as side rail of the Muscle Ladder, 7, 10

minimalist training, 217–218

momentum, minimizing, 61–62

most muscular, progress photos for, 41

multijoint muscle, 356

multivitamins, 313–314

muscle confusion, 193–194

muscle damage, 184

muscle gain/growth

    with excess fat gain, 46, 47

    factors influencing rate of, 31–35

    meal frequency for, 307

    reasons for, 179–182

    setting science-based goals for, 36–39

    strength and, 194

Muscle Ladder

    about, 4

    building, 5–6

    structure of, 7–10

muscular fat, 44

music, listening to, 17

myo-reps, 260–261, 356

N

National Sleep Foundation, 22

neck

    about, 161–162

    adjusting volume for, 212, 214

neck extensors

    Head Harness Neck Extension for, 138

    Plate-Loaded Neck Extension for, 137

neck flexors, Plate-Loaded Neck Curl for, 136–137

negative, controlling the, 25, 59

neural signals, for triggering muscle growth, 180–182

newbie period, 6

no pain, no gain, 55–56, 179, 180

nocebo effect, 173–174

noncompetitive lifter, macrocycle for, 276

non-exercise activity thermogenesis (NEAT), 291, 292, 293

Nordic Ham Curl, 89

Norton, Layne, 231

nutrition, cardio, and supplements

    about, 290

    calories-in, calories-out (CICO), 291–293

consuming alcohol, 305

doing cardio, 310–311

drinking water, 304

fiber, 301

flexibility, 302

managing micronutrients, 305–306

managing peri-workout nutrition, 307–309

managing supplements, 311–315

planning meal frequency, 306–307

refeeds, 298

setting up calories, 294–297

setting up carbs, 300–301

setting up fats, 300

setting up protein, 299

using nontracking approaches to diet, 303–304

nutrition labels, 303

O

obliques, 166

Long-Lever Pelvic Tilt (LLPT) Plank for, 143

Plank for, 142

one-rep max (1RM)

about, 235

defined, 356

determining, 244–245

percentage of, 243–246

outcome-oriented goals, process-oriented goals vs., 38–39

Overhead Cable Triceps Extension, in double-split routines, 232

Overhead Triceps Extension, 130, 203

overloading

about, 193

via mind-muscle connection, 202–203

via shorter rest periods, 203–204

via technique, 201

via velocity, 202

overtraining, 356

P

pacing, proper, 28–29

pain, handling, 25–26

partial reps, 60–62, 257–259, 356–357

patience, for pain and injuries, 26

Pec Deck, 114, 226

pectorals, 158

Banded Push-Up for, 115

Barbell and Overhead Press for, 116–117

Bench Press for, 102–106

Cable Fly for, 113

Close-Grip Bench Press for, 107

Decline Bench Press for, 108

Deficit Push-Up for, 115

Dip for, 111

Dumbbell Bench Press for, 109

Dumbbell Fly for, 112

Dumbbell Incline Press for, 110

horizontal pushing movements and, 152, 155

Incline Bench Press for, 107

Pec Deck for, 114

Push-Up for, 114

Pendlay Row, 97

percentage of one-rep max (%1RM), 243–246

periodization

about, 268–269

defined, 357

macrocycle, 270–276

mesocycle, 277–285

microcycle, 286–289

as a rung of the Muscle Ladder, 9

peri-workout nutrition, managing, 307–309

placebo effect, 173

Plank, 142

plateaued, advanced trainee (specialization phases), macrocycle for, 275

Plate-Loaded Decline Sit-Up, 140

Plate-Loaded Neck Curl, 136–137

Plate-Loaded Neck Extension, 137

podcasts, listening to, 17

positive, staying, 26

post-workout nutrition, 309

powerbuilding, macrocycle for, 273

powerlifting, macrocycle for, 272

practical hypertrophy rep range, 238–239

pre-workout nutrition, 307–308

primary exercises
    about, 146
    defined, 357
    hard sets for, 208

prioritization, microcycle and, 286–287

process-oriented goals, outcome-oriented goals vs., 38–39

professional help, for pain and injuries, 26

progress
    measuring, 39–49
    photos for measuring progress, 39–43

progression scheme, 193

progressions
    basic for mesocycle, 277–279
    expectations of, 195–196

progressive overload
    about, 192–193
    defined, 357
    general approaches to, 194–204
    muscle confusion, 193–194
    muscle growth and strength, 194
    rotating exercises, 205
    as a rung of the Muscle Ladder, 8

proper ROM, 59–60

proper technique, practicing, 25–27

protein
    for body recomposition, 35
    requirements for, 23
    setting up, 299

protein powder, 312

Pull-Up, 92–93, 224

pushing it, 184–186

Push/Pull/Legs (PPL) Split, 228–230
    with leg prioritization, 286
    6x/week, 348–351, 352–353

Push-Up, 114

Q

quadriceps
    about, 162–163
    adjusting volume for, 212, 213
    Barbell Back Squat for, 65–66
    Barbell Front Squat for, 67–68
    Barbell Lunge for, 70
    Conventional Deadlift for, 74–76
    Dumbbell Lunge for, 71
    exercises for, 65–73
    Goblet Squat for, 69
    Leg Extension for, 73
    Leg Press for, 71–72
    squat-type movements and, 149, 155
    Sumo Deadlift for, 77–78

quantity, of volume, 210–211

quick and dirty method, for calories, 294

R

range of motion (ROM), 25, 59–60, 257

rate of perceived exertion (RPE)
    about, 186–190, 241–243
    defined, 357
    early set, 317
    increasing, 278

rear delts. *See* deltoids

rear double biceps, progress photos for, 42

rear lat spread, progress photos for, 41

rear relaxed, progress photos for, 42

recent tough set, 245

recommendations, for rest periods, 250–251

recording sets, as a strategy for estimating RPE, 187

recovery
    about, 21–22, 249
    defined, 357
    diet, 23–24
    ensuring adequate, 21–24
    rest, 24
    sleep, 22–23

rectus abdominis, 166

rectus femoris, 162

refeeds, 298

remaining frequency, high-frequency, full-body training, 226–227

rep ranges. *See* load and rep ranges

repair-oriented training, 179–180

reps
    cheat, 263–264
    effective, 260
    forced, 262

increasing, as a strategy for progressive overload, 196

myo-, 260–261

partial, 60–62, 257–259

volume of, 207

reps in reserve (RIR), 186–190, 357

research

on rep ranges, 235

on rest periods, 249

resistance exercise, 249

rest periods

about, 248

"the burn," 254

importance of, 249–250

overloading via shorter, 203–204

recommendations for, 250–251

recovery and, 24

research on, 249

as a rung of the Muscle Ladder, 9

short, 253

supersets, 252–253

tracking, 251

resting energy expenditure (REE), 291, 292, 293

results, getting, 17

return to baseline, 21, 26

reverse linear periodization, 280–281, 357

Reverse Pec Deck, 122, 232

rhomboids

about, 159

Band Pull-Apart for, 123

Barbell Row for, 96

Chest-Supported T-Bar Row for, 99

Chin-Ups for, 94

Dumbbell Bent-Over Reverse Fly for, 121–122

Dumbbell Row for, 98

Lat Pulldown for, 94–95

Pendlay Row for, 97

Pull-Ups for, 92–93

Reverse Pec Deck for, 122

Rope Face Pull for, 123

Romanian Deadlift (RDL), 83–84

Rope Face Pull, 123

in body-part split for advanced, 222

in body-part split for beginners, 221–222

in body-part split for intermediates, 222

in four-day-per-week upper/lower split, 223

in six-day-per-week upper/lower split, 224

rotating exercises, 205

rotator cuff, Rope Face Pull for, 123

routines and habits, building, 50–54

rungs, of the Muscle Ladder, 8–10

S

safety

about, 18

ensuring adequate recovery, 21–24

of leg extensions, 162

managing total workload, 20–21

practicing proper technique, 25–29

risk of injury from lifting, 19–20

saunas, 24

Schoenfeld, Brad, 237, 309

science-based goals, setting for building muscle, 36–39

Seated Cable Row

in body-part split for advanced, 222

in six-day-per-week upper/lower split, 224

Seated Calf Raise, 91

Seated Leg Curl, 87, 200

secondary exercises

about, 146–147

defined, 357

hard sets for, 208

incorporating RPE and RIR in training with, 189

self-trust, acceptance and, 56–57

semimembranosus muscle, 163

semitendinosus muscle, 163

separated supersets, 252

set volume, 207–208

sets

adding, as a strategy for progressive overload, 200

extending, as a strategy for progressive overload, 204

mesocycle and adding, 279

sex, as a factor influencing rate of muscle gain, 31, 32

shoulder exercises, 116–123

shoulder stabilizers, Long-Lever Pelvic Tilt (LLPT) Plank for, 143

shoulders
    about, 156–158
    adjusting volume for, 212, 213

Shrugs, for progressive overload, 203

side chest, progress photos for, 42

side delts. *See* deltoids

side rails, of the Muscle Ladder, 7

side triceps, progress photos for, 42

Single-Arm Pulldown, in six-day-per-week upper/lower split, 224

skinfold calipers, 48

Skull Crusher, 128–129

sleep
    recovery and, 22–23
    sleep disorders, 23
    sleep-extension studies, 22

specialization phases, incorporating, 216

spinal erectors
    Barbell Back Squat for, 65–66
    Barbell Front Squat for, 67–68
    Conventional Deadlift for, 74–76
    45-Degree Back Extension for, 80
    Goblet Squat for, 69
    Good Morning for, 84–85
    hip-hinge movements and, 150, 155
    Romanian Deadlift (RDL) for, 83–84
    Sumo Deadlift for, 77–78

splits and frequency, as a rung of the Muscle Ladder, 9

squat-type movements, 149, 155, 162

Standing Calf Raise, 90–91

Steele, James, 182

sternal head, of pectorals, 158

steroids, 294

Straight-Arm Lat Pullover, 100

strategies
    for estimating RPE, 186–189
    for progressive overload, 194–204

strength
    hypertrophy vs., 224
    incorporating RPE and RIR in training for gain in, 190

    linear periodization for focus on, 280
    muscle growth and gain in, 194
    performance of, for measuring progress, 39
    reverse linear periodization for focus on, 280
    as a specific adaptation, 240
    weekly undulating periodization for focus on, 282

stretching, 264–265

subjective factors, 49

subordinate goals, 37–38

sugary beverages, 303

Sumo Deadlift, 77–78

superordinate goals, 37

supersets, 252–253, 317

supplements, managing, 311–315

supportive communities, 52

sustainability
    about, 12
    enjoyment as a factor in, 13–18
    safety as a factor in, 18–24
    as side rail of the Muscle Ladder, 7, 10
    technique as a factor in, 25–29

systemic recovery, 21

T

technical failure, 182–183

technique. *See also* advanced techniques
    about, 58
    breathing, 62–63
    controlling the negative, 59
    exercise, 64–143
    overloading via, 201
    partial reps, 60–62
    practicing proper, 25–27
    proper range of motion, 59–60
    as a rung of the Muscle Ladder, 8

tempo training, 267, 357

temptation bundling, 50

teres major
    about, 159
    horizonal pulling movements and, 154, 155
    vertical pulling movements and, 153, 155

terminology, for training programs, 317–318

tertiary exercises
    about, 147
    defined, 357
    hard sets for, 208
thermic effect of food (TEF), 291, 292, 293
thighs, progress photos for, 40
tier 1 supplements, 312–313
tier 2 supplements, 313–314
tier 3 supplements, 314–315
time-restricted feeding, 303
total daily energy expenditure (TDEE), 291–292
total workload, managing, 20–21
tracking
    rest periods, 251
    sample of, 317
training. *See also* volume
    accentuated eccentric, 266–267, 355
    age, as a factor influencing rate of muscle gain, 31, 32
    consistency of, as a factor influencing rate of muscle gain, 31, 32
    environments for, 17
    frequency of, 16, 220, 233
    minimalist, 14–15, 217–218
    optimization of, as a factor influencing rate of muscle gain, 31, 32
    partners for, 17
    status of, 5
training log, 246
training programs
    about, 316
    Full Body Split 2x/week, 319–320
    Full Body Split 3x/week, 321–323
    Full Body Split 4x/week, 330–335
    Full Body Split 5x/week, 336–339
    Push/Pull/Legs Split 6x/week, 348–353
    terminology for, 317–318
    Upper/Lower 6x/week, 344–347
    Upper/Lower Split 4x/week, 324–329
    Upper/Lower/Push/Pull/Legs 5x/week, 340–343
    warm-up protocol, 318
training splits
    about, 220
    body-part splits, 221–222
    defined, 357
    double-split routines, 232
    full-body splits, 225
    hybrid splits, 231
    push/pull/legs (PPL) splits, 228–230
    upper/lower splits, 223–224
transverse abdominis, 166
trapezius, 159
    adjusting volume for, 212, 214
    Band Pull-Apart for, 123
    Barbell Row for, 96
    Barbell Shrug for, 134–135
    Barbell Upright Row for, 120
    Cable Upright Row for, 121
    Chest-Supported T-Bar Row for, 99
    Chin-Ups for, 94
    Dumbbell Bent-Over Reverse Fly for, 121–122
    Dumbbell Lateral Raise for, 119
    Dumbbell Row for, 98
    Dumbbell Shrug for, 135–136
    Head Harness Neck Extension for, 138
    Lat Pulldown for, 94–95
    Pendlay Row for, 97
    Plate-Loaded Neck Extension for, 137
    Pull-Ups for, 92–93
    Reverse Pec Deck for, 122
    Rope Face Pull for, 123
trend, in tour progress, 49
triceps
    about, 160–161
    adjusting volume for, 212, 213
    Banded Push-Up for, 115
    Barbell and Overhead Press for, 116–117
    Bench Press for, 102–106
    Cable Triceps Kickback for, 131
    Close-Grip Bench Press for, 107
    Decline Bench Press for, 108
    Deficit Push-Up for, 115
    Dip for, 111
    Dumbbell Bench Press for, 109
    Dumbbell Incline Press for, 110
    exercises for, 128–131
    horizontal pushing movements and, 152, 155
    Incline Bench Press for, 107

triceps *(continued)*
    Overhead Triceps Extension for, 130
    Push-Up for, 114
    Skull Crusher for, 128–129
    Straight-Arm Lat Pullover for, 100
    Triceps Pressdown for, 130
    vertical pushing movements and, 151, 155
Triceps Pressdown, 130, 197–198
true one-rep-max test, 245

U

undulating, 281
upper trap and neck exercises, 134–138
Upper/Lower Split, 223–224
    with chest prioritization, 287
    5x/week, 344–347
    4x/week, 223, 324–329
    6x/week, 223–224
Upper/Lower/Push/Pull/Legs, 5x/week, 340–343
urine, water consumption and, 304

V

Valsalva maneuver, 62–63
variation
    about, 287
    daily undulating periodization (DUP), 287–288
    in exercise, 168–170, 289
vastus intermedius, 162
vastus lateralis, 162
vastus medialis, 162
velocity, overloading via, 202
vertical pulling movements, 153, 155
vertical pushing movements, 151, 155
volume
    about, 206–208
    adjusting according to body part, 212–214
    cycling, 216
    defined, 357
    effect of on muscle growth, 185
    hard sets, 208
    importance of, 209
    incorporating volume cycling and
      specialization phases, 216
    individualizing, 214–215
    minimalist training, 217–218
    quantity of, 210–211
    relationship with effort and frequency, 219
    as a rung of the Muscle Ladder, 8
volume load, 207, 237

W–Z

waist measurements, 48
warm-up
    importance of, 26–28
    protocol for, 318
    set for, 208, 242
warning signs, of injury, 20–21
water
    consuming, 304
    fluctuations in, 292
weak point prioritization, 176
weekly undulating periodization (WUP), 281–283, 357
weight
    for lifting, 241–246
    risk of injury from training, 19–20
    of weights, 25
Weighted Dip, for high-frequency, full-body training, 226
women, rates of muscle gain in, 33–34
work capacity
    defined, 357
    reverse linear periodization for focus on, 280
working set, 208, 242
workload, managing total, 20–21
workouts, length of, 15–16
wrist extensors
    about, 161
    Dumbbell Wrist Extension for, 133
wrist flexors
    about, 161
    Dumbbell Wrist Curl for, 132
Yates, Dorian, 184, 206